Monitoring and Evaluation in Health and Social Development

New approaches are needed to monitor and evaluate health and social development. Existing strategies tend to require expensive, time-consuming analytical procedures. A growing emphasis on results-based programming has resulted in evaluation being conducted in order to demonstrate accountability and success, rather than how change takes place, what works and why. The tendency to monitor and evaluate using log frames and their variants closes policy makers' and practitioners' eyes to the sometimes unanticipated means by which change takes place.

Two recent developments hold the potential to transcend these difficulties and to lead to important changes in the way in which the effects of health and social development programming are understood. First, there is growing interest in ways of monitoring programmes and assessing impact that are more grounded in the realities of practice than many of the 'results-based' methods currently utilised. Second, there are calls for the greater use of interpretive and ethnographic methods in programme design, monitoring and evaluation.

Responding to these concerns, this book illustrates the potential of interpretive methods to aid understanding and make a difference in real people's lives. Through a focus on individual and community perspectives, and locally grounded explanations, the approaches explored in this book offer a potentially richer way of assessing the relationships between intent, action and change in health and social development in Africa, Asia, Europe and the Americas.

Stephen Bell is a senior research fellow at the Kirby Institute, UNSW Australia, where he undertakes qualitative and ethnographic sexual health research with young people and other marginalised populations in rural and remote settings. His current interests involve examining how the youth-led design of culturally and socially attuned sexual health programmes might evolve from, and be centred on, young people's own everyday strategies of sexual health risk assessment and harm reduction.

Peter Aggleton is Scientia Professor in Education and Health in the Centre for Social Research in Health at UNSW Australia, where he is also Director of the Arts and Social Sciences Practical Justice Initiative. He has worked internationally in health and development for over 30 years, with a focus on health education and health promotion. He is an adjunct professor in the Australian Research Centre in Sex, Health and Society at La Trobe University, Australia, and holds visiting professorial positions at the UCL Institute of Education in London, UK, and at the University of Sussex, UK. Alongside his academic work, Peter has served as a senior adviser to numerous international agencies including UNAIDS, UNESCO, UNICEF and WHO.

Monitoring and Evaluation in Health and Social Development

Interpretive and ethnographic perspectives

Edited by Stephen Bell and Peter Aggleton

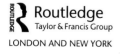

LONDON AND NEW YORK

First published 2016
by Routledge
2 Park Square, Milton Park, Abingdon, Oxon OX14 4RN

and by Routledge
711 Third Avenue, New York, NY 10017

Routledge is an imprint of the Taylor & Francis Group, an informa business

© 2016 S. Bell and P. Aggleton

The right of Stephen Bell and Peter Aggleton to be identified as the authors of the editorial material, and of the authors for their individual chapters, has been asserted in accordance with sections 77 and 78 of the Copyright, Designs and Patents Act 1988.

All rights reserved. No part of this book may be reprinted or reproduced or utilised in any form or by any electronic, mechanical, or other means, now known or hereafter invented, including photocopying and recording, or in any information storage or retrieval system, without permission in writing from the publishers.

Trademark notice: Product or corporate names may be trademarks or registered trademarks, and are used only for identification and explanation without intent to infringe.

British Library Cataloguing-in-Publication Data
A catalogue record for this book is available from the British Library

Library of Congress Cataloging in Publication Data
Monitoring and evaluation in health and social development : interpretive and ethnographic perspectives / edited by Stephen Bell and Peter Aggleton.
p. ; cm.
Includes bibliographical references and index.
I. Bell, Stephen (Social researcher), editor. II. Aggleton, Peter, editor.
[DNLM: 1. Health Care Evaluation Mechanisms. 2. Social Change. 3. Cultural Characteristics. 4. Public Health Practice. 5. Quality Assurance, Health Care-- methods. 6. Social Conditions. W 84.41]
RA427
362.1–dc23
2015031609

ISBN: 978-1-138-84415-5 (hbk)
ISBN: 978-1-138-84418-6 (pbk)
ISBN: 978-1-315-73059-2 (ebk)

Typeset in Gill Sans and Goudy
by GreenGate Publishing Services, Tonbridge, Kent

Contents

List of illustrations viii
Contributors x
Acknowledgements xvi
Abbreviations xvii

1 Interpretive and ethnographic perspectives: alternative approaches to monitoring and evaluation practice 1
STEPHEN BELL AND PETER AGGLETON

PART I
The present challenge 15

2 The political economy of evidence: personal reflections on the value of the interpretive tradition and its methods 17
ANGELA KELLY-HANKU

3 Measurement, modification and transferability: evidential challenges in the evaluation of complex interventions 32
HELEN LAMBERT

4 What really works? Understanding the role of 'local knowledges' in the monitoring and evaluation of a maternal, newborn and child health project in Kenya 47
ELSABÉ DU PLESSIS AND ROBERT LORWAY

PART II
Programme design 63

5 Permissions, vacations and periods of self-regulation: using consumer insight to improve HIV treatment adherence in four Central American countries 65
KIM LONGFIELD, ISOLDA FORTIN, JENNIFER WHEELER AND DANA SIEVERS

6 Generating local knowledge: a role for ethnography in evidence-based programme design for social development 81
RUTH EDMONDS

7 Interpretation, context and time: an ethnographically inspired approach to strategy development for tuberculosis control in Odisha, India 95
JENS SEEBERG AND TUSHAR KANTI RAY

8 Designing health and leadership programmes for vulnerable young women using participatory ethnographic research in Freetown, Sierra Leone 110
NAANA OTOO-OYORTEY, ELIZABETH GEZAHEGN KING AND KATE NORMAN

PART III
Monitoring processes 125

9 Using social mapping techniques to guide programme redesign in the Tingim Laip HIV prevention and care project in Papua New Guinea 127
LOU McCALLUM, JENNIFER MILLER, SCOTT BERRY AND CHRISTOPHER HERSHEY

10 Pathways to impact: new approaches to monitoring and improving volunteering for sustainable environmental management 143
JODY AKED

11 Ethnographic process evaluation: a case study of an HIV prevention programme with injecting drug users in the USA 159
YAN ALICIA HONG, SHANNON GWIN MITCHELL, JAMES A. PETERSON, CARL LATKIN AND KARIN TOBIN

12 Using the Reality Check Approach to shape quantitative findings: experience from mixed method evaluations in Ghana and Nepal 172
DEE JUPP

PART IV
Understanding impact and change   185

13 Innovation in evaluation: using SenseMaker to assess the inclusion of smallholder farmers in modern markets   187
IRENE GUIJT

14 The use of the Rapid PEER approach for the evaluation of sexual and reproductive health programmes   203
ELEANOR BROWN, RACHEL GRELLIER AND KIRSTAN HAWKINS

15 Using interpretive research to make quantitative evaluation more effective: Oxfam's experience in Pakistan and Zimbabwe   219
MARTIN WALSH

16 Can qualitative research rigorously evaluate programme impact? Evidence from a randomised controlled trial of an adolescent sexual health programme in Tanzania   232
MARY LOUISA PLUMMER

Index   247

Illustrations

Figures

2.1	'We don't have a proper market'	26
2.2	'LNG money is everywhere'	27
4.1	Maternal, Newborn and Child Health and Nutrition Project overview	50
4.2	Excerpt from the 1994–1996 District Development Plan for Taita Taveta	55
4.3	Question in survey tool eliciting reasons for not attending an antenatal clinic	58
5.1	A new framework for treatment adherence for people living with HIV	70
6.1	Key stages of a typical programme cycle in social development contexts	82
7.1	Issues related to health providers	106
7.2	Overall strategic framework	107
9.1	The Tingim Laip STEPS Model	135
9.2	Mapping the context of HIV risk and impact along the Highlands Highway in Papua New Guinea. © DFAT	137
10.1	Systemic action research as an approach to understanding and enhancing volunteer action	147
10.2	A small group of volunteers create a systems map with community-generated insights	150
12.1	Chatting and hanging out with a range of villagers, Sulawesi, East Indonesia, 2014	175
13.1	A triad question about autonomy in the value chain	190
13.2	A slider about the degree of shared decision making	191
13.3	A 'stones' question about risk sharing	191
13.4	Smallholder story trends for production, trade and processing	196
14.1	Self-reported changes by male and female PEER researchers pre- and post-programme intervention	208
14.2	PEER researcher's drawings illustrating the impact of the intervention on their lives	210

Tables

6.1 Comparing and contrasting programme goals and girls' goals 89
10.1 Tools and techniques included in the volunteer training 148

Contributors

Peter Aggleton is Scientia Professor in Education and Health in the Centre for Social Research in Health at UNSW Australia, where he is also director of the Arts and Social Sciences Practical Justice Initiative. He has worked internationally in health and development for over 30 years, with a focus on health education and health promotion. He is an adjunct professor in the Australian Research Centre in Sex, Health and Society at La Trobe University, Australia, and holds visiting professorial positions at the UCL Institute of Education in London, UK, and at the University of Sussex, UK. Alongside his academic work, Peter has served as a senior adviser to numerous international agencies including UNAIDS, UNESCO, UNICEF and WHO.

Jody Aked is a doctoral researcher in the Participation Cluster at the Institute of Development Studies, UK, and is an associate with the consulting arm of the New Economics Foundation, UK. Her work facilitates social and organisational change using well-being insights, systems thinking, social network mapping tools and action research. In 2012–2014, Jody carried out two years' research in the Philippines exploring how social relationships and personal well-being influence the effectiveness of volunteering as a strategy for environmental management. She has published on the role of volunteering in sustainable development.

Stephen Bell is a senior research fellow at the Kirby Institute, UNSW Australia, where he undertakes qualitative and ethnographic sexual health research with young people and other marginalised populations in rural and remote settings. His current interests involve examining how the youth-led design of culturally and socially attuned sexual health programmes might evolve from, and be centred on, young people's own everyday strategies of sexual health risk assessment and harm reduction.

Scott Berry is an HIV technical practitioner for APMGlobal Health and a regional advisor for the HIV Foundation Asia based in Bangkok, Thailand. With over 25 years' experience in HIV, he designs programmes and services to promote innovation in the scale-up of HIV services in high prevalence settings across Asia and the Pacific. In Australia, Scott has worked for peak state and national AIDS organisations, as well as a term as the President of Positive Life NSW.

Eleanor Brown has over 15 years' experience working as an applied anthropologist with a focus on qualitative and participatory methodologies, particularly in the health sector. She is a technical specialist at Options Consultancy Services in London, UK, and has led ethnographically informed research projects in maternal, sexual and reproductive health, typically examining sensitive issues such as women's access to safe abortion services and addressing violence against women.

Ruth Edmonds is a social development consultant at Keep Your Shoes Dirty, UK, where she uses local knowledge to help understand people and their lives from their own vantage points to inform programme and policy design. In academic and consultancy roles, Ruth has designed and managed ethnographic research with street and working children, ex-combatants, child-headed households and child sex workers, and has edited a special issue of the journal *Children's Geographies* entitled, 'Ambiguous Agency: critical perspectives on social interventions with children and youth in Africa'.

Isolda Fortin serves as qualitative researcher for the PASMO (Pan-American Social Marketing Organisation) Regional Office, which is PSI's network member in Central America. Isolda is an anthropologist with a background in intercultural relationships, gender and health, and a specific interest in qualitative research and medical anthropology. She has published work on drug use and HIV risk in Guatemala.

Rachel Grellier is a senior gender and social inclusion specialist for Options Consultancy Services, based in Johannesburg, South Africa. She has a background in medical sociology and has a particular interest in participatory research methods. Rachel has led a number of rapid ethnographic research studies, including in Papua New Guinea, and has also lectured about the use of this approach as a participatory research method for the Consortium for Advanced Research Training in Africa (CARTA) at the University of Witwatersrand, South Africa.

Irene Guijt has worked globally in rural development for 25 years, focusing on participatory processes in planning, monitoring and evaluation. Irene recently started as Head of Research at Oxfam Great Britain. Before that she worked independently, including for the Overseas Development Institute, London, to build impact evaluation capacity in the Australian Department of Foreign Affairs and Trade. She has recently co-edited a book entitled *The Politics of Evidence and Results in International Development* (Practical Action Publishing, 2015).

Kirstan Hawkins is an anthropologist and writer. She is a technical director at Options Consultancy Services, London, and is the co-designer of PEER methodology. Kirstan has worked extensively on the application of this technique in different contexts. She has published on research findings relating to young women's constructions of identity, power and risk in transactional sexual relationships in Mozambique, and on the use of the PEER methodology for health research.

Christopher Hershey is a human rights activist living in Papua New Guinea since 1989. His work is committed to social inclusion, gender equality and other expressions of human rights. He has worked with Save the Children PNG, and the Tingim Laip Project, and has contributed to the formation or strengthening of national networks representing sex workers, people living with HIV, and men of diverse sexuality in PNG.

Yan Alicia Hong is an associate professor in the Department of Health Promotion and Community Health Sciences at the Texas A&M University School of Public Health. Her expertise is in the development and evaluation of culturally appropriate behavioural interventions, and she has worked with female sex workers, drug users, migrant workers, AIDS orphans and cancer survivors. She has published more than 60 peer-reviewed articles in these areas.

Dee Jupp has been an independent social development and participation advisor for more than 28 years. She is currently working as the Technical Team Leader for the Reality Check Approach Project in Indonesia, and as an advisor to Reality Check Approach research in Ghana, Mozambique, Ethiopia, Uganda, Nepal and Bangladesh. She is a passionate promoter of mixed methods research, and has contributed chapters to edited collections including *Knowledge from the Margins: An Anthology from a Global Network on Participatory Practice and Policy Influence* (Institute of Development Studies, 2014), and *Who Counts? The Power of Participatory Statistics* (Practical Action Publishing, 2013).

Angela Kelly-Hanku is Senior Principal Research Fellow and Head of the Sexual, Reproductive and Maternal Health Unit at the Papua New Guinea Institute of Medical Research. She is also a senior research fellow in the School of Public Health and Community Medicine at UNSW Australia. Angela has 20 years' experience in HIV-related work covering care and support training and service provision, as well as research and policy development. She lives in Papua New Guinea where most of her work takes place.

Elizabeth Gezahegn King has worked as Africa Programme Manager in the Foundation for Women's Health Research and Development (FORWARD) since 2008. She has spent the last 12 years working as an activist and frontline worker on sexual and reproductive health and rights of women and girls, in Africa and the UK. Over the past five years, she has coordinated and participated in programme-related ethnographic research studies addressing issues such as child marriage, female genital mutilation, obstetric fistula and teenage pregnancy in Tanzania, Sierra Leone, Liberia and Ethiopia.

Contributors xiii

Helen Lambert is Reader in Medical Anthropology in the School of Social and Community Medicine at Bristol University, UK. She has conducted extensive ethnographic, qualitative and interdisciplinary health research mostly in India and the UK. Her current work focuses on HIV, suicide prevention, medical pluralism, treatment-seeking practices and notions of evidence in public health and the social sciences. She recently guest-edited a special issue of the journal *Evidence & Policy* on the role of qualitative and ethnographic evidence in evaluating health interventions, and is currently ESRC Research Champion for social science research on Antimicrobial Resistance.

Carl Latkin is a professor in the Department of Health Behavior and Society and Department of Epidemiology in the Johns Hopkins University Bloomberg School of Public Health, USA. His research interests focus on HIV prevention and care among disadvantaged populations, domestic and international approaches to behaviour change, social and personal network analysis, neighbourhood factors and health behaviours. He has more than 20 years' research experience in HIV prevention and has published more than 250 articles.

Kim Longfield is Director for Strategic Research and Evaluation at PSI, USA, and has worked for the organisation since 2001. She leads a research unit that provides evidence about the effectiveness of PSI's work and uses that evidence to inform internal strategy as well as global best practices. Kim has always had a passion for qualitative research and has published work on interpretive research with hard-to-reach populations in journals including *Culture, Health & Sexuality, Sexual Health* and *Studies in Family Planning*.

Robert Lorway is an associate professor at the Centre for Global Public Health at the University of Manitoba, Canada. A medical anthropologist, he is interested in the critical ethnographic study of long-term, large-scale global health interventions in parts of Asia and Africa. He recently published a book, *Namibia's Rainbow Project: Gay Rights in an African Nation* (Indiana University Press, 2014), which is based on fieldwork conducted among a group of gay and lesbian youth living in an impoverished township in Namibia.

Lou McCallum is a health and development worker based in Sydney, Australia, working on projects that focus on connecting people from marginalised populations with the full range of health services, education and employment opportunities that are their right. He is a Director of APMGlobal Health and has been Technical Director and Contractor Representative for the Tingim Laip Project in Papua New Guinea for the last five years.

Jennifer Miller is a public health specialist, with expertise in sexual and reproductive health including HIV, key populations, monitoring and evaluation, youth, development and capacity building. Since 2007, her work has focused on evidence-informed, community-centred, peer-led interventions in Papua New Guinea. She has been part of numerous research studies on key populations, and is a member of Papua New Guinea's Strategic Information Technical Working Group, providing technical inputs for the development of a national unique identifier code.

Shannon Gwin Mitchell is a senior research scientist at Friends Research Institute in Baltimore, Maryland, USA. She is a community psychologist whose research focuses on prevention, early intervention, and treatment for substance use disorders. With expertise in qualitative and mixed methods research, Shannon has authored or co-authored over 60 peer reviewed publications, including papers in *Addiction*, *AIDS Education & Prevention* and *Health & Justice*.

Kate Norman is a freelance consultant and researcher based in the UK. She has spent the last 15 years supporting international organisations and foundations, national government departments of health, and bilateral health programmes in the areas of community health programming and research, behaviour change communication and capacity building and training. Kate works closely with FORWARD on participatory research that focuses on giving voice to girls and women from marginalised communities across Africa and ensuring they are involved in designing the programmes that affect them.

Naana Otoo-Oyortey is the Executive Director of FORWARD, a not-for-profit African-led organisation based in the UK that tackles female genital mutilation, child marriage, and sexual and reproductive health inequality. She has over 20 years' experience working on sexual and reproductive health and rights, which includes providing expert advice to the UK government on women and girls and the European Parliament on female genital mutilation. Naana is an activist, championing the rights of African girls and young women in rural and marginalised communities. She is a board member of ACORD and President of the Board of the End FGM European Network, based in Brussels.

James A. Peterson is research professor in the Department of Epidemiology and Biostatistics, The Milken Institute School of Public Health, George Washington University, USA. He has significant experience of ethnographic fieldwork in urban settings, and has conducted ethnographic research among substance abusers, men who have sex with men, HIV positive people, and hard-to-reach populations. James has authored and co-authored numerous publications in this area, including recent community-based work with HIV positive prison re-entrants.

Elsabé du Plessis is a doctoral candidate in the Department of Community Health Sciences at the University of Manitoba, Canada, where she is affiliated with the Centre for Global Public Health. Elsabé has been involved in various global health research projects since 2004, and is interested in the critical social study of global health as a field of social practices.

Mary Louisa Plummer is currently working as a UNICEF adolescent and youth technical advisor seconded to the Tanzanian government institution that coordinates the national response to HIV/AIDS (TACAIDS). She is interested in the potential of qualitative research to evaluate the impact of sexual health programmes. Mary is the author of *Young People's Lives and Sexual Relationships in Rural Africa* (Lexington Books, 2011) and *Promoting Abstinence, Being Faithful, and Condom Use with Young Africans* (Lexington Books, 2012).

Tushar Kanti Ray is a public health consultant with over 25 years of experience working in Asia and Africa. This included the planning and implementation of tuberculosis control programmes in India, Bhutan, Myanmar and Nigeria. He has worked as an independent consultant to the Stop TB Partnership, WHO and other international agencies in more than 25 countries. He is also a strong patient advocate.

Jens Seeberg is an associate professor in the Department of Anthropology at Aarhus University, Denmark, where he is also head of department. He has worked as a medical anthropologist in South Asia for 25 years, and as an advisor to Danida and the WHO. He is currently the director of several research projects on epidemics and migration. He has recently published on tuberculosis in India in *Cambridge Anthropology* (2014) and in an edited book called *Navigating Social Exclusion and Inclusion in Contemporary India and Beyond* (eds Skoda, Nielsen and Fibiger, Anthem, 2013).

Dana Sievers is a research assistant in the Strategic Research and Evaluation department at PSI. She provides support on PSI's studies and publications, and is responsible for knowledge management and data sharing agreements.

Karin Tobin is an associate professor in the Department of Health Behavior and Society at Johns Hopkins University Bloomberg School of Public Health, USA. Her research interests are in the development and evaluation of behavioural interventions that aim to reduce disparities in HIV risk, specifically as this affects adult populations in urban environments including drug users and men who have sex with men. Her research has been continuously funded by the US National Institutes of Health and she has published more than 100 articles.

Martin Walsh is Global Research Adviser at Oxfam GB, where he edits (2012–) Oxfam's online *Research Guidelines* and is working on a series of in-depth programme evaluations. He has lectured on the anthropology of development and research methods in the University of Cambridge, UK, and written extensively about gender and development issues and East African ethnography.

Jennifer Wheeler is PSI's Regional Researcher for Latin America and the Caribbean. She manages and provides technical assistance to the region's research portfolio, including qualitative and quantitative studies in the areas of HIV, family planning and gender violence. She has recently published an article in *Global Health Action* about HIV risk behaviour among men who have sex with men in nine cities in Central America.

Acknowledgements

We would like to thank our partners, Annie and Preecha, for their understanding and support while preparing this book, and Rakhi Kabawala for her assistance in preparing the manuscript for publication.

Abbreviations

CAD	community action day
CARTA	Consortium for Advanced Research Training in Africa
DFID	Department for International Development
DMSC	Durbar Mahila Samanwaya Committee
DOTS	Directly Observed Treatment, Short-course
ESSENCE	Enhancing Support for Strengthening the Effectiveness of National Capacity Efforts
FGM	female genital mutilation
FORWARD	Foundation for Women's Health Research and Development
ICS	International Citizen Service
PEER	Participatory Ethnographic Evaluation and Research
PNG	Papua New Guinea
PPI	Public and Patient Involvement
PSI	Population Services International
RCT	randomised controlled trial
SAR	systemic action research
STEP	Stand up and be positive
TB	tuberculosis
USAID	United States Agency for International Development
VECO	Vredeseilanden
VSO	Voluntary Services Overseas
WE-Care	Women's Empowerment and Care
WHO	World Health Organisation

Interpretive and ethnographic perspectives

Alternative approaches to monitoring and evaluation practice

Stephen Bell and Peter Aggleton

Introduction

Interpretive and ethnographic approaches have long been used in research to monitor and evaluate programmes in social development and health. The successful use of these approaches has been documented in relation to schooling and community (Dorr-Breme 1985, Erickson 1977), drug and substance use (Singer 1993, Singer et al. 1995, Hong et al. 2005, Needle et al. 2008, McNeil et al. 2015), rural livelihoods (Niehof and Price 2008, Siyoum et al. 2012, Harrison 2015), peacebuilding and justice (Miller and Rudnick 2010, 2012, Mieth 2013), adolescent marriage (White 2015), and the delivery of a range of health care services (Diamond 1986, Bentley et al. 1988, Shawyer et al. 1996, Price and Pokharel 2006, Savage 2006, Jain and Jadhav 2009, Brewer and Sparkes 2011, Millard and Ladia 2015), among other topics. In recent times, the fields of HIV and sexual health have perhaps benefitted the most from the application of interpretive and ethnographic approaches to programme monitoring and evaluation across a diverse range of social and cultural global settings (e.g. Clatts 1989, Schensul and Weeks 1989, Ingstad 1990, Schensul and Schensul 1990, Carrier and Magana 1991, Farmer 1992, Green 1992a, 1992b, Singer 1994, Obot et al. 1997, Waterston 1997, Parker 2001, Price and Hawkins 2002, Green et al. 2009, Leclerc-Madlala 2009, Mignone et al. 2009, Turkon et al. 2009, Simmons 2011, Bell and Aggleton 2012).

Despite this activity, interpretive and ethnographic approaches are side-lined in much contemporary evaluation work, and current monitoring and evaluation practice remains heavily influenced by more positivist approaches (Eyben 2010, 2013, Natsios 2010, Bell and Aggleton 2012, Harrison 2015, White 2015, Winther 2015). These not infrequently seek to specify in advance what will be measured and how predetermined outcomes will be brought about. This style of work, while popular, is problematic in several respects, not only because of cost (the analytic frameworks advocated for by development agencies often suggest that expensive experimental and quasi-experimental attribution analyses are required to identify whether a programme has had its intended effect), but also because it often occurs at the expense of sensitive, in-depth qualitative research documenting community perspectives on impact and change (Bell and Aggleton 2012).

The emphasis given to results-based programme reporting also means that monitoring and evaluation are usually undertaken for upward accountability purposes and to demonstrate success (Batliwala and Pittman 2010), rather than to learn how change happens, what went wrong, what works within a particular context, and how best to refine programmatic approaches. The tendency to monitor and evaluate health programmes using a 'logical framework' (or log frame) or a 'theory of change' can flatten complex processes of growth, development and change into overly simple linear models of cause and effect (Batliwala and Pittman 2010, Grove and Zwi 2008). Within these models, programme impact and success are often measured against external programme goals, rather than against the more local changes that have occurred in people's lives.

This book emerges from a growing sense of concern about the challenges faced in knowing how best to intervene to improve health and social development. The current preference for outsider-led, top-down quantitative studies tends to be driven by concerns that are external to the affected communities. All too often, local people are involved in programmes as 'participants' or 'beneficiaries', rather than as informed, local experts capable of ensuring that programmes are relevant and achieve the desired results. Responding to these concerns, this book seeks to counter the marginalisation of qualitative perspectives resulting from the prevailing 'methodological triumphalism' (Barrett and Carter 2010: 516), which assumes that quantitative approaches to evaluation are superior, more robust and more scientifically valid. Chapters seek to illustrate the potential of interpretive and ethnographic methods to improve understanding and make a difference to communities on the ground. Through a focus on individual and community perspectives and locally grounded explanation, we aim to offer a richer way to assess the relationship between intent, action and change in health and social development.

Current trends in monitoring and evaluation

Monitoring and evaluation serves a range of purposes including learning what works, refining and redesigning programme approaches, and attributing cause and effect. When implemented effectively, it involves reporting downwards to local communities and upwards to development agencies and funders for the purpose of accountability and credibility (Batliwala and Pittman 2010, O'Flynn 2010, Bell and Aggleton 2012).

Most often the focus is on measuring the 'impact' of specific programmes and interventions. However, as is explained elsewhere (Bell and Aggleton 2012: 796–798), confusion abounds concerning two rather different understandings of what impact evaluation might involve (White 2009). The first approach prioritises the use of studies that aim to attribute changes in selected outcomes to a specific intervention using 'scientifically valid' designs. These studies should more accurately be called 'attribution analyses' (White 2009). Proponents of this approach argue that carefully designed experimental and quasi-experimental research can determine whether (and to some degree why) an intervention had its intended effect.

A number of concerns can be raised about this way of working (Bell and Aggleton 2012: 797). First, while attribution analyses have their place, attribution is not the only purpose of impact evaluation, and there are important ethical concerns relating to the use of 'control groups' as counterfactuals who do not benefit from programmes or interventions. Second, these approaches are costly and often beyond the budgets of national and local programmes in developing countries. Third, the methods used tend to rely on a level of expertise that excludes important local and professional programme stakeholders, including community members, from being involved in the evaluation. Finally, efforts to understand context and engage with community members in order to develop a theory of change to guide programme design, implementation and quantitative evaluation tend to be weak, instead relying on the expertise of programme managers and/or external evaluators.

A second approach to impact evaluation advocates that monitoring and evaluation research should centre on the programme implementation cycle. This type of research attempts to understand whether expected programme outcomes have been achieved, as well as their resulting long-term effects. It aims to evaluate success as an integral dimension of programme design and implementation, answering questions such as 'what should we do?', 'are we on track?' and 'did it work, and how?' (Collumbien *et al.* 2006: 155). Typically, information is gathered in line with a monitoring and evaluation framework – an integrated system blending monitoring research with evaluation research that collects experiences and information during and after programme delivery – to assess programme delivery, progress and impact. This tends to involve four rather different things: (i) needs assessment and insight research to inform programme planning, (ii) the monitoring of programme delivery, (iii) impact assessment and evaluation, and (iv) the analysis of the information collected to document best practice.

Monitoring, or process evaluation, is an ongoing programme management activity that assesses the implementation of programme activities and progress towards meeting target programme outcomes. Ideally, it should take place periodically and systematically throughout the programme cycle to determine whether work is proceeding as planned. In doing this, it generates information that enables managers to make improvements or put programmes back on track (Batliwala and Pittman 2010, Collumbien *et al.* 2006). Evaluation research, on the other hand, is designed to assess the overall impact of a programme, typically against an explicit set of predetermined goals and objectives. It involves the systematic collection and analysis of data to help discover if, how and why a particular intervention or set of interventions worked (Batliwala and Pittman 2010). It usually takes place less often than monitoring, is more comprehensive in character, and tries to capture impact at particular moments in time. Evaluation research can take several different forms. For example, summative evaluation may occur at the end of a given programme cycle and focuses in on programme outcomes, strengths and weaknesses (Batliwala and Pittman 2010). In contrast, impact evaluations offer an analysis of lasting or significant change – positive or negative, intended or not – in people's lives brought about by an action or a series of actions (O'Flynn, 2010).

A recent review (Batliwala and Pittman 2010) highlights a number of weaknesses in current evaluation practice. For example, the log frame approach heavily promoted by some funding agencies frequently flattens complex change processes into overly simple causes and effects. It prioritises attention to programme goals or a theory of change, rather than the changes taking place in ordinary people's lives. Likewise, too keen an interest in individual behaviour change (again, a much loved focus of health and development work) can blind us to the influence of social, cultural, economic and political factors in bringing about change. Finally, too close a focus on what it is that a programme seeks to achieve can cause us to ignore or misrecognise negative change, reversals and unexpected outcomes, and the longer-term changes that may take place beyond a programme itself.

Lack of familiarity with qualitative approaches to evaluation by programme staff and donor agencies also influences the preference for quantitative methods in monitoring and evaluation work (Bell and Aggleton 2012). At donor level, this tendency is compounded by a lack of space to talk about alternatives to conventional monitoring and evaluation approaches, and the benefits of using evaluation as a learning device rather than as an accountability tool. Chapters in this book provide the opportunity for practitioners, donors and policy makers to learn about the benefits of using these kinds of strategies.

Interpretive and ethnographic approaches

Some forty years ago, the social sciences witnessed a major epistemological shift – from hitherto predominantly positivist ways of understanding social life to more interpretive approaches. Often referred to as 'the interpretive turn in social science' (e.g. Geertz 1973, Rabinow and Sullivan 1979), researchers sought to modify the methodological logic underpinning social enquiry. Methodologically, positivist research tends to be *hypothetico-deductive* in character. Hypotheses are created from existing theory in advance of data collection, and research is conducted to test whether or not these 'hunches' are supported by the data. This type of enquiry tends to employ quantitative methods, using either comparative designs (comprising experimental and control groups) or surveys involving large and representative samples. The goal of this style of research is to come up with generalisations in the form of 'law-like' statements relating to human behaviour across a range of settings.

Interpretivist social scientists were quick to reject these ideas, arguing that reality is constructed in multiple ways, by people who build their understandings of the world through experience and interaction with others (Willis 2007).

In contrast to positivist approaches, the goal of much interpretive research is to access subjective understandings, recognising that how people see themselves and others is heavily contextual (Willis 2007, Schwartz-Shea and Yanow 2012). Interpretive research often adopts more qualitative approaches to data collection, paying attention to local detail and the 'social situatedness' of knowledge. Its methodology is generally *inductive* rather than hypothetico-deductive, with meanings and understandings being built upwards from the ground rather than in a top-down manner informed by existing theory and predetermined hypotheses.

This book focuses on this latter approach and in particular on inductive and interpretive approaches to information gathering for programmatic purposes. The chapters it contains describe a variety of qualitative methods that have been used to access insider perspectives on the design and monitoring of social development and health programmes, and to understand impacts and changes. Much of the work focused upon aims to be emic ('insider' or 'experience-near') (Geertz 1973, 1983, Parker 2001) in character, generating understandings as seen through the eyes of a specific community or culture. In contrast, a more etic (or 'outsider' or 'experience-distant') approach draws on concepts and categories derived from the more theoretical understandings already written about by researchers.

However, our focus here is also on *ethnographic* styles of work. Ethnography can be defined in different ways, and more detailed analyses of the various forms it takes both within and across disciplines can be found elsewhere (e.g. Delamont and Atkinson 1980, Atkinson et al. 2001). Traditionally, for anthropologists, ethnography promoted a concern to open up and understand how human beings live in culturally unique settings around the world. In sociological studies, it has involved an interest in the life worlds of those living on the margins of 'modern' and urban societies, as well as the exploration of social processes in specific institutional settings (e.g. in the classroom or on the street). More recently in development studies, ethnography has been used to explore the internal workings of international agencies and development organisations (e.g. Hilhorst 2003) and development practice (e.g. Crewe and Harrison 1998, Mosse 2004), as well as the impact of development interventions, national policies and governance processes in different realms (e.g. social, cultural, economic, legal) and at different scales (e.g. household, community, national) in society. Crucially, ethnography aims to understand and describe cultures and the belief systems and social rules that motivate action within them (Hammersley and Atkinson 2007). Rather than describing any one form of research that aims to make sense of individual life experiences from participants' own point of view, ethnography stresses the importance of taking into account the role that social and cultural relations play in enabling people to interpret life experiences in a particular way (Atkinson 2015).

A number of well-established texts outline the specific principles and practices of ethnography as a research approach (e.g. Marcus 1998, Crang and Cook 2007, Hammersley and Atkinson 2007, Fetterman 2009, Lecompte and Schensul 2010, Emerson et al. 2011), and several key principles distinguish ethnographic research approaches from other forms of qualitative enquiry (Atkinson 2015: 3–7). First, it demands a distinctive way of 'knowing', in which close attention is given to the particularities of social life, and in which there is reflexive concern for an ethnographer's own position and work. Second, it requires a degree of participation, engagement and observation in the everyday lives of the social actors whose lives we want to understand. Third, it involves a distinctive set of methods – including participant observation, key informant interviews and in-depth interviews, as well as other approaches to build understanding from the grassroots upwards. The role of the ethnographer is to watch, listen, take part in daily life and ask questions to throw light on a particular research issue.

Interpretive and ethnographic evaluation

Interpretive and ethnographic approaches to monitoring and evaluation seek to apply the analytic methods of interpretive researchers and ethnographers to the purposes of programmatic decision making. They strive to be emic rather than etic in character, focusing in on how participants and stakeholders interpret a programme and its effects in the light of local realities and meaning systems (Dorr-Bremme 1985, Bell and Aggleton 2012). They struggle to be context-sensitive, in recognition of the fact that individuals' systems of perceiving, believing and acting vary depending on where they are, who they are with, and the life experiences they have had (Dorr-Bremme 1985, Bell and Aggleton 2012). They encourage reflexivity and critical self-awareness on the part of researchers. Monitoring and evaluation specialists need to question their own behaviour, attitudes, values and beliefs in the light of the influence these may have on others (Hammersley and Atkinson 2007). Finally, this type of evaluation requires findings, interpretations and inferences to be cross-checked against one another through processes of 'triangulation' (Hammersley and Atkinson, 2007).

Several barriers exist to undertaking interpretive or ethnographic evaluation. The fieldwork involved can be time consuming, and training and experience is required for researchers to enter a cultural setting and feel comfortable questioning their own assumptions and beliefs. Developing an emic understanding is not always easy, especially for those who find it hard to 'bracket' their own academic and professional training and who feel sure they know in advance the solutions to the problems local communities face. Openness of mind, the ability to separate dominant social values from local perspectives, the ability to build rapport and empathy with other people, a willingness to learn, and a strong and patient work ethic are among the many skills required to undertake this type of work.

Evaluators using interpretive and ethnographic methods regularly grapple with the request to collect data in circumstances where time and budgetary constraints require the use of a rapid methodological approach. As a result, there is a growing literature on what have been called rapid ethnographic approaches (Shawyer et al. 1996, Needle et al. 2005). Examples include the use of rapid ethnographic assessment for the dietary management of diarrhoea in Peru and Nigeria (Bentley et al. 1988), for the development of assessment tools predictive of HIV infection in rural India (Mignone et al. 2009), and to elicit emic perspectives from inmates and administrators concerning HIV prevention in correctional facilities in the USA (Obot et al. 1997). Rapid approaches are best deployed by researchers who have long-standing experience in a particular field site, within a specific culture, or with the population groups under study.

Summary of contributions

In this book, we have brought together a number of chapters that aim to offer the reader a sense of how interpretive and ethnographic approaches to monitoring and evaluation can be used to deliver successful programmes in health and social development. To illustrate how these approaches can enhance current monitoring and evaluation, we have organised chapters so as to provide insight into current challenges, and then to demonstrate how these methods can be used at three different stages of the programme and policy cycle: *programme design*, including needs assessment and baseline survey research; *programme delivery*, including research to monitor the delivery of particular programme activities, and outputs and outcomes arising from these; and *programme evaluation*, including research to examine impact and change resulting from programmes.

With these goals in mind, Part I, 'The present challenge', focuses first on overviews and critiques of current evaluation practice and the challenges that can arise in trying to use interpretive and ethnographic methods.

In Chapter 2, 'The political economy of evidence: personal reflections on the value of the interpretive tradition and its methods', Angela Kelly-Hanku draws on her personal experience working in Papua New Guinea with a focus on HIV and sexual health. She discusses the difficulties encountered in an environment where a research politics of ignorance and conflicting agendas privileges numerically driven evaluation. She describes experiences illustrating how value judgements on the part of researchers and evaluators mean that more traditional survey-based evaluation practices are no more likely to generate neutral or 'valid' evidence than interpretive approaches to monitoring and evaluation research.

In Chapter 3, 'Measurement, modification and transferability: evidential challenges in the evaluation of complex interventions', Helen Lambert draws on examples from HIV prevention interventions in India to examine the tensions between 'outward-facing' (quantitative, outcome-focused measurement) and 'inward-facing' (qualitative, process-focused explanation) modes of evaluation. She argues that experimental designs may appear to hold out the promise of generalisability, but controlled outcome measurement necessarily renders invisible the local conditions conducive to success or failure. Instead, ethnography and qualitative case studies can help document the context-specific adaptations and local adjustments required to help replicate or scale up complex social change interventions that have proven successful in other settings.

In Chapter 4, 'What really works? Understanding the role of 'local knowledges' in the monitoring and evaluation of a maternal, newborn and child health project in Kenya', Elsabé du Plessis and Robert Lorway reflect on the limitations of a narrow understanding of 'evidence' in the form of knowledge generated through standardised project monitoring indicators. This chapter examines the ways in which historically situated local knowledges – i.e. experiential and contextual understandings, such as those adhered to by project staff – are generated over time and operate throughout the life history of global health projects. The authors illustrate how ethnographic evaluation can highlight how conflicting ways of knowing interact to undermine survey-based programme impact evaluation efforts, but also allow project staff to address monitoring and evaluation tensions before these derail project activities.

In Part II of this volume, 'Programme design', we turn our attention to settings in which interpretive and ethnographic research has been applied most commonly to date. Authors in this section illustrate how interpretive and ethnographic research may be used to generate and apply local knowledge to the design of specific health and social development programmes and policies. In Chapter 5, 'Permissions, vacations and periods of self-regulation: using consumer insight to improve HIV treatment adherence in four Central American countries', Kim Longfield and colleagues illustrate how one ethnographic method – the life history interview – helped social marketers gather improved consumer insight, subsequently shaping the marketing planning process and programme design for a campaign to improve adherence to HIV treatment in Costa Rica, El Salvador, Nicaragua and Panama.

In Chapter 6, 'Generating local knowledge: a role for ethnography in evidence-based programme design for social development', Ruth Edmonds illustrates how an ethnographic approach revealed important cultural constructs that were used to underpin the design of a locally meaningful girls' empowerment programme in Rwanda.

In Chapter 7, 'Interpretation, context and time: an ethnographically inspired approach to strategy development for tuberculosis control in Odisha, India', Jens Seeberg and Tushar Kanti Ray describe the use of interpretive analysis during the development of a health programme for tuberculosis control. They discuss the challenge of delivering results speedily and the time required to develop an adequate interpretation of perspectives in the field, and stress the importance of systematic interpretive analysis to understand the complexity of local context in programme development.

Finally, in Chapter 8, 'Designing health and leadership programmes for young vulnerable women using participatory ethnographic research in Freetown, Sierra Leone', Nanna Otoo-Oyortey, Elizabeth Gezahegn King and Kate Norman describe how formative ethnographic research led to the implementation of a new programme and a registered girl-led community organisation that aimed to equip young girls with skills to advocate against harmful social values that marginalise young mothers, and community practices including female genital mutilation and other forms of gender-based violence.

Chapters in Part III, 'Monitoring processes', focus on the least documented area of use of interpretive or ethnographic evaluation approaches – namely, research undertaken to monitor the implementation of health and social development programmes. Contributors examine how these approaches can be used to generate both process data (with a focus on programme delivery) and longitudinal impact data (with a focus on community perspectives of change) to assess the appropriateness of programme implementation. For example, in Chapter 9, 'Using social mapping techniques to guide programme redesign in the Tingim Laip HIV prevention and care project in Papua New Guinea', Lou McCallum and colleagues describe the use of ethnographic and social mapping techniques to inform ongoing implementation of the largest community-based HIV project in Papua New Guinea.

In Chapter 10, 'Pathways to impact: new approaches to monitoring and improving volunteering for sustainable environmental management', Jody Aked explores the value of interpretive research in reviewing and improving the design of volunteer interventions to influence pro-environmental behaviour in communities in the Philippines to support the management of a watershed, and to build capacity for local youth action and engagement in decision making.

In Chapter 11, 'Ethnographic process evaluation: a case study of an HIV prevention programme with injecting drug users in the USA', Yan Alicia Hong and colleagues illustrate how participant observation and key informant interviews were used to adapt HIV prevention education materials and programme activities. The authors highlight how ethnographic methods provided vital local insight to adjust the intervention to local people's specific practices.

In Chapter 12, 'Using the Reality Check Approach to shape quantitative findings: experience from mixed method evaluations in Ghana and Nepal', Dee Jupp presents the use of an ethnographically informed methodology called the Reality Check Approach, which involved participant observation and in-depth interviews during extended home stays. This was used to monitor and understand the change experienced by households in Ghana and Nepal as a result of a planned and integrated set of health, education and rural access interventions.

In the final Part of this book, 'Understanding impact and change', contributors examine how interpretive and ethnographic approaches to evaluation can generate understandings of impact and change from a range of individual and community perspectives. In Chapter 13, 'Innovation in evaluation: using SenseMaker to assess the inclusion of smallholder farmers in modern markets', Irene Guijt discusses the application of an interpretive, micro narrative-based research approach used to assess local perspectives of change among banana chip farmers in Equador and farmers involved in tea production in Vietnam.

In Chapter 14, 'The use of the Rapid PEER approach for the evaluation of sexual and reproductive health programmes', Eleanor Brown and colleagues examine the use of a participatory, ethnographic method to understand community perspectives on change resulting from a female genital mutilation prevention programme in the UK and an HIV behaviour change programme in Papua New Guinea. The examples chosen illustrate the benefits of involving programme participants and community members in a socioculturally sensitive examination of change.

In Chapter 15, 'Using interpretive research to make quantitative evaluation more effective: Oxfam's experience in Pakistan and Zimbabwe', Martin Walsh documents Oxfam International's evolving practice employing in-depth qualitative and other interpretive research methods to deepen the findings of effectiveness reviews based on the use of a quasi-experimental survey design.

Finally, in Chapter 16, 'Can qualitative research rigorously evaluate programme impact? Evidence from a randomised controlled trial of an adolescent sexual health intervention in Tanzania', Mary Louisa Plummer examines the use of multi-method, representative interpretive research to evaluate the impact of a large-scale sexual health programme in rural Tanzania, which was also evaluated quantitatively as part of a randomised controlled trial. Triangulation between the quantitative and qualitative findings suggests that the qualitative research produced more consistent and valid programme impact data than did the biomedical and interview survey methods, and also delivered behavioural data with greater meaning and depth.

In bringing together these different contributions, we have worked hard to illustrate how high quality ethnographic and interpretive evaluation research can seriously strengthen contemporary quantitative monitoring and evaluation practice. Throughout the book, contributors highlight the importance of using these approaches to ensure that local people's socially constructed views, meanings, explanations and interpretations become central to processes of programme design, monitoring and evaluation. Using these principles, programme monitoring and evaluation holds the potential to enable practitioners to learn more about programme impact and, through local feedback, improve programme design and delivery.

Both individually and together, contributors to this volume share a commitment to working with local people to promote health and social development. By listening carefully and respectfully to what individuals and communities have to say, it is possible to lay secure foundations for a successful programmatic response. We hope the contributions in this book inspire you to try out some of these methods and approaches for yourself, and to document their application across additional contexts. Join us, as we work towards securing a step-change in international monitoring and evaluation practice in relation to social development and health.

References

Atkinson, P. (2015) *For Ethnography*, London: SAGE.

Atkinson, P., Coffey, A., Delamont, S., Lofland, J. and Lofland, L. (eds) (2001) *Handbook of Ethnography*, London: SAGE.

Barrett, C.B. and Carter, M.R. (2010) 'The power and pitfalls of experiments in development economics: some non-random reflections', *Applied Economic Perspectives and Policy*, 32(4): 515–548.

Batliwala, S. and Pittman, A. (2010) *Capturing Change in Women's Realities: A critical overview of current monitoring and evaluation frameworks and approaches*, Toronto: AWID.

Bell, S.A. and Aggleton, P. (2012) 'Integrating ethnographic principles in NGO monitoring and impact evaluation', *Journal of International Development*, 24: 795–907.

Bentley, M.E., Pelto, G.H., Straus, W.L., Schumann, D.A., Adegbola, C., de la Pena, E., Oni, G.A., Brown, K.H. and Huffman, S.L. (1988) 'Rapid ethnographic assessment: applications in a diarrhea management program', *Social Science & Medicine*, 27(1): 107–116.

Brewer, J.D. and Sparkes, A.C. (2011) 'Young people living with parental bereavement: insights from an ethnographic study of a UK childhood bereavement service', *Social Science & Medicine*, 72: 283–290.

Carrier, J. and Magaña, R. (1991) 'Use of ethnosexual data on men of Mexican origin for HIV/AIDS prevention programs', *Journal of Sex Research*, 28(2): 189–202.

Clatts, M. (1989) 'Ethnography and AIDS intervention in New York City: life history as an ethnographic strategy', in National Institute of Drug Abuse (ed.) *Community-Based AIDS Prevention, Studies of Intravenous Drug Users and their Sexual Partners*, Rockville, MD: National Institute of Drug Abuse, pp. 225–233.

Collumbien, M., Douthwaite, M. and Jana, L. (2006) 'Using evaluation to improve sexual health of young people', in Ingham, R. and Aggleton, P. (eds) *Promoting Young People's Sexual Health: International perspectives*, London: Routledge, pp. 155–173.

Crang, M.A. and Cook, I. (2007) *Doing Ethnographies*, Norwich: Geobooks.

Crewe, E. and Harrison, E. (1998) *Whose Development? An ethnography of aid*, London: Zed Books.

Delamont, S. and Atkinson, P. (1980) 'The two traditions in educational ethnography: sociology and anthropology compared', *British Journal of Sociology of Education*, 1(2): 139–152.

Diamond, T. (1986) 'Social policy and everyday life in nursing homes: a critical ethnography', *Social Science & Medicine*, 23(12): 1287–1295.

Dorr-Bremme, D.W. (1985) 'Ethnographic evaluation: a theory and method', *Educational Evaluation and Policy Analysis*, 7(1): 65–83.

Emerson, R.M., Fretz, R.I. and Shaw, L.L. (2011) *Writing Ethnographic Fieldnotes*, Chicago, IL: University of Chicago Press.

Ericksen, F. (1977) 'Some approaches to inquiry in school-community ethnography', *Anthropology & Education Quarterly*, 8(2): 58–69.

Eyben R. (2010) *The Political and Ideological Context of Assessing and Reporting on Making a Difference in Development*. Available at: www.ids.ac.uk/index.cfm?objectid=832D48DD-0914-1D37-483AAAA9480E7 (accessed 19 June 2015).

Eyben, R. (2013) *Uncovering the Politics of 'Evidence' and 'Results': A framing paper for development practitioners*. Available at: http://bigpushforward.net/wp-content/uploads/2011/01/The-politics-of-evidence-11-April-20133.pdf (accessed 19 June 2015).

Farmer, P. (1992) *AIDS and Accusation: Haiti and the geography of blame*, Berkeley, CA: University of California Press.

Fetterman, D.M. (2009) *Ethnography: Step-by-step*, Thousand Oaks, CA: SAGE.

Geertz, C. (1973) *The Interpretation of Cultures*, New York: Basic Books.

Geertz, C. (1983) *Local Knowledge: Further essays on interpretive anthropology*, New York: Basic Books.

Green, E.C. (1992a) 'The anthropology of sexually transmitted disease in Liberia', *Social Science & Medicine*, 35(12): 1457–1468.
Green, E.C. (1992b) 'Sexually transmitted disease, ethnomedicine and health policy in Africa', *Social Science & Medicine*, 35(2): 121–130.
Green, E.C., Dlamini, C., D'Errico, N.C., Ruark, A. and Duby, Z. (2009) 'Mobilising indigenous resources for anthropologically designed HIV-prevention and behaviour-change interventions in southern Africa', *African Journal of AIDS Research*, 8(4): 389–400.
Grove, N.J. and Zwi, A.B. (2008) 'Beyond the logframe: a new tool for examining health and peacebuilding initiatives', *Development in Practice*, 18(1): 66–81.
Hammersley, M. and Atkinson, P. (2007) *Ethnography: Principles in practice*, Abingdon: Routledge.
Harrison, E. (2015) 'Anthropology and impact evaluation: a critical commentary', *Journal of Development Effectiveness*, 7(2): 146–159.
Hilhorst, D. (2003) *The Real World of NGOs: Discourses, diversity and development*, London: Zed Books.
Hong, Y., Mitchell, S.G., Peterson, J.A., Latkin, C.A., Tobin, K. and Gann, D. (2005) 'Ethnographic process evaluation: piloting an HIV prevention intervention program among injection drug users', *International Journal of Qualitative Methods*, 4(1). Available at: http://ejournals.library.ualberta.ca/index.php/IJQM/article/view/4450 (accessed 19 June 2015).
Ingstad, B. (1990) 'The cultural construction of AIDS and its consequences for prevention in Botswana', *Medical Anthropology Quarterly*, 4(1): 28–40.
Jain, S. and Jadhav, J. (2009) 'Pills that swallow policy: clinical ethnography of a community mental health program in Northern India', *Transcultural Psychiatry*, 46(1): 60–85.
Leclerc-Madlala, S. (2009) 'Cultural scripts for multiple and concurrent partnerships in southern Africa: why HIV prevention needs anthropology', *Sexual Health*, 6: 103–110.
LeCompte, M.D. and Schensul, J.J. (2010) *Designing and Conducting Ethnographic Research*, Lanham, MD: AltaMira Press.
McNeil, R., Kerr, T., Lampkin, H. and Small, W. (2015) '"We need somewhere to smoke crack": an ethnographic study of an unsanctioned safer smoking room in Vancouver, Canada', *International Journal of Drug Policy*, 26: 645–652.
Marcus, G.E. (1998) *Ethnography through Thick and Thin*, Princetown, NJ: Princetown University Press.
Mieth, F. (2013) 'Bringing justice and enforcing peace? An ethnographic perspective on the impact of the special court for Sierra Leone', *International Journal of Conflict and Violence*, 7(1): 10–22.
Mignone, J., Hiremath, G.M., Sabnis, V., Laxmi, J., Halli, S., O'Niel, J., Rmaesh, B.M., Blanchard, J. and Moses, S. (2009) 'Use of rapid ethnographic methodology to develop a village-level Rapid Assessment tool predictive of HIV infection in rural India', *International Journal of Qualitative Methods*, 8(3): 52–67.
Millard, A.V. and Ladia, M.A.J. (2015) 'TB meets IE: contributions of ethnography', *Journal of Development Effectiveness*, 7(2): 175–191.
Miller, D.B. and Rudnick, L. (2010) 'The case for situated theory in modern peacebuilding practice', *Journal of Peacebuilding & Development*, 5(2): 62–74.

Miller, D. and Rudnick, L. (2012) *A Framework Document for Evidence-Based Programme Design on Reintegration*. Available at: www.unidir.org/files/publications/pdfs/a-framework-document-for-evidence-based-programme-design-on-reintegration-396.pdf (accessed 16 March 2015).

Mosse, D. (2004) *Cultivating Development: An ethnography of aid policy and practice*, London: Pluto Press.

Natsios, A. (2010) *The Clash of the Counter-bureaucracy and Development*. Available at: www.cgdev.org/content/publications/detail/1424271 (accessed 18 June 2015).

Needle, R., Kroeger, K., Belani, H., Achrekar, A., Parry, C.D., and Dewing, S. (2008) 'Sex, drugs and HIV: rapid assessment of HIV risk behaviors among street-based drug using sex workers in Durban, South Africa', *Social Science & Medicine*, 67: 1447–1455.

Niehof, A. and Price, L.L. (2008) 'Etic and emic perspectives on HIV/AIDS impacts on rural livelihoods and agricultural practice in Sub-Saharan Africa', *NJAS*, 56(3): 139–153.

Obot, E.G., Braithwaite, R.L., Mayberry, R., Gunn, E.L., Harris, B., Harrison, A., Murdaugh, H. and Cozza, S. (1997) 'Ethnographic assessment of HIV risk reduction programs in correctional facilities', *Journal of Health Education*, 28(Suppl. 1): S38–S43.

O'Flynn, M. (2010) 'Impact assessment: understanding and assessing our contributions to change', *M&E Paper 7*. Available at: www.intrac.org/resources.php?action=resource&id=695 (accessed 18 June 2015).

Parker, R. (2001) 'Sexuality, culture and power in HIV/AIDS research', *Annual Review of Anthropology*, 30: 163–179.

Price, N. and Hawkins, K. (2002) 'Researching sexual and reproductive behaviour: a peer ethnographic approach', *Social Science & Medicine*, 55: 1325–1336.

Price, N. and Pokharel, D. (2006) 'Using key informant monitoring in safe motherhood programming in Nepal', *Development in Practice*, 15(2): 151–164.

Rabinow, P. and Sullivan, W.M. (1979) *Interpretive Social Science: A reader*, Berkeley, CA: University of California Press.

Savage J (2006) 'Ethnographic evidence: the value of applied ethnography in healthcare', *Journal of Research in Nursing*, 11(5): 383–393.

Schensul, J.J. and Schensul, S.L. (1990) 'Ethnographic evaluation of AIDS prevention programs: better data for better programs', *New Directions for Program Evaluation*, 46: 51–62.

Schensul, J.J. and Weeks, M. (1989) 'Ethnographic evaluation of AIDS-prevention programs', in National Institute of Drug Abuse (ed.) *Community-based AIDS Prevention, Studies of Intravenous Drug Users and their Sexual Partners*, Rockville, MD: National Institute of Drug Abuse, pp. 110–120.

Schwartz-Shea, P. and Yanow, D. (2012) *Interpretive Research Design: Concepts and processes*, London: Routledge.

Shawyer, R.J., bin Gani, A.S., Punufimana, A.N. and Seuseu, N.K.F.S. (1996) 'The role of clinical vignettes in rapid ethnographic research: a folk taxonomy of diarrhoea in Thailand', *Social Science & Medicine*, 42(1): 111–123.

Simmons, D. (2011) 'The role of ethnography in STI and HIV/AIDS education and promotion with traditional healers in Zimbabwe', *Health Promotion International*, 26(4): 476–83.

Singer, M. (1993) 'Knowledge for use: anthropology and community-centered substance abuse research', *Social Science & Medicine*, 37: 1337–1346.

Singer, M. (1994) 'Community-centered praxis: toward an alternative non-dominative applied anthropology', *Human Organization* 53: 336–344.

Singer, M., Romero-Daza, N., Weeks, M. and Pelia, P. (1995) 'Ethnography and the evaluation of needle exchange in the prevention of HIV transmission', in Lambert, E.Y., Ashery, R.S. and Needle, R.H. (eds) *Qualitative Methods in Drug Abuse and HIV Research. National Institute on Drug Abuse Research Monograph Series*, 157: 231–257.

Siyoum, A.D., Hilhorst, D. and Pankhurst, A. (2012) 'The differential impact of microcredit on rural livelihoods: case study from Ethiopia', *International Journal of Development and Sustainability*, 1(3): 957–975.

Turkon, D., Himmelgreen, D., Romero-Daza N. and Noble, C. (2009) 'Anthropological perspectives on the challenges to monitoring and evaluating HIV and AIDS programming in Lesotho', *African Journal of AIDS Research*, 8(4): 473–480.

Waterston, A. (1997) 'Anthropological research and the politics of HIV prevention: towards a critique of policy and priorities in the age of AIDS', *Social Science & Medicine*, 44(9): 1381–1391.

White, H. (2009) 'Some reflections on current debates in impact evaluation', *International Initiative for Impact Evaluation, Working Paper 1*. Available at: www.3ieimpact.org/media/filer_public/2012/05/07/Working_Paper_1.pdf (accessed 19 June 2015).

White, S (2015) 'Qualitative perspectives on the impact evaluation of girls' empowerment in Bangladesh', *Journal of Development Effectiveness*, 7(2): 127–145.

Willis, J.W. (2007) *Foundations of Qualitative Research: Interpretive and critical approaches*, London: SAGE.

Winther, T. (2015) 'Impact evaluation of rural electrification programmes: what parts of the story may be missed?', *Journal of Development Effectiveness*, 7(2): 160–174.

Part I

The present challenge

2

The political economy of evidence

Personal reflections on the value of the interpretive tradition and its methods

Angela Kelly-Hanku

> Personally, being an indigenous local researcher and being bred within my own culture, I can now assess my culture, its negative and positive segments and impacts on the society, through my study in this project. It is like climbing up to the top of a hill for the first time in my life with a binocular and watching a tribal fight in my own village in the valley below. I feel different being on the hilltop. I can observe some of the things I have never seen before while being in that valley for my entire life. I now can observe the fight with my own eyes and know exactly what is happening; which directions the arrows are traveling, who is going to get killed, who is the bravest and, which side is winning. Being on the hilltop with the binocular gives me a clear and closer view. This observation gives me the opportunity to plan my next course of action, all because I moved away from that valley.
>
> (Martha Kupul,[1] HIV Social Research Cadet, 8 May 2008)

Introduction

When I first met Martha in December 2006, she had just given birth to her third daughter who was carefully positioned on her babysitter's lap in a traditional Papua New Guinean *bilum* (a traditional bag to carry babies, food and other value items). Martha looked like any other woman of her culture, dressed in a *meri blouse* (a blouse worn by women that was introduced through missionalisation), a *laplap* (a sarong) tied around her waist, with dusty old thongs adorning her feet. As her daughter lay, swaddled in her *bilum*, she and I were blissfully unaware how her life would unfold, and how unconventional it would be. That lack of convention lay in part due to the research capacity programme in which Martha was involved, and the ongoing research she led that examined issues of health, sexuality, gender and development in Papua New Guinea.

Martha has played an important role in my life and work in Papua New Guinea, most significantly with respect to how and what I have learned of Papua New Guinean cultures, of building research capacity and of undertaking research in this context. Through her, I have come to further understand the importance of witnessing that which is not measured or indeed even measurable, which is a key challenge for any monitoring and evaluation process. The reason this newborn's life was to be different was not because Martha had married a wealthy businessman, politician or landowner, nor was it because she had completed a degree in geological sciences at the national university. Her life was to be different because her mother had moved away from the valley (at least metaphorically) and returned transformed. Using the binoculars she referred to in her 'most significant change' story (Davies and Dart 2005), she now possessed the skills to observe, reflect and assess her community's practices in ways previously unimaginable. The binocular offers an important metaphor for privileging interpretive, rather than quantifiable, methods for programme evaluation. Unlike excel spreadsheets, interpretive methods offer a means by which to see, view and witness, rather than measure, record and decontextualise.

Having lived on the largest of the Pacific Island nations for almost a decade, and having started working there five years earlier, I have sought to build the long-term research capacity of Papua New Guineans to examine issues as diverse as male circumcision for HIV prevention, male and female sex work, gender minorities and sexual diversity, violence, masculinity and prevention of parent to child transmission of HIV. During this time, I have come to understand more fully and value the importance of the personal cultural and religious changes brought about by people's involvement in such research programmes. Drawing upon these experiences, in this chapter I explore the importance of interpretive approaches to data collection, and long-term engagement in this social setting, to understand and assess the impact of social development, health and capacity building initiatives and programmes.

Interpretive methods are not the primary concern here. However, they are reflective of a wider theoretical paradigm, sometimes called the interpretive turn in social science (Geertz 1973, Rabinow and Sullivan 1979). 'The interpretive turn [and therefore their methods] refocuses attention on the concrete varieties of cultural meaning, in the particularity and complex texture but without falling into the traps of historicism or cultural relativism' (Rabinow and Sullivan 1979: 4). Within this tradition, the goal is to understand 'how people conceptualise, understand their world, what they are doing, how they are going about doing it, to get an idea of their world' (Geertz in Panourgia 2002: 422). I am informed by a commitment to this interpretive tradition, especially as advanced by phenomenologically informed social sciences (Jackson 1989) and anthropology of experience (Turner and Bruner 1986). In these approaches all five senses are valued as means by which we come to know and understand our social worlds; in this way, I do not believe that complex life worlds can be reduced only to understanding via log frames.

Although I make my theoretical and epistemological stance clear, I do not aim to provide new theoretical insights into evaluation practices in this chapter. Instead, through 'thick description' (Geertz 1973) I want to reflect candidly on some of the challenges I have encountered in my experiences of monitoring and evaluation practices in one local context. While my stories relate to Papua New

Guinea, they reflect broader concerns in monitoring and evaluation praxis and transcend, at least conceptually, the local context with which I am most familiar. By focusing on events and issues where monitoring and evaluation would have (or did) benefit from a close-focus interpretive lens, I detail my own anxieties about the use of numerically driven, predetermined and top-down logical framework-based methods of understanding change and impact.

The politics of evidence

In late 2006, I was appointed as the team leader of Papua New Guinea's first HIV Social Research Cadetship Programme, a joint initiative of the Papua New Guinea Institute of Medical Research and the former National Centre in HIV Social Research at UNSW Australia. The programme was funded by an HIV capacity building grant scheme from AusAID (now the Australian Department of Foreign Affairs and Trade). I was employed to support the development of an evidence-informed response to the epidemic, which was lacking at that time in Papua New Guinea. The programme involved training a group of early career researchers in Papua New Guinea in the field of HIV, which had not yet happened in a formal and systematic fashion. Since then, we have undertaken more than 20 separate studies in Papua New Guinea in the areas of sexual, reproductive and maternal health, including several evaluations using both quantitative and qualitative methods.

The need for interpretive approaches to monitoring and evaluation is not new (see Greene 2000, Patton 1990, 1997). More than 15 years ago, Nastasi and Berg (1999: 2) posited that an ethnographic approach (which relies on interpretive methods) provides 'a better understanding of the local conditions, culture, meaning, and facilitators and barriers to carrying out the program successfully'. A renewed and rigorous examination of monitoring and evaluation practices across the globe, and across diverse thematic areas (e.g. health and education) is timely, given the current preference for use of Excel spread sheets – or *spredsitim* (Pondrelei and Bainton 2015) as it is now referred to in Tok Pisin in Papua New Guinea – to assist with the demands from funding bodies and development partners to developing a quantifiable and economic rationale for decision making.

Programme evaluation has three primary purposes: to facilitate improvements, render judgements and/or generate knowledge (Patton 1997). The ability to address these features is not the sole domain of numerical indicators. Rather, interpretive methods are equally able to generate knowledge, render judgements and facilitate improvements. The issue here I suggest is not one of methodological superiority per se, but of the politics of evidence. This is also a politics of ignorance, stigma and conflicting agendas whereby qualitative methods are rendered the lowest grade of evidence (Sackett 1993) and not recommended to inform practice and policy (Morse 2006). This political economy of evidence is intimately entwined with values placed on what and how we know; in other words, the epistemological frameworks used to guide research and monitoring and evaluation practices.

As stated by Greene (2000: 983), 'evaluators do not just claim to know something, they claim to know how good it is from a selected vantage point'. In my work I am guided by interpretive as well as critical social sciences epistemologies. These paradigms value, among other things, the multiplicity of voices, contextualisation, empowerment, social action and change. In the following sections, I use two examples to illustrate the need for measuring and understanding impact outcomes in locally contextualised, culturally meaningful ways. The first relates to the importance of narratives in understanding programmatic success. The second examines issues to do with method selection. To highlight these issues I focus largely on Papua New Guinea's largest liquefied natural gas project, known as the 'LNG Project'.

'Let me tell you a story'

Although I had already worked in Papua New Guinea alongside development practitioners building the capacity of health care workers, when I began as team leader I was naïve to the magnitude of work required to develop ten cadets as HIV social researchers. The challenge I was to learn did not lie in the domain of intellectual skill per se, although that posed its own difficulties as well. The real challenge I faced lay in developing what the Brazilian educator Paulo Freire (1974/2006) has called 'critical consciousness'.

For Freire, critical consciousness involves people learning to become aware of the social, cultural, political and economic circumstances that systematically structure their lives, leading to everyday experiences of marginalisation and vulnerability. In becoming critically aware of these issues, a person becomes better able to struggle against these aspects of daily life in order to take action and bring about social change. Having worked in adult education for many years, I was accustomed to asking people to think, reflect and consider possibilities as implied by building critical consciousness. My approach was deeply embedded in adult learning practices and traditional Papua New Guinea ways of learning – by doing, sharing experiences, internal and external reflection, interacting and observing.

I have been told on repeated occasions that Papua New Guinea is 'not a learning culture'; that it does not take to looking critically at itself. Moments that invite or demand such critiques are often rebutted with phrases such as 'that's not the Melanesian way'; a term used and advanced by the late Papua New Guinean public servant and philosopher Narokobi (1983). In this context, the phrase creates a distance, a sense of othering and of not needing to critically reflect on practices, attitudes and ways of being. This resistance to critical self-reflection would in time be central to what was, at one stage, looking like the demise of the research training programme. Yet these skills in learning to be reflective – whereby the distinction between insider and outsider is problematised – are precisely what others say are needed in the training of indigenous researchers (Tuhiwai Smith 2003). In time, and in a supportive and empowering context, the cadets became able to reflect critically on their lives, and therefore participate in a culture of learning. But, as Martha said, this requires first leaving the valley.

More than data collectors

As I experienced first-hand, the cadets were implicated personally, and not just professionally, in every aspect of the HIV social research cadetship programme. In Papua New Guinea, where HIV is almost exclusively a sexually transmitted infection, it was inevitable that understandings of both local and global sexualities would be central to the programme. The cadets knew how HIV was transmitted and were happy to talk about people dying in their villages, of accusations of sorcery and witchcraft, of blaming people for immorality. But the notions of sex and sexuality, particularly sexual and gender diversity, were constrained, and anything other than what they knew – or wanted to know – was deemed un-Papua New Guinean. Without an understanding of and sensitivity towards the diversities of sexual and gendered experiences and expressions, it is not possible, at least from my perspective, to undertake any research on HIV.

The implication of the types of judgements most, if not all, of the cadets embodied might have jeopardised the quality and reliability of any of the research findings we achieved. More significant, however, was the adverse impact such attitudes were likely to have had on the people who participated in our studies, including people living with HIV, sex workers and men with diverse sexual practices. Addressing the moralisation of the epidemic, and those living with HIV and most vulnerable to infection, was both urgent and critical.

Not wanting to reinforce highly stereotypical cultural representations of men's attraction to other men, as typified for example in productions such as *The Adventures of Priscilla, Queen of the Desert* (1994), I hosted a film event at my home showing *Brokeback Mountain* (2005). There were no locally produced films at that time to share. For the few weeks after the viewing, and as I dealt with the consequences of the film, I wished I had not shown it. But without addressing entrenched homophobia, as well as any other gender and sexual differences that did not conform to the conservative Christian teachings prevalent in Papua New Guinea, this cadetship programme would have been a complete failure.

The next day at our team film analysis discussion, one of the cadets said that homosexuality was 'against the natural order'. Rather than argue with her, I wanted to use this to invite the cadets to develop arguments and ideas, to develop critical reflexivity. I asked this cadet to explain the term used, including where this belief came from and what she meant by 'the natural order'. Frustrated, and no doubt angry with me, she yelled and stormed out from the room. She remained absent for some time. I later found her in the medical research institute's library reading a book on Christian healing. Christianity has a complicated but deeply important role in the lives of Papua New Guineans and the ways in which they view, but not necessarily act, in the world, with understandings of sexuality and HIV intimately implicated (Kelly *et al.* 2009b).

Time went on and the cadets continued to use non-sociological terms to describe behaviours, practices and sexual relationships. For example, they kept referring to extra marital relations as 'adultery', pre-marital sex as 'fornication', and having more than one sexual partner, paid or not, as 'promiscuous'. No matter how skilled or confident a person is to design and implement a survey or an in-depth interview, the judgemental attitudes of the cadets, as reflected in their language at that time, was always going to pose a risk to any participant in a future HIV-related study. It got to a point in the programme where I was compelled to hold up two books – the Bible and a social science dictionary. Realising the extent to which the former informed participants' worldview, I guided them to use the Bible and its terminology when at home and at church, but not in the context of research. The same was true in reverse for the latter. In time, the changes were notable. For example, we employed an openly HIV-positive gay man to work as part of our research team in a study on the social impacts of antiretroviral therapies, who was respected and treated as a valuable team member (Kelly et al. 2009a). The way the HIV social research cadets interviewed people with HIV also reflected a change in judgement. These transformations were not insignificant, and it was these types of change that were made evident in the 'most significant change' stories – a form of participatory monitoring and evaluation that involves the collection of stories of significant change that are then later collectively analysed for domains of programmatic impact (Davies and Dart 2005) – that I collected from the cadets as part of the programme evaluation. Such narratives offer an important means of monitoring without indicators (Sigsgaard 2002).

This issue of value judgement is important. Data results and data collection are not apolitical. Even if one were to rely on collecting numerical data for research or monitoring and evaluation, the ways in which questions are written (*and* translated), as well as the tone and body language the person employs when asking the question, can impact on the quality of data collected. All these issues can lead to social desirability bias, whereby a person answers what they think the person asking the question wants to hear. The implication of this is that the researchers and enumerators used in monitoring and evaluation practices are no more likely to generate neutral, 'valid' or objective evidence than the approaches I concern myself with in this chapter. Experiences with this programme taught me that the values, morals and attitudes of researchers and enumerators cannot be separated from the collection of information. This is rarely discussed as important in monitoring and evaluation practice.

Changing endpoints

We made enormous progress in addressing issues of homophobia and gender, including understanding the implications of bride wealth exchanges commonly referred to (and misappropriated) as bride price. But questions about these changes were not asked of cadets during evaluation of the programme. Instead, based on the grant application, they were assessed on their confidence to design and implement a survey, and the amount of time devoted to different research methods, among other things. But these endpoints (or outcomes) were no longer my or the programme grant holder's sole driving force. Something far more significant was taking place in the lives of the individual cadets and their families, which was obscured from the evaluation because such change was not envisaged as an indicator, outcome or endpoint of the project at the time it was originally designed.

Martha valued these endpoints as much as she did the specific skills of research design and methods. At the cadets' graduation, Martha gave an expanded version of her most significant change story. In her graduation speech she denounced bride price and said that, as the single mother of three daughters, she was making it publicly known to all, including her elderly parents who were in attendance, that she would not subject her daughters to this cultural practice. Predetermined measures of programmatic success cannot account for the impacts Martha spoke of. It would be rare to expect a programme of teaching research methods to evoke the types of changes we saw in the cadets. Yet, as a programme designed to address HIV, it would have been inadequate not to support and provoke the types of changes needed to bring about an enabling environment for HIV prevention and address the powerful social and cultural structures that increase vulnerability or result in marginalisation.

Ensuring that these research cadets could move between insider and outsider – holding onto and valuing their culture while also critically examining it, and where appropriate, seeking change – became enormous, unsung achievements of the programme. This is particularly important for research and evaluation, which relies on researchers or survey enumerators who are embedded, along with their families, in the social, cultural and moral communities that they study. The evaluation of the cadet training programme that was conducted six months prior to the programme end was not designed in such a way as to account for (and therefore value) the profound individual, social and spiritual changes that the cadets underwent. This important limitation of that evaluation is not unique to that programme but is a universal issue with evaluations of programmes that require significant personal and social transformation. This is why methods to monitor and evaluate without indicators are so important (Sigsgaard 2002).

Seeing that which is not measured

Over the past few years, the medical research institute at which I work has been provided with funding from the resource extraction companies to conduct health 'impact' studies. In reality, very few of those commissioned were designed to actually assess impact. For example, in 2009, we offered to design a 'gold-standard' sophisticated randomised controlled bio-behavioural survey among villages in the province where Papua New Guinea's largest LNG Project was to begin. The survey design was stratified by degree of physical and financial impact: physical impact with royalty/compensation payments; no physical impact but with royalty/compensation payments; and neither physical impact nor royalty/compensation payments. Our offer was rejected, I believe, not because of its poor design, but because it was designed to actually measure the impact of the project on sexual practices and thus changes in incidence of HIV and other sexually transmitted infections. If measured, such impacts would have suggested liability; those involved in the operation could be shown to have impacted negatively upon the health of Papua New Guineans in the affected areas. This is of course not ideal from the perspective of the resource extraction companies. Rather, they more usually seek to promote the positive impacts brought about by the project, including employment and skills training.

Later, I was afforded an opportunity to apply for funding from a grant scheme offered within the same institute, which was being paid directly by the gas company to do impact assessment studies. We designed a study that relied entirely on interpretive methodologies to assess the impacts of resource development on the socio-sexual and gendered relations in areas affected by the LNG Project. I was warned by a senior colleague that, because our institute received direct funding from the resource extraction company involved in the LNG Project, the Institute's Director might not want to risk that funding mechanism by supporting a proposal that was designed to elicit a very different picture of impact to that which the company wanted to illustrate. The Director resisted such politics of evidence and granted us funding.

On arrival in Hela Province where LNG extraction is occurring – with my team of Papua New Guinean researchers, an Australian colleague and my husband – we were welcomed into people's homes where we saw how their lives and traditions had transformed. We were met at the gates of one of the larger processing and accommodation compounds by my husband's *papa* – any older man in Papua New Guinea can be called '*papa*' as a sign of respect for seniority, but in this case my husband had been officially brought into this man's family during his years working in the area. He was an older man dressed in traditional *bilas* (costume); a leader of his people. He was standing at the gates surrounded by workmen, large transport trucks and countless four wheel drive vehicles, CD (music and movie) houses and trade stores selling cans of Coca-Cola for 8 PNG Kina (GBP1.91, which would cost GBP 0.48 where I live in Goroka).

Sitting in his home, made from tin roofing, my husband's *papa* and his younger brother shared stories of how the LNG Project had changed everything (*olgeta santing sensim*). In order to reflect the extent of change, my husband's *papa* held my arm and invited me to sit next to him. Among the Huli people, notions of 'pollution' have long prevailed, whereby women are feared and controlled in order to ensure men's strength and health. As a result of these cultural beliefs, strict highly sanctioned and regulated gendered divisions in all aspects of life ensued. To have his son's wife sit next to him in this way spoke volumes about change. He went on to describe degradation of the local water supply, and his frustration at the company for deceiving and taking advantage of him and his people. He then took me outside and placed the well-known Huli wig on my head. I, not he, was mortified by such a cultural transgression, as was my female Papua New Guinean colleague. For him, the LNG Project was a cultural transgression that had destroyed much that had once been held important to the people of the area, including strict gender segregation. His deliberate sharing of his wig with me, as a woman and as his daughter-in-law (*tambul meri*), illustrated the type of structural changes occurring as a result of the LNG Project.

The importance of the visual

Monitoring and evaluation activities that accommodate interpretive methods can detail important impacts that are not easy to understand through the use of timely, reliable and responsive statistics (NSO/NPM 2015). Powerful in and of themselves, these methods need not be denigrated to complementing numerical indicators, but can also be used independently.

As well as anthropological methods such as participant observation and formal and informal interviews, we complemented the study on the impacts of the LNG Project with the participatory action research method called Photovoice (Wang and Burris 1997).[2] This method uses photography and videography as tools to encourage critical reflection and dialogue about particular issues among people in marginalised communities who are typically excluded from research and consultation processes (Mamary et al. 2007). Photovoice method is designed to elicit social action within and beyond communities, through newly created lines of dialogue between local people and leaders and policy makers. The approach requires training participants to equip them with skills in photography and videography that create visual stimuli around which local narratives of matters important to those who are marginalised and silenced are gathered. Photovoice is an established method used in diverse contexts – such as South Africa (Mitchell et al. 2005), the USA (Mamary et al. 2007) and Bolivia (Velasco et al. 2014) – to address public health and other social issues.

All participants in the study described ways in which the LNG Project had changed their lives, and the impacts were diverse. For example, Tepei (not her real name) reflected on the enduring unhygienic state of the local market where food is prepared and sold in the provincial capital of Hela Province.

> We don't have a proper market in Tari Town and that is my concern. That is the current situation of our market in Hela. Tari market has no proper shelter or a market place. We do our marketing beside the road, outside the shops, government buildings and police station, and everywhere at any corner. When it rains, the place is wet and muddy and when it is sunny, the place is dusty. We don't have a proper market house or tables for us to sit and sell our food. This is a common sight everywhere on how we do our marketing and it is upsetting me.
>
> (Tepei, female Photovoice participant, Hela Province)

In this quotation, and in the photograph in Figure 2.1, she highlights the inequality in development and challenges of resource development, and associated impacts on improving the lives of ordinary Papua New Guineans.

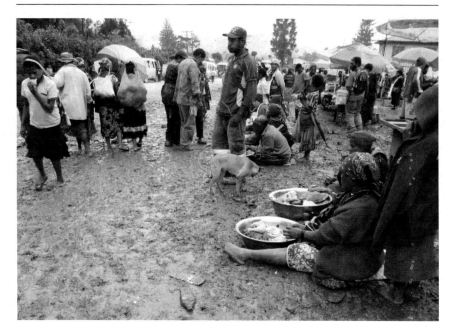

Figure 2.1 'We don't have a proper market'

As illustrated in the quote below, Bertha (not her real name) described how the LNG Project had resulted in her 'economic empowerment'.

> In the past I used to make gardens, look after pigs, chicken and sell these things to get money. Then, when LNG project started I gave up gardening and I always sit on the road from 6am to 6pm, doing marketing by selling store goods only. I see money. There is money so when I do marketing I always make a lot of money. When I sit like this, I hold my mobile [phone]. So I arrange my goods on display for sale on the table and sit with my phone switched on for any calls to come in. [If a call comes in] for someone to come for pick up, that is for me to go and stay overnight at the guest house or wherever I go and sleep and get money. I go to do sex work to get money and the next morning, come and feed my children. This is done through mobile phone network. LNG was started, mobile phone came and money floats [too much cash flows]. Why should I worry and work hard in the garden?
> (Bertha, female Photovoice participant, Hela Province)

As a rural area heavily dependent on agriculture for food and livelihoods, Bertha made an important decision to 'leave the garden', traditionally the domain of women, to pursue urban income generating activities where more money could be made more readily. Facilitated by the advent of the mobile phone in this

The political economy of evidence 27

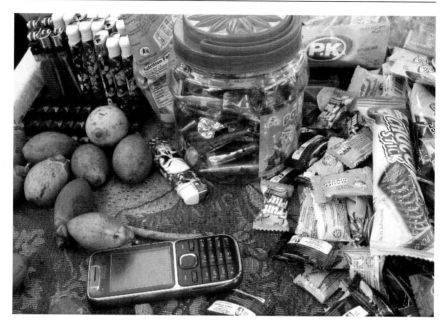

Figure 2.2 'LNG money is everywhere'

remote area as a result of the LNG Project, as illustrated in Figure 2.2, she came to realise that she could complement her income from street sales by taking money for sexual favours. Yet these impacts are not represented in official documentation of the LNG Project. By allowing those who are marginalised a vehicle by which to show and describe their lives and the impacts of the programme, we were able to appreciate the diverse ways in which local people experienced the impacts of resource extraction in this context. At the same time they are given voice and recognised as valued citizens.

These stories highlight the highly political nature of evidence more generally, and monitoring and evaluation more specifically. Visual sociologists and anthropologists have long argued that the visual is 'a neglected dimension in our understanding of social life' (Harrison 2002: 856). As examples of material culture, these images and their narratives offer an important counter narrative to 'spredsitim' (Pondrelei and Bainton 2015) in which targets are sought, recorded and represented as if objective facts that speak for themselves. There is an increasing emphasis in Papua New Guinea on the importance of visual methods in programme evaluation, largely pioneered by the Centre for Social and Creative Media at the University of Goroka. It is currently unclear how influential such methods will be in the medium to long term and whether the attraction of them will be a fleeting, rather than enduring approach in monitoring and evaluation.

Binoculars as a metaphor

In this chapter I have addressed an often-overlooked aspect of monitoring and evaluation – the politics of evidence. While focusing on examples from my work in one Pacific country, these are issues and challenges relevant to other diverse cultural, political, geographic and economic settings.

Seeing through photos, and listening to narratives, are primary senses that guide daily life. They are key tenets of interpretive traditions, particularly as advanced within the traditions of phenomenological social sciences and anthropology of experience. Despite this, they remain underutilised when it comes to monitoring and evaluation practices, as well as in research praxis more generally. Log frame-based approaches to monitoring and evaluation are predetermined, and are often designed and agreed upon in advance of a programme. Log frames imply a deductive rather than an inductive logic, yet the types of change that can be understood through interpretive methods cannot by their very nature be deduced prior to their taking place.

My work does involve working with outcome numbers and statistics, and I can see the attraction to numerically driven methods. Although I do not believe that they offer more valid evidence, I appreciate that they can offer a seemingly simple answer to what is in reality a complex life world. For example, it is less challenging to address the number of condoms distributed than it is to understand the ways in which condoms are incorporated (or not as the case may be) into sexual choreographies and the reasons underpinning this. As colleagues and I have reflected elsewhere: 'Social life is frequently more complex than even the most sophisticated clinical trials or the lengthiest program guidelines can capture. Put simply, there are many factors influencing the way we are, how we think, and how we behave' (Paiva *et al.* 2015: 479).

An interpretive approach to monitoring and evaluation is needed now more than ever. The social contexts in which people live and operate are moving at a pace of unprecedented change. As long as we rely solely on methods and approaches to knowledge production that are deductive and rigid rather than inductive and flexible, our ability to monitor and understand change will be hindered. By adopting interpretive approaches (either alone or with numerically driven approaches) to research, and to the monitoring and evaluation of health and social development programmes, it is possible to understand programmatic impacts more comprehensively. For countries such as Papua New Guinea, where there are endless obstacles to success, the in-depth insights needed to understand challenges in context are not often gathered using normative approaches.

I have illustrated the tensions that exist between epistemological approaches to knowledge, where some methods are valued and considered more valid than others. But as I detailed through examples of the HIV Social Research Cadetship programme, the very idea of an objective data collector is questionable as the social values of enumerators and researchers can negatively bias data collection in any given setting. These issues relating to the influence of social values on data collection are important in assessing bias in many numerical data sets. Recognising and engaging with moralisation, prejudice, stigma, discrimination and homophobia are crucial when undertaking research and monitoring and evaluation in the contexts of HIV, sexuality and sexual behaviour.

Interpretive approaches to knowledge production are not universally or widely applied in monitoring and evaluation activities, but do offer important benefits in contrast to deductive numerically driven normative methods. These advantages include being able to account for the complexity of social life, cater for the temporal nature of life and programmatic impacts, more readily understand and respond to unforeseen impacts, allow for changing programmatic endpoints, interests and priorities, and validate the voice and lives of often marginalised, vulnerable and powerless programme participants. In short, interpretive practices offer us the ability to address some of the 'confusing and chaotic problems that are too difficult to tackle quantitatively' (Morse 2006: 403).

The binoculars Martha described in her most significant change story highlighted the importance of *seeing*, of developing critical consciousness and reflexivity, of leaving the valley and returning transformed. Without the use of interpretive approaches it would not have been possible to understand the value Martha placed on the binoculars and of seeing in a new way. No measures, however well designed and intended, can foresee and predict the complexity of social life in advance. By taking a more encompassing and interpretive approach to monitoring and evaluating health and social development programmes, it becomes possible to value the successes that ensue or, more despondently, that do not, as programmes unfold and come to a close. The challenge that remains for those of us who resist normative and deductive approaches is that of the *political economy of evidence*: it 'is not a question of evidence or no evidence, but who controls the definitions of evidence and what kind is acceptable to whom' (Larner 2004: 20). Nowhere does evidence ever speak for itself.

Note

1 I use her real name here with both her permission and her blessing.
2 This part of the study was led by Agnes Mek, who gave permission to the author to report on the results and use the photographs presented in Figures 2.1 and 2.2.

References

Brokeback Mountain (2005) motion picture, Focus Features, Los Angeles.
Davies, R. and Dart, J. (2005) *The 'Most Significant Change' (MSC) Technique: A guide to its use*. Online. Available at: www.mande.co.uk/docs/MSCGuide.pdf (accessed 22 May 2015).
Freire, P. (1974/2006) *Education for Critical Consciousness*, London: Continuum.
Geertz, C. (1973) *The Interpretation of Cultures*, New York: Basic Books.

Greene, J.C. (2000) 'Understanding social programs through evaluation', in Denzin, N.K. and Lincoln, Y.S. (eds) *Handbook of Qualitative Research*, Thousand Oaks, CA: SAGE, pp. 981–1000.

Harrison, B. (2002) 'Seeing health and illness worlds – Using visual methodologies in a sociology of health and illness: a methodological review', *Sociology of Health & Illness*, 24(6): 856–872.

Jackson, M. (1989) *Minima Ethnography: Intersubjectivity and the anthropological project*, Chicago, IL: University of Chicago Press.

Kelly, A., Frankland, A., Kupul, M., Kepa, B., Cangah, B., Nosi, S., Emori, R., Walizopa, L., Mek, A., Pirpir, L., Akuani, F., Frank, R., Worth, H. and Siba, P. (2009a) *The Art of Living: The social experience of treatments for people living with HIV in Papua New Guinea*, Goroka: PNG IMR.

Kelly, A., Walizopa, L., Pirpir, L., Emori, R., Akuani, F., Kupul, M., Nosi, S., Kepa, B., Cangah, B., A., M., Keleba, K., Worth, H. and Siba, P. (2009b) 'Christian discourses in young people's narratives of sex, condoms and HIV in the Eastern Highlands Province, Papua New Guinea', *Catalyst*, 39(2): 102–114.

Larner, G. (2004) 'Family therapy and the politics of evidence', *Journal of Family Therapy*, 26(1): 17–30.

Mamary, E., McCright, J. and Roe, K. (2007) 'Our lives: an examination of sexual health issues using photovoice by non-gay identified African American men who have sex with men', *Culture, Health & Sexuality*, 9(4): 359–370.

Mitchell, C., Delange N., Moletsane R., Stuart, J. and Buthelezi, T. (2005) 'Giving a face to HIV and AIDS: on the uses of photo-voice by teachers and community health care workers working with youth in rural South Africa', *Qualitative Research in Psychology*, 2(3): 257–270.

Morse, J.M. (2006) 'The politics of evidence', *Qualitative Health Research*, 16(3): 395–404.

Narokobi, B. (1983) *The Melanesian Way*, Port Moresby: Institute of PNG Studies.

Nastasi, B. and Berg, M. (1999) 'Using ethnography to strengthen and evaluate intervention programmes', in Schensul, J., LeCompte, M., Hess, G.A., Nastasi, B., Berg, M., Williamson, L., Brecher, J. and Glasser, R. (eds) *Using Ethnographic Data: Interventions, public programming and public policy. Ethnographer's Toolkit 7*. Walnut Creek, CA: Altammira Press, pp. 1–56.

NSO/NPM (2015) *Why Papua New Guinea Needs Good Statistics?* Port Moresby: National Statistics Office and National Planning and Monitoring.

Paiva, V., Ferguson, L., Aggleton, P., Mane, P., Kelly-Hanku, A., Giang, L.M., Barbosa, R.M., Caceres, C.F. and Parker, R. (2015) 'The current state of play of research on the social, political and legal dimensions of HIV', *Cadernos de Saúde Pública*, 31(3): 477–486.

Panourgia, N. (2002) 'Interview with Clifford Geertz', *Anthropological Theory*, 2(4): 421–431.

Patton, M.Q. (1990) *Qualitative Evaluation and Research Methods*, Newbury Park: SAGE.

Patton, M.Q. (1997) *Utilization-Focused Evaluation: The next century text*, Newbury Park, CA: SAGE.

Pondrelei, W. and Bainton, N. (2015) 'Spredsitim: social data collection, storage and use at the Lihir gold mine', paper presented at Resource Development and Human well-being in Papua New Guinea: Issues in the measurement of progress Conference, Port Moresby, Papua New Guinea, 17–19 March 2015.

Rabinow, P. and Sullivan, W.M. (1979) *Interpretive Social Science: A reader*, Berkeley, CA: University of California Press.

Sackett, D.L. (1993) 'Rules of evidence and clinical recommendations', *Canadian Journal of Cardiology*, 9(6): 487–489.

Sigsgaard, P. (2002) 'Monitoring without indicators: An ongoing testing of the MSC approach', *Evaluation Journal of Australasia*, 2(1): 8–15.

The Adventures of Priscillia, Queen of the Desert (1994) motion picture, Gramercy Pictures, New York.

Tuhiwai Smith, L. (2003) *Decolonizing Methodologies: Research and indigenous peoples*, Dunedin, New Zealand: University of Otago Press.

Turner, V. and Bruner, E. (eds) (1986) *The Anthropology of Experience*, Urbana, IL: University of Illinois Press.

Velasco, M.L., Berckmans, I., O'Driscoll, J.V. and Loots, G. (2014) 'A visual narrative research on photographs taken by children living on the street in the city of La Paz – Bolivia', *Children and Youth Services Review*, 42: 136–146.

Wang, C. and Burris, M.A. (1997) 'Photovoice: concept, methodology, and use for participatory needs assessment', *Health Education & Behavior*, 24(3): 369–387.

3

Measurement, modification and transferability

Evidential challenges in the evaluation of complex interventions

Helen Lambert

Introduction

Evaluation comes in a multiplicity of forms, but all of these entail the production of different varieties of evidence. Monitoring and evaluation activities are usually seen as essential to the implementation of health and development programmes, but the purpose of evaluation – what the evidence produced is to be used for – is often left unclear or not fully explicated.

There are several rationales for monitoring and evaluation (World Bank 2007). Funders may insist on monitoring for reasons of accountability, in order to ensure that funds are being disbursed efficiently and appropriately for their intended purpose, objectives are being met, and implementation is occurring in accordance with programme design within a designated time frame. Implementers may undertake 'process' evaluation for programme improvement, to document and explore what is and is not working and to identify where activities need modification in order to achieve objectives. In turn, 'outcome' (as well as 'process') evaluation may be used to appraise the overall effectiveness of a programme or intervention, justify funding expenditures, secure further resources and/or ascertain whether it has sufficient value to warrant duplication elsewhere.

There are inherent tensions between the evidentiary requirements associated with these differing rationales for evaluation. This is particularly so with respect to 'outward-facing' and 'inward-facing' modes of evaluation. The former focus on measurable outcomes for reasons of external accountability and verification of effect and can thus be seen as outward-facing. In contrast, inward-facing modes are designed to gather information for enhancing intervention effectiveness by identifying flaws in programme design and implementation to enable operational adjustments.

In this chapter, I explore how the specific need to produce measurable and standardised evaluative indicators and outcomes in order to demonstrate accountability and document efficacy inhibits the deployment of inductive, context-based modifications to intervention design. The use of ethnographic and interpretive research to evaluate projects and document as well as inform such modifications can provide key insights for the potential transferability of successful interventions. Incorporated into evaluation activities, these approaches can maximise the potential effectiveness of interventions deemed successful in one setting when rolled out or scaled up elsewhere, by ensuring that they are appropriately modified to fit the social context and the daily lives of local populations. In experimental interventions too, these forms of study can provide invaluable insights for enhancing fidelity in implementation. The chapter therefore centres around two key issues: the transferability of different evidentiary forms (i.e. the extent to which evidence produced in one setting is generalisable to another); and the respective roles and value of experientially and statistically based varieties of evidence.

Qualitative research and the character of evaluation

While monitoring and evaluation is frequently regarded as entirely discrete from 'research', evaluation activities are, nonetheless, fundamentally forms of enquiry. Such activities entail the systematic investigation of an object of enquiry, including the development or application of a methodology, data gathering, analysis and interpretation. The understanding of monitoring and evaluation as a routinised and discrete technical exercise among many agency and programme staff working in health and social development projects reveals the implicit dominance of the accountability function over all others in conventional approaches to evaluation, especially among non-governmental organisations whose spending is generally dependent on external funding. This contrasts with the learning function emphasised by bilateral agencies, particularly with regard to complex interventions. For example, guidelines produced by Enhancing Support for Strengthening the Effectiveness of National Capacity Efforts (ESSENCE, an international initiative between major funding agencies to coordinate investments into research capacity) states, 'monitoring and evaluation activities should ultimately lead to improved practice' (ESSENCE on Health Research 2011: 5) and that, 'PM&E [planning, monitoring and evaluation] systems that accompany the process of capacity strengthening should enhance continuous learning' (ibid.: 6).

In an overview of shifts in the purpose of evaluation over time, Levin-Rosalis (2003) points to certain fundamental similarities between anthropologically informed ethnographic research and evaluation. Noting that like ethnographers, evaluators cannot choose the participants, setting or variables of the project, she argues that evaluation instruments and methods (e.g. interviews, observations, analysis of protocols, questionnaires) must be chosen to fit the requirements of the evaluation, taking account of situation-specific issues such as the population, funding available and nature of evaluation contract. Likewise she asserts that evaluators do not deal with isolated variables but with events, 'which include most of the possible variables, together with their interconnections and contexts, as well as factors that are not variables (the type of neighbourhood or the character of the school, for example)' (ibid.: 15–16).

As in ethnographic and other qualitative research, the evaluator is seen as the research instrument and, given the complexity of interactions between innumerable variables in any project and the pre-eminent requirement to appraise that specific project, the evaluator is concerned only with internal validity. Drawing on Campbell (1986), who argues that cause-and-effect relationships may appear in the field that are unaccounted for by pre-existing theory, it is suggested that – as in other interpretive research – casual relationships observed in the field may be used inductively to generate new theory, reversing the usual direction of the relationship between theory and activity.

Levin-Rosalis asserts that due to these similarities, evaluation and research are distinguished only by their ultimate aims – research is conducted in order to contribute to general knowledge, whereas evaluation aims to produce feedback useful to a project. This distinction relies on an assumption that research cannot be designed for immediate application and that conversely, evaluation is always designed solely to serve the short-term needs of the project or programme within which it is conducted. Over the past decade this assumption has partially ceased to hold as the rationales and methodologies for both research and evaluation have shifted; the distinctions between them increasingly rest on more mundane features such as levels of investment and differentiated communities of expertise and practice. In the health research arena, demands on funders especially in the public sector to demonstrate that their activities and investments are producing results have grown in response to increasingly stringent requirements for institutional transparency and accountability (Lambert 2006). Funders in turn have increased requirements of researchers to demonstrate the relevance and utility of their research. This is manifest in the growing expectation that researchers involve participants and publics in their studies and foster 'public engagement' with their findings; thus Public and Patient Involvement or PPI (INVOLVE 2014) has been made a mandatory requirement for all health researchers working in the UK National Health Service who apply for funding from the National Institute of Health Research. Likewise, publicly funded research in the UK must now demonstrate that it has direct benefits (by influencing policy or changing practice, for example), as signalled by the addition of a new 'impact' indicator in the latest statutory quinquennial appraisal of research quality that determines governmental funding allocations to all higher education departments in the UK (HEFCE 2014).

Reciprocal shifts have occurred over the same period in global health and development that have led to the introduction of prominent research techniques into approaches to evaluation. Similar concerns about accountability have produced a heightened emphasis on the need to generate evidence of the effectiveness and cost-effectiveness of health and social development interventions in order to justify expenditure. Increasingly rigorous approaches to outcome measurement are being adopted that draw on experimental designs developed within clinical and public health research, development economics and education, foremost among them the randomised controlled trial (RCT). As evidence of effectiveness becomes a fundamental requirement in formulating health and development policy, experimental designs such as the RCT and systematic reviews to appraise the evidence base for use in policy-making have increasingly been favoured by major funders, including agencies such as the World Bank (Deaton 2010: 438).

These approaches contrast with the kind of project- and situation-specific inductive evaluation described above in which context-dependent issues, accessed through the evaluator's detailed field investigations, are prioritised in data collection. Such inward-facing, inductive evaluation activities have become less central as 'implementation science' has developed and evaluations designed to document behavioural interventions are increasingly expected to specify 'programme theory' and the 'logic models' associated with them prior to implementation. Conventional research paradigms including systematic reviews, mathematical modelling and trial methodologies to decide on 'what works' are being embraced by funders and policy makers in fields as diverse as education, income generation and public health; see, for instance, examples of 'rigorous impact evaluations' involving randomisation conducted under the auspices of MIT's Poverty Action Lab (Poverty Action Lab n.d.).

Evidence transfer and the limitations of RCTs

The criteria developed to evaluate the quality of research evidence in evidence-based medicine, such as the 'evidence pyramid' favoured by organisations such as the Cochrane Collaboration (Lambert 2013: 43), assume standardisation and control to be indicative of rigour and hence give primacy to method (Lambert 2006). This is why positive findings from RCTs are widely assumed to demonstrate not only the efficacy but the effectiveness of the intervention being trialled. This understanding has, as described above, become influential in a range of other fields. Critics, among them economists and philosophers of science (e.g. Cartwright 2013, Deaton 2010), have argued against the precept that the RCT is uniquely capable of producing unbiased and objective evidence of effectiveness, on the grounds that demonstration of effect (efficacy) in one setting does not logically entail that similar effects will be seen elsewhere (effectiveness). The problem of transferability, particularly in complex interventions, is exemplified in various public health initiatives such as using participatory women's groups to reduce neonatal mortality that failed in Bangladesh (Azad et al. 2010) having succeeded in Nepal (Manandhar et al. 2004).

The assumption that RCT results are broadly generalisable rests on two logical errors: that the contextual dimensions or 'support factors' (Cartwright 2013: 99) that contributed to the observed effectiveness of the intervention in its original setting will also be present in a different setting; and that the causal pathways that produced effectiveness in the first setting will obtain in the new setting (Lambert 2013). In order to judge the true transferability of such evidence to different settings, specific information regarding the conditions obtaining in these new settings is required. Such contextual information cannot be obtained through RCTs but may be accessed through the kinds of qualitative and ethnographic data-gathering that are employed in inward-facing modes of formative and process evaluation.

While demonstrating effects through the measurement of standardised, rigorously comparable, quantified outcomes may be the ultimate goal of evaluation research, there are especially significant methodological and ethical challenges to achieving this for complex interventions that by their nature entail social or environmental change or modifications in human behaviour (MRC n.d.). This is all the more so because enabling such change tends to require on-going context-responsive adaptation of interventions in order to achieve their goals. Such adaptations undermine the scientific principle that requires conditions to be held stable and comparable throughout an intervention so that changes from baseline to completion can be measured.

Techniques for gathering quantitative evidence of effectiveness depend on defining appropriate outcomes, which need to be specific and isolated in order to measure statistically observable effects. However, the health outcomes of complex social interventions are rarely isolable in this manner, nor are these necessarily outcomes for which such interventions are primarily designed. Housing improvement, micro-credit initiatives, social insurance and poverty alleviation strategies are just a few examples of social interventions that may have important effects on the health of recipients. Using the example of urban regeneration, Petticrew (2013) demonstrates how seeking to impose an experimental design in order to obtain the most putatively robust form of evidence may not be appropriate, even if it is feasible. The character of such interventions and the complexity of the social and environmental influences at work during a programme's implementation mean that health effects are not readily attributable to the intervention itself, even if they can be measured accurately.

Inward- and outward-facing evaluation

There is an inherent tension between modes of evaluation that are outward-facing (designed for the purpose of demonstrating value and effectiveness to funders, researchers, policy makers and other audiences external to the programme) and those that are inward-facing (undertaken in order to inform programme implementers and recipients how well the intervention is working). Outward-facing modes of evaluation are generally outcome-focused and employ quantitative analysis of measurement indicators (such as vaccination rates) developed by implementers or specified by external funding agencies to ensure comparability with baseline data and/or with similar interventions elsewhere. Inward-facing modes of evaluation often employ qualitative and case study data to document, for example, community perspectives on the effectiveness of an intervention and participants' perceptions of its strengths and weaknesses (such as mothers' assessments of the accessibility of vaccination camps held on particular days). These inward-facing approaches have the potential to generate findings that are of practical value to implementers in improving intervention effectiveness but outward-facing modes are more likely to produce results that are perceived as generalisable, robust and reliable, though they may lack internal validity.

Below, I illustrate this tension through the example of community-focused targeted interventions for HIV prevention in India. Through this example I want to explore the potential value of what can loosely be seen as a focus on plausibility (Habicht et al. 1999, Auerbach et al. 2011, Lambert 2012), rather than reliability or validity, in analysing why interventions do or do not 'work' and discerning their potential transferability to new populations and settings.

Community engagement in HIV prevention offers a useful exemplar through which to illustrate the tensions between measurement (enumeration) and meaning (interpretation) in evaluation work. HIV prevention programmes targeted at high risk populations have considerable potential for limiting the spread of HIV, although clear evidence for the effectiveness of conventional targeted intervention components for preventing HIV infections in populations such as sex workers remains surprisingly limited (Shahmanesh et al. 2008). There is growing consensus that targeted interventions require attention to the 'structural drivers' (Auerbach et al. 2011) that render certain populations particularly vulnerable to infection, and that active community engagement is needed if prevention initiatives are to succeed (Campbell and Cornish 2010). 'Community mobilisation' or 'collectivisation' has been shown to be associated with indicators of risk-reduction involving behavioural change (Saggurti et al. 2013). Furthermore, community-led structural interventions have been shown to be effective in specific settings, although structural interventions themselves are not necessarily community-based (Evans et al. 2010). The latest set of guidelines for HIV prevention among sex workers highlights the need for community empowerment (WHO 2012) and comparisons between effective and ineffective community mobilisation programmes in contrasting settings suggest that the broad social environment within which interventions take place strongly influences their success (Campbell and Cornish 2010, Campbell 2003).

Community-based HIV prevention in India

Unlike sub-Saharan Africa, HIV in India has not become widespread in the general population but remains 'concentrated' in high-risk populations and in particular geographical regions (NACO 2012). Prevention efforts have remained focused on particular populations known to be at special risk of HIV infection, including sex workers and their clients, injecting drug users, men who have sex with men, truckers and male migrant workers. The States with higher overall prevalence in the south and north-east of the country have been the main focus of targeted prevention programmes. As elsewhere, HIV has recently shown a downward trend in national prevalence, but certain States that are classified by the National AIDS Control Organisation (NACO) as low-prevalence overall have been found to have pockets of high and increasing prevalence. Male migrant workers are receiving increasing attention as possible 'bridges' between urban high- and rural low-prevalence regions of the country (NACO 2012, Rai et al. 2014).

One of the best-known and longest-running targeted interventions in India is an HIV prevention project with sex workers in Kolkata, West Bengal (Wheeler et al. 2012). The Sonagachi project has been widely viewed as a model for effective community-led structural intervention (Jana et al. 2004). Initiated by NACO as a conventional public health intervention and implemented by a government medical institute with funding support from the UK government, its content and approach evolved organically in response to the expressed needs and concerns of sex workers engaged as peer educators and participants in the project. Initially literacy classes were offered to the salaried peer educators at their behest and sex workers themselves gradually became increasingly central to its orientation, with a gradual shift in focus towards social and economic interventions that could influence the underlying determinants of sex workers' vulnerability to infection. For example, the project and its beneficiaries successfully lobbied the State government to overturn discriminatory banking policies that required husbands' signatures on forms to open bank accounts, thus preventing sex workers from availing themselves of financial services; this change allowed sex workers to save money and improve their economic security, thereby enabling them to refuse unsafe sex. They mounted collective protests against violent clients and negotiated with police and local gangs who exploited and perpetrated violence against sex workers (Evans et al. 2010). In 1999 Durbar Mahila Samanwaya Committee (DMSC), a sex workers' collective, assumed management of the project and continues to run several interventions across West Bengal including a cooperative, education services, HIV prevention and other health programmes and rights-based activities (DMSC n.d).

The situational particularities of sex work and community structures in Kolkata are difficult to encapsulate in accounts of the project designed to offer a replicable model of the Sonagachi project for utilisation elsewhere. Generic components recommended in guidelines for use in other settings include peer education, condom distribution, free clinic services and community involvement (e.g. WHO 2012; see Evans and Lambert 2008 for discussion and further examples). In reality the success of these elements in Sonagachi often depended on informal processes that remain largely undocumented in project evaluations, papers and reports (Jana et al. 2004). Qualitative research, however, has identified some of these less readily itemised aspects. A long-term ethnographic study identified as crucial the project's success in navigating the internal politics of the local sex industry to recruit or marginalise influential leaders who might have otherwise jeopardised the project (Evans and Lambert 2008). Another essential element was the articulation of sex workers' demands through a political ideology – workers' rights – that had long-standing governmental and regional support in a specific setting where the communist party had dominated regional politics for decades (Evans and Lambert 2008, Campbell and Cornish 2010). Insights of this kind emerging from detailed qualitative study can help develop deeper understanding about why this particular intervention worked, as well as identify which components may, because of their contextually specific resonance, require reformulation if similar approaches are implemented in different settings.

Launched in 2003 and funded by the Bill & Melinda Gates Foundation, the Avahan programme sought to prevent HIV in vulnerable communities in India on a larger scale. Avahan supported the development of targeted interventions through local implementing partners and non-governmental organisations in the five highest-prevalence states of India. Four in southern India had a particular focus on sex work and men who have sex with men, and one in Manipur targeted injecting drug use as the main mode of transmission in this north-eastern State. The Avahan approach combined conventional preventative interventions – condom promotion and where appropriate, needle exchange, treatment of sexually transmitted infections, and referral to HIV and tuberculosis testing and care – with peer-led health education, outreach and efforts to 'mobilise' high-risk communities.

The community mobilisation component of the Avahan programme drew explicitly on the example of Sonagachi (Laga and Vyulsteke 2011), but implementers soon realised that they could not impose a uniform 'model'. That local partners needed flexibility to develop their own designs became clear as they sought to involve sex workers, men who have sex with men and other communities targeted for HIV prevention across a wide range of localities and social environments (Wheeler et al. 2012). Contextually appropriate structural interventions subsequently evolved, such as crisis response teams to tackle incidents of violence against sex workers and work with police to 'sensitise' them. While such work does have public health implications – violence has been associated with poorer outcomes relating to HIV prevention in various studies – such initiatives were necessary to the building of trust and a greater sense of security that are prerequisites for community mobilisation (Wheeler et al. 2012). This observation reinforces the point made earlier that broadly health-promoting interventions that tackle distal determinants of risk may not have direct or rapidly measurable effects on health outcomes.

Unfortunately community mobilisation was not included in the Avahan programme's evaluation design from the start (Laga and Vyulsteke 2011), but programme implementers progressively tried to incorporate evaluation into this component. Avahan activities and findings are documented in many published papers (including special issues of *BMC Public Health* in 2011 and *Journal of Epidemiology and Community Health* in 2012) and attempts to evaluate its community mobilisation activities usefully exemplify some of the tensions between inward- and outward-facing modes of evaluation. Not only were there difficulties in developing common indicators to measure outcomes – inevitable given the 'dynamic and multi-dimensional nature' of community mobilisation (Jana 2012: 6) which is difficult to capture using standardised methodologies – but the imposition of certain routine indicators for monthly monitoring had adverse effects on community mobilisation processes (Wheeler et al. 2012). These adverse effects resulted from the need to report identical indicators across widely varying implementation sites in an effort to measure change over time consistently. Where local implementers are allowed the necessary flexibility in project implementation to accommodate widely varying local contextual circumstances (an example of inward facing evaluation), it can be difficult to find universal indicators that accurately measure intervention progress and effects in each site while enabling strict comparison between them (an example of outward-facing evaluation). Second, once such standardised indicators are adopted, they may inadvertently distort implementation activities. Thus, after 'Number of Community-Based Organisations' was finalised as a routine indicator across Avahan sites in 2007, the number of community-based organisations reported as active increased rapidly, but the indicator had the effect of diverting efforts away from actual community-building activities in favour of registering new organisations that were not really functional in order to meet reporting requirements (Wheeler et al. 2012). Similarly, 'Number of incidents of violence' also proved problematic, since crisis response teams lacked a standardised definition for such incidents and cases often went unreported when they were resolved rapidly, so this indicator did not accurately capture the effectiveness of the approach (ibid.).

Measuring the relationship between community change and health outcomes was also difficult. Towards the end of the committed funding period, implementers focused on institutionalising programme activities prior to their transfer to government control. To this end another indicator, the Community Preparedness Index, was successfully developed through participatory monitoring and planning. However analysis of the Community Preparedness Index (Narayanan et al. 2012) showed that in at least one programme area, organisational readiness, as demonstrated through the development of functioning management and governance structures in organisations participating in the programme, was correlated with a decline in the networking activities that are indicative of actual community engagement and participation. Thus, outward-facing modes of evaluation in the form of measurement requirements and institutional development associated with the demands of monitoring, governance and accountability, may be counterproductive to the primary aims of the intervention (Lambert 2012).

Theory and interpretation in intervention design and evaluation

The Avahan example demonstrates how, even in a programme widely deemed to have been successful at population level (Laga and Vuylsteke 2011), assumptions enshrined in the community mobilisation component can lead to distortions both in effectiveness and in the measurement of these effects. Thus the initial precept that membership in community-based organisations was a necessary prerequisite for community mobilisation inadvertently resulted in energies and resources being diverted away from actual community-based activities to the formation and recruitment of community-based organisations, because the measurement indicator selected to monitor output was interpreted as a target. Target setting has a lengthy and unhappy history in Indian health programmes and has had distorting effects (Lambert 2012). However, ethnographic research that was conducted in one Avahan site demonstrated that membership of a community group was neither a prerequisite for, nor an indicator of, individual empowerment (Wheeler et al. 2012).

Thus the increasingly common requirement that a 'theory of change' to drive an evaluation must be formulated prior to its development (Michie et al. 2011) can constitute something of a problem for the successful implementation of complex and community-led programmes that entail behavioural change. Enshrining programme goals and objectives in a logic model undoubtedly assists in arriving at a clearer sense of the purpose(s) of evaluation, through articulating explicitly the often embedded hypotheses or assumptions about the pathways and mechanisms through which an intervention will effect change (Michie et al. 2011). Yet these models and the measures of behavioural change rest on individualist assumptions about what drives alterations in people's actions and practices, while collective change is social, and the more complex an intervention, the greater the uncertainty as to the drivers for such change. This is ultimately why interventions need to be tailored to the particular social, cultural and economic structures into which they are being introduced and why as-yet-untheorised cause–effect relationships may emerge during implementation that cannot be captured in pre-specified logic models.

The unexpected findings described above concerning relationships between community organising and behavioural change illustrate the potential value of ethnographic research in the design of programmes, as well as in the development of programme evaluation models. They also highlight the risks of relying exclusively on outward-facing modes of evaluation, since without ethnographic and other qualitative research taking place during the life of the programme, quantitative analysis based on the use of inappropriate indicators would not accurately capture what is actually happening. The imposition of predefined indicators can, as described by the Avahan programme leaders, have adverse effects on achieving programme objectives.

One underlying reason for these effects is that in the Avahan conceptual framework, as in many other community-based HIV prevention initiatives, community participation is conceived as necessary for community mobilisation (Galavotti et al. 2012). These terms are frequently used interchangeably and directionality is hard to discern (Lambert 2012), but such terminologies nonetheless imply that the communities being targeted already exist as entities, so the work of implementers is simply to mobilise them. However, as ethnographic and qualitative evidence from Avahan and at Sonagachi, as well as in other settings (Campbell 2003) shows, the *formation* of collective identity is key to both community participation and mobilisation (Evans et al. 2010; Gaikwad et al. 2012). The emphasis on community-based organisation formation in Avahan was driven by the adoption of the Sonagachi project as a model for emulation, but interpretive ethnographic study of the project revealed that even in Sonagachi, community empowerment did not develop straightforwardly from the formation of a community-based organisation. Rather, it resulted from combining a culturally appropriate patron-based model of leadership with a relatively egalitarian organisational structure, together with the fostering of political and moral values that enabled the gradual development of ownership by the sex workers (Evans and Lambert 2008). The complex processes entailed in developing a collective identity that is essential to effective community-led development inevitably become invisible retrospectively and can only be documented accurately through ethnographic or other contemporaneous interpretive work.

The implications of this issue are not confined solely to the way in which intervention activities are (mis)represented (as where community mobilisation is understood as an 'input') but extend to their reproducibility, because different high-risk populations vary significantly in the extent to which they have developed, or are able to develop, a communal identity that facilitates collective action. In the programme logic of most health interventions, disease categories rather than social entities are the ultimate focus of programme objectives and outcome evaluations. Consequently, a key objective such as reduction in HIV transmission risk may obscure the importance of correctly characterising social relationships within target populations, leading to unsuitable models of community mobilisation or participation being advanced in programme planning. For example, evaluation literature on India's targeted intervention programmes mostly focuses on sex workers and the conceptual framework retrospectively formulated to evaluate community mobilisation in Avahan relates solely to this population (Galavotti *et al.* 2012). Community mobilisation that is reported to be effective in HIV prevention programme evaluations tends to be construed as demonstrating the success of community mobilisation per se, but the evidence for its appropriateness and effectiveness among other vulnerable communities in south Asia – including the injecting drug users, transgender communities and men who have sex with men who were also targeted in Avahan and other NACO programmes – is relatively sparse. In reality the existence of a shared occupational identity among sex workers may make community formation and mobilisation easier to initiate among sex workers than among injecting drug users or men who have sex with men, whose only necessary common characteristic is a set of behavioural practices that places them at high risk of HIV infection.

Commensurability between different evaluation regimes: the role of the plausible

The sources of tension between 'measurement' and 'meaning' illustrated by the examples described ultimately rest on issues of inference and plausibility. Habicht *et al.* (1999) offer a tripartite characterisation of evaluation of health interventions, distinguished in terms of their focus on 'adequacy', 'plausibility' or 'probability'. In this typology 'adequacy evaluations' describe whether or not expected changes have taken place as a means to assess how well programme activities have met expected objectives. Indicators used are those conventionally employed in monitoring impact, such as number of children vaccinated or enrolled in school or, at larger scale, percentage change over the duration of the intervention (such as proportion of mothers breastfeeding, or increases in average exam grades achieved). The limitation of adequacy evaluations is that it is not possible to link these observed changes causally to programme activities. 'Plausibility evaluations' use methodological approaches that incorporate the additional step of trying to exclude other possible causes of the observed change through the use of comparison. Examples include historical comparison, the use of case-control methods, and comparison between communities or geographical areas with and without the intervention. Causality still cannot be unequivocally demonstrated in plausibility evaluations because the comparison groups or situations (i.e. context) will inevitably differ in some respects. In turn, 'probability evaluations' such as RCTs incorporate randomisation of the intervention to (presumptively) similar groups or individuals to minimise the likelihood that observed changes are due to anything other than the intervention itself. However, the artificially stringent conditions required to achieve true randomisation mean that they rarely reflect the reality to which the results of such trials are subsequently extrapolated. The external validity of such trials and their pertinence to policy decisions thus become questionable and plausibility evaluation is recommended wherever possible, even where probability evaluation is undertaken, particularly since qualitative evidence is often more persuasive to policy makers than statistical results alone (Habicht et al. 1999). Such reasoning resonates with that of social science researchers who have called for greater consideration of what is socially and culturally, as well as biologically, plausible when gathering and interpreting evidence concerning the effectiveness of social and behavioural interventions (Auerbach et al. 2011, Lambert 2012).

Conclusion

If an intervention's success relies on the creation of a highly artificial situation or on situation-specific elements extraneous to the components of the intervention as originally designed, this will limit its applicability in other settings and its potential for replication or 'scaling up'. The holy grail in health and social development is to discover effective interventions that are widely replicable, but the complex combination of influences that makes interventions work is often resistant to easy measurement, and requires ethnographic and interpretive approaches to gather and analyse relevant forms of evidence. Moreover, meeting the need for quantification to demonstrate measurable effects can come at the cost of maximising actual effectiveness through real-time adjustment to modify intervention elements to better fit emerging circumstances. The potential value of such grounded adjustments is now being recognised in evaluative health research, for example in the growing use of ethnographic approaches embedded in RCTs to enhance their veracity (Smith-Morris et al. 2014, Donovan et al. 2014).

The claims to universality of statistical evidence produced by, say, a group of RCTs are rooted in different epistemological assumptions from context-specific qualitative evidence that can inductively generate theories to explain how and why an intervention does or does not work in a specific setting. When operationalised discretely in evaluation, these outward-facing and inward-facing modes of enquiry may be in tension. However, they have great value when used in conjunction, for although data produced through the use of rigorous experimental methods carries particular weight as offering putatively context-independent and hence generalisable 'evidence', the extent to which such findings are applicable or even relevant to settings other than the one in which the evidence was initially gathered, rests largely on the analysis and utilisation of other, non-epidemiological forms of evidence.

References

Auerbach, J.D., Parkhurst, J.O. and Caceres, C.F. (2011) 'Addressing social drivers of HIV/AIDS for the long-term response: conceptual and methodological considerations', *Global Public Health*, 6(Suppl. 3): S293–S309.

Azad, K., Barnett, S., Banerjee, B., Shaha, S., Khan, K., Rego, A.R., Barua, S., Flatman, D., Pagel, C., Prost, A., Ellis, M. and Costello, A. (2010) 'Effect of scaling up women's groups on birth outcomes in three rural districts in Bangladesh: a cluster-randomised controlled trial', *Lancet*, 375: 1193–1202.

Campbell, C. (2003) *'Letting Them Die': Why HIV/AIDS prevention programmes fail*, Oxford, Bloomington, IN and Wetton: International African Institute: James Currey, Indiana University Press and Double Storey.

Campbell, D. (1986) 'Relabelling internal and external validity for applied social scientists', *New Directions for Program Evaluation*, 31: 67–77.

Campbell, C. and Cornish, F. (2010) 'Towards a "fourth generation" of approaches to HIV/AIDS management: creating contexts for effective community mobilisation', *AIDS Care*, 22(Suppl. 2): 1569–1579.

Cartwright, N. (2013) 'Knowing what we are talking about: why evidence doesn't always travel', *Evidence & Policy*, 9(1): 97–112.

Deaton, A. (2010) 'Instruments, randomization, and learning about development', *Journal of Economic Literature*, 48(June): 424–455.

DMSC (n.d.) *Durbar Mahila Samanwaya Committee*, http://durbar.org (accessed 28 January 2015).

Donovan, J.L., Paramasivan, S., de Salis, I.O. and Toerien, M.G. (2014) 'Clear obstacles and hidden challenges: understanding recruiter perspectives in six pragmatic randomised controlled trials'. *Trials*, 15(5). Available at: www.trialsjournal.com/content/15/1/5 (accessed 28 January 2015).

ESSENCE on Health Research (2011) 'Planning, monitoring and evaluation: Framework for capacity strengthening in health research', *ESSENCE Good Practice Document Series*, Geneva: TDR/WHO.

Evans, C. and Lambert, H. (2008) 'Implementing community interventions for HIV prevention: insights from project ethnography', *Social Science & Medicine*, 66: 467–478.

Evans, C., Jana, S. and Lambert, H. (2010) 'What makes a structural intervention? Reducing vulnerability to HIV in community settings, with particular reference to sex work', *Global Public Health*, 5(5): 449–461.

Gaikwad, S.S., Bhenda, A., Nidhi, G., Saggurti, N. and Ranebennur, V. (2012) 'How effective is community mobilisation in HIV prevention among highly diverse sex workers in urban settings? The Aastha intervention experience in Mumbai and Thane districts, India', *Journal of Epidemiology & Community Health*, 66: ii69–ii77.

Galavotti, C., Wheeler, T., Kuhlmann, A.S., Saggurti, N., Narayanan, P., Kiran, U. and Dallabetta, G. (2012) 'Navigating the swampy lowland: a framework for evaluating the effect of community mobilization in female sex workers in Avahan, the India AIDS initiative', *Journal of Epidemiology & Community Health*, 66: ii9–ii15.

Habicht, J.P., Victora, C.G. and Vaughn, J.P. (1999) 'Evaluation designs for adequacy, plausibility and probability of public health program performance and impact', *International Journal of Epidemiology*, 28: 10–18.

HEFCE (2014) *Home: REF [Research Excellence Framework] 2014*. Available at: www.ref.ac.uk/ (accessed 30 January 2015).

INVOLVE (2014) *INVOLVE supports public involvement in NHS, public health and social care research*. Available at: www.invo.org.uk (accessed 25 January 2014).

Jana, S. (2012) 'Community mobilisation: Myths and challenges', *Journal of Epidemiology & Community Health*, 66: ii5–ii6.

Jana, S., Basu, I., Rotheram-Borus, M. J. and Newman, P. (2004) 'The Sonagachi project: a sustainable community intervention program', *AIDS Education and Prevention*, 16: 405–414.

Laga, M. and Vyulsteke, M. (2011) 'Evaluating AVAHAN's design, implementation and impact: lessons learned for the HIV prevention community', *BMC Public Health*, 11(Suppl. 6): S16.

Lambert, H. (2006) 'Accounting for EBM: contested notions of evidence in medicine', *Social Science & Medicine*, 62(11): 2633–2645.

Lambert, H. (2012) 'Balancing community mobilisation and measurement needs in the evaluation of targeted interventions for HIV prevention', *Journal of Epidemiology & Community Health*, 66: ii3–ii4.

Lambert, H. (2013) 'Plural forms of evidence in public health: tolerating epistemological and methodological diversity', *Evidence & Policy*, 9(1): 43–48.

Levin-Rosalis, M (2003) 'Evaluation and research: differences and similarities', *Canadian Journal of Program Evaluation*, 18(2): 1–31.

Manandhar, D.S., Osrin, D., Shrestha, B.P., Mesko, N., Morrison, J., Tumbahangphe, K.M., Tamang, S., Thapa, S., Shrestha, D., Thapa, B., Shrestha, J.R., Wade, A., Borghi, J., Standing, H., Manandhar, M., Costello, A.M. and members of the MIRA Makwanpur trial team (2004) 'Effect of a participatory intervention with women's groups on birth outcomes in Nepal: cluster-randomised controlled trial', *Lancet*, 364: 970–979.

Michie, S., Van Stralen and West, R. (2011) 'The behaviour change wheel: a new method for characterising and designing behaviour change interventions', *Implementation Science*, 6: 42. Available at: www.implementationscience.com/content/6/1/42 (accessed 28 January 2015).

MRC (n.d.) 'Developing and evaluating complex interventions: new guidance'. Available at: www.mrc.ac.uk/documents/pdf/complex-interventions-guidance (accessed 1 January 2015).
NACO (2012) *Annual Report 2011–2012*, New Delhi: Ministry of Health and Family Welfare, Government of India.
Narayanan, P., Moulasha, K., Wheeler, T., Baer, J., Bharadwaj, S., Ramanathan, T.V. and Thomas, T. (2012) 'Assessing community mobilisation and organizational capacity among high-risk groups in an HIV prevention programme in India: findings using a Community Ownership and Preparedness Index', *Journal of Epidemiology & Community Health*, 66: ii34–ii41.
Petticrew, M. (2013) 'Public health evaluation: epistemological challenges to evidence production and use', *Evidence & Policy*, 9(1): 87–95.
Poverty Action Lab (n.d.) *The Abdul Lateef Jameel Poverty Action Lab*. Available at: www.povertyactionlab.org (accessed 30 January 2015).
Rai, T., Lambert, H., Borquez, A., Saggurti, N., Mahapatra, B. and Ward, H. (2014) 'Circular labor migration and HIV in India: exploring heterogeneity in bridge populations connecting areas of high and low HIV infection prevalence, *Journal of Infectious Diseases*, 210(11): S556–S561.
Saggurti, N., Mishra, R.M., Proddutoor, L., Tucker, S., Kovvali, D., Parimi, P. and Wheeler, T. (2013) 'Community collectivization and its association with consistent condom use and STI treatment-seeking behaviors among female sex workers and high-risk men who have sex with men/transgenders in Andhra Pradesh, India', *AIDS Care*, 25(Suppl. 1): S55–S66.
Shahmanesh, M., Patel, V., Mabey, D. and Cowan, F. (2008) 'Effectiveness of interventions for the prevention of HIV and other sexually transmitted infections in female sex workers in resource poor settings: a systematic review', *Tropical Medicine & International Health*, 13: 659–679.
Smith-Morris, C., Lopez, G., Ottomanelli, L., Goetz, L. and Dixon-Lawson, K. (2014) 'Ethnography, fidelity, and the evidence that anthropology adds: supplementing the fidelity process in a clinical trial of supported employment', *Medical Anthropology Quarterly*, 28(2): 141–161.
Wheeler, T., Kiran, U., Dallabetta G, Jayaram, M., Chandrasekaran, P., Tangri, A., Menon, H., Kumta, S., Sgaier, S., Ramakrishnan, A., Moore, J., Wadhwani, A. and Alexander, A. (2012) 'Learning about scale, measurement and community mobilisation: reflections on the implementation of the Avahan HIV/AIDS initiative in India', *Journal of Epidemiology & Community Health*, 66: ii16–ii25.
WHO (2012) *Toolkit for targeted HIV prevention and care in sex work settings*. Available at: www.who.int/hiv/topics/vct/sw_toolkit/en (accessed 20 March 2015).
World Bank (2007) *Monitoring and Evaluation* [World Bank Small Grants Program] Available at: http://siteresources.worldbank.org/INTBELARUS/Resources/M&E.pdf (accessed 31 January 2015).

4

What really works?

Understanding the role of 'local knowledges' in the monitoring and evaluation of a maternal, newborn and child health project in Kenya

Elsabé du Plessis and Robert Lorway

Introduction

'We know that does not work!' the field officer exclaimed one hot Wednesday afternoon in Taita Taveta County, Kenya, during a staff meeting the first author was attending in late 2014. Working on a Canadian government-funded maternal, newborn and child health and nutrition project, the staff members were in the midst of planning the final project activities. The field officer who, like many of the other staff had grown up in the region where the project was being implemented, continued to argue against a food security strategy that was under consideration. It was a strategy that had been tried 'many times before' in the region and never succeeded. Distribution of livestock to groups, rather than individuals, did not work, he explained, because no one took responsibility for the goats and they benefitted no one. The group did not argue with him as he had belonged to the organisation that employed them much longer than they had. The staff recognised the authority of the field officer because of his familiarity with the numerous health and development projects that had come and gone in Taita Taveta over decades.

The field officer's exclamation stands in sharp contrast to the declaration, 'we know what works!' re-asserted by the technical team who were tasked with the selection and implementation of interventions and the supervision of the monitoring and evaluation components of the project. Articulated by the governing academics and scientists (both Canadian and Kenyan alike), this refrain often accompanied the lament that too many health programmes and interventions were not 'evidence-based'. The notion of 'evidence' here narrowly refers to the forms of knowledge that can be generated through universalistic, standardised project monitoring indicators. In other words, 'legitimate' knowledge is assumed to be limited to that which can be articulated in quantitatively measurable terms (Erikson 2012). This assumption calls to mind the words of medical anthropologist Vincanne Adams with respect to evidence-based global health: 'for evidence to say anything valid … it must speak the language of statistics and epidemiology' (Adams 2013: 57).

Based on this type of evidence, the World Health Organisation (WHO) (2005) asserted that global knowledge pertaining to maternal, newborn and child health has reached a critical mass in which 'technically appropriate, effective interventions for reducing child mortality and improving child health are available. It is now necessary to implement these on a much larger scale' (WHO 2005: xxii). Implicit in such declarations, is the universalistic idea that expert forms of knowledge can be regarded as part of a singular, unified epistemological system that is closed to differing interpretations. In this chapter, we challenge the narrowness of this view by arguing that there is no single knowledge system that operates in contemporary global health interventions. Certainly one knowledge system is privileged and seen as legitimate, carrying 'more weight than others, either because … [it] explain[s] the state of the world better for the purposes at hand (efficacy) or because they are associated with a stronger power base (structural superiority), and usually both' (Jordan 1997: 56). But with respect to the day-to-day decision making in the Kenyan maternal, newborn and child health project, it very much operated through an on-going process of negotiation through which shared understandings and priorities were contested, negotiated and mutually transformed (Mosse 2004).

This chapter focuses less on the primacy or 'constitution of authoritative knowledge', per se, and instead examines more the ways in which 'local knowledges' – i.e. experiential and contextual understandings, such as those claimed by the field officer – invariably come to operate throughout the life history of global health projects like this one in Taita Taveta. Even though local forms of knowledge may be discounted and dismissed within reigning global health discursive arenas, we argue that they nevertheless play a vital role in how interventions unfold – how they are implemented and the kinds of health outcomes they yield. This perspective is not intended to diminish the utility of the quantitative approaches more routinely employed in monitoring and evaluation procedures. Rather, by drawing upon eight months of intensive fieldwork, we demonstrate how ethnographic methodology, when used alongside more conventional project monitoring and tracking systems, can reveal the complex and integral role that local knowledges play in the everyday workings of interventions, even when they are rendered invisible. Attention to locally situated epistemologies, as we will show, holds important implications for scaling up interventions or attempts to replicate them across varied human geographies.

Project background

In June 2010, Canada's Prime Minister, Stephen Harper, announced the Muskoka Initiative for Maternal, Newborn and Child Health, committing $2.85 billion dollars over 5 years (2010–2015). Nutrition was a focus area of the Muskoka Initiative. According to Bhushan (2014), 28.1 per cent of funds channelled through the Muskoka Initiative went to basic nutrition services. It builds on commitments made during a meeting at the 2010 United Nations summit in New York where leaders from across the globe pledged support to programmes focusing on 'the 1000 days window of opportunity' – that is, the period of time from conception to a child's second birthday (Horton 2008, Maternal and Child Nutrition Study group 2013). To qualify for these funds, Canadian organisations submitting proposals had to partner with non-governmental organisations (NGOs) in the country of implementation (IDRC 2014). Funds were administered through the Canadian International Development Agency (which later became the Department of Foreign Affairs, Trade and Development). Additional funding was made available through the Canadian Food Grains Bank which provided funds to the food security initiative by matching Canadian International Development Agency's financial contributions.

Through the Muskoka Initiative, the University of Manitoba received project funding to integrate maternal and child health with nutrition, addressing nutrition through food security initiatives in Taita Taveta County, Kenya. The project logic followed on the assumption that previous projects addressing maternal, newborn and child health, nutrition, and food security in Kenya have done so in a vertical manner with few linkages between the areas. Project partners included the University of Manitoba, in Canada, and Kenyan faith-based organisations, World Renew Kenya and the Anglican Development Services Pwani, as the implementing partners. A baseline assessment that collected both quantitative and qualitative data was conducted late in 2012. Based on the assessment findings, the project team selected what they considered to be a critical package of interventions for implementation. Interventions were considered if they addressed a gap identified by the baseline, were in concordance with Government of Kenya strategic priorities, were supported by 'sound evidence', and were not being implemented by other organisations. These interventions targeted four specific groups: pregnant women, women who were breastfeeding, women with children under five, and women of reproductive age not included in the previous categories.

Project activities could be divided into two components: health and nutrition interventions (targeting approximately 22,000 women of reproductive age across the four categories) and food security interventions (targeting 1,600 of the beneficiaries). Figure 4.1 provides an overview of the project activities.

The project provided community health volunteers with training so that they could deliver counselling services to the different 'target groups'. The training modules were developed by the project staff and student interns in conjunction with the local community health staff, including community health assistants and the Community Health Strategy focal persons. The project followed the current Government of Kenya Community Health Volunteer curriculum, providing more in-depth information on topics identified as critical by the maternal, newborn and child health technical team. During the volunteer training, time was devoted to dispelling 'local misconceptions' (e.g. uvula cutting in childhood as prevention for coughs and colds) and conveying the 'correct' western biomedical knowledge. This information was captured in 'care cards': a collection of laminated, A4 sheets (and colour coded by target group) designed by project staff (also with assistance from student interns) to assist volunteers with their daily service delivery activities. Volunteers were also trained in using the project's assessment

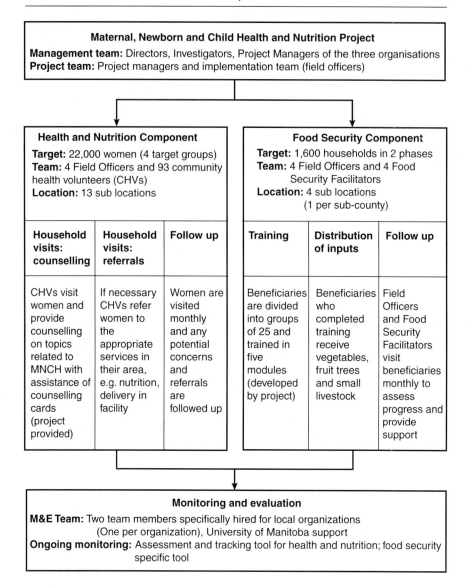

Figure 4.1 Maternal, Newborn and Child Health and Nutrition Project overview

and tracking tool. In its final iteration the tracking tool took the form of a book in which volunteers were expected to document what services they delivered to women and which counselling topics they covered; it facilitated the tracking of women to ensure that they had received the necessary services. The information collected was the backbone of the project's monitoring system, serving the dual purposes of collecting quantitative information on the care women had received, as well as monitoring individual volunteers' performance. The health and nutrition field officers followed up with the project's volunteers, 'shadowing' them regularly to provide supervision, support and feedback on any performance issues.

Exploring the contexts and practices of the project

Alongside the maternal, newborn and child health project was a Students for Development internship programme that provided support to ten senior students from the University of Manitoba to gain the experience of working with a global maternal, newborn and child health project. On 1 September 2012, the first author arrived in Kenya through this programme to assist with the initial set-up of the maternal, newborn and child health project, and to assist with the design of the qualitative component of the baseline assessment. Being part of the initial set up of the project allowed her to witness the challenges that emerged as new global health partnerships were forged. Sometimes incommensurable and competing knowledge systems and organisational structures contributed to the formation of uneven partnerships. But the effect that these tensions had on project activities certainly would not be captured in formal 'process evaluation' (Steckler and Linnan 2002) or conventional monitoring practices.

The first author returned to the project in 2014 to follow the final months of the project for her doctoral research using a 'project ethnography' approach (Evans and Lambert 2008). Central to this approach is a conceptualisation of projects

> as social arenas made up of different social actors and intersecting ideologies, relationships, interests, and resources. The interactions between different actors (including the project and its staff) and the changes that occur over time as a result of these interactions form the focus for understanding intervention processes.
>
> (Evans and Lambert 2008: 469)

Project ethnography attends to context, implementation practices, the agency of those involved in the project and the distribution of power within projects as the focus of research (Lewis *et al.* 2003, Evans and Lambert 2008). This approach is similar to institutional ethnography, which investigates the effect that the activities and work practices of one group of people have on the coordination and organisation of activities of another group of people (Smith 2001, Mykhalovskiy and McCoy 2002). This research went beyond a project ethnography approach, in a sense, by also including a more in-depth exploration of the historical context of global health and development projects in the region through primary and secondary archival research. This exploration was based on the assumption that the historical development of intervention policies has a profound effect in shaping local intervention knowledges and the concomitant willingness of local individuals to participate in the project under study.

During the research, the first author split her time between observing project implementation in Taita Taveta and tracking down historical materials at the National Archives in Nairobi. She attended project meetings, spent time in the offices of the local partner organisations with their staff and participated in project activities. In all these activities she kept detailed field notes (Emerson *et al.* 2011) focusing specifically on those everyday tasks of the project that 'made it work'. Participant observation of these everyday implementation practices and organisational relationships can reveal aspects of implementation the project staff may not be aware of, or find difficult to articulate (Evans and Lambert 2008), but that nevertheless affect 'the design, presentation and implementation of projects, and the assumptions embedded within them' (Markowitz 2001: 42).

At the Kenya National Archives, the documents the first author reviewed included Ministry of Health files for Taita Taveta, beginning with those files that included monthly reports from district nutritionists and public health nurses. As the librarian discerned the interest in Taita Taveta County, he provided the Taita Taveta Annual Reports from 1948 to 1990, as well as the District Development reports from 1974 to 1996. These reports were not yet catalogued at the time, and without the librarian's help would have remained elusive. These reports offered a rich source of information for understanding the context in Taita Taveta County, highlighting the history of external funding and the array of projects in the area.

Taita Taveta County

A five hour drive along the Nairobi–Mombasa highway brings you to Voi – the largest town in Taita Taveta County. It is also the centre of one of the four sub-counties, the others being Mwatate, Taita and Taveta. Almost two thirds (62 per cent) of the area is covered by the Tsavo East and Tsavo West National Parks; of the 284,657 people estimated to live in the county, the majority practice agriculture and raise livestock (Taita Taveta County Government 2014). As a semi-arid region, water is of great concern. In interviews and focus group discussions conducted for the project (both at baseline and during the project evaluation), the availability of water was a major concern in all sub-counties and it contributes significantly to food insecurity in the area. According to the County Government, over half the population (57.2 per cent) are living in absolute poverty (Taita Taveta County Government 2014).

Taita Taveta County was recently listed as one of the 14 counties in Kenya with the worst maternal, newborn and child health indicators (Maina 2014). Maternal mortality is estimated at 603 per 100,000 births, infant mortality at 71 deaths per 1,000, and under five mortality at 93 per 1,000. Slightly more than two thirds (68.1 per cent) of infants are considered to be fully immunised (Taita Taveta County Government 2014). Based on these statistics, the County was the first to receive a mobile clinic through the Kenyan First Lady's Beyond Zero campaign (Rugene 2015). The stated goal of the Beyond Zero Campaign is to mobilise and provide leadership towards zero new HIV infections and reduce the number of deaths among women and children in Kenya (Republic of Kenya 2013). One of the major activities of the programme is to donate mobile clinics to the counties, that will provide integrated HIV, maternal and child health outreach services in the country (UNAIDS 2014).

A number of NGOs work concurrently in the area, most visibly World Vision Kenya. Others include Action Aid, and Wildlife Works. The United Nations World Food Programme and the United States Agency for International Development (USAID) are also prominent actors in the area (Taita Taveta County Government 2014). Historically, because of periodic drought, food shortages and poor health outcomes, Taita Taveta County became a vibrant site of various foreign and locally funded interventions over many decades. Most recently, the County Government signed a memorandum of understanding with the University of Maryland with the goal of improved health outcomes by focusing on health systems support, addressing communicable diseases such as HIV and tuberculosis (TB), and education and training (Taita Taveta County Government 2015). Thus, the University of Manitoban-led maternal, newborn and child health project operated as one vessel within this much larger sea of projects.

A history of projects

In late 2014 the first author attended the training for the second group of community health volunteers recruited into the maternal, newborn and child health project. Training was facilitated jointly by project staff, and public health officers and community health assistants from the sub-counties. On the first day, one of the impeccably dressed public health officers was wearing a light blue polo shirt bearing the USAID logo. On the second day, another public health officer was wearing a t-shirt from a previous project that focused on families and health. All across the county, these signifiers of previous and ongoing projects abounded. Public health officers, staff employed by the project, community health volunteers and community members could all be spotted sporting t-shirts or carrying tote bags or messenger bags and *lessos* (also called *kangas*, these colourful, rectangular pieces of cotton are most often worn by women, or used to carry babies, and sometimes used to mobilise communities, especially women, in political and public health campaigns) with various project logos and slogans. Those related to health ranged in topic from 'HIV prevention' to 'healthy communities' to 'health literacy'. Traces of the multitude of foreign-funded health and development programmes that had descended on the area were also evident in the labelling of infrastructure with funder's and organisational branding.

During the project's evaluation the first author travelled across the county to conduct interviews and focus groups. In one sub-county the field officer who showed her team around wore two different project t-shirts on consecutive days: on the first day she wore a World Water Day t-shirt, and on the second a t-shirt related to a TB project funded by the International Medical Corps. When asked about the t-shirts the field officer replied that she worked closely with the government, and as a result of her involvement she was invited to training sessions and special events where she had been given the t-shirts. These were her 'field clothes', she explained, and she complained about not having a t-shirt for the maternal, newborn and child health project.

The proliferation of these t-shirts is not only emblematic of a lively contemporary history of health and development projects in the area. The pride with which people were wearing them as field uniforms, both in their daily activities and during training sessions and meetings, allowed them to display their knowledge and thus make epistemological claims; they served as a visual reminder that they possessed specialised knowledge and experience in the field. The contemporary history of projects in the area and people's participation in multiple projects over time (in whatever capacity) had cultivated local knowledge systems – that is, an understanding of health and development projects, how they work, and what one can expect in the course of implementing development projects on the ground. Associated with the work of anthropologist Clifford Geertz, local knowledge is described as 'local ways of knowing, perspectives and understandings over and against cosmopolitan, assumed to be universal, forms of knowledge' (Good 1992: 1359). In this chapter, we work from this understanding of 'local knowledge' but we argue that as people repeatedly participate in development or research projects over extended periods of time, universalistic knowledge interacts with local knowledge systems and unfolds in locales to become grounded epistemologies. In other words we want:

> to avoid any radical dichotomy between local and universal knowledge. Little is purely local, less is truly universal. I argue for a plurality of intelligible contexts, all of which involve some interplay between levels of knowledge, depending on the nature of the sources and the aims of the inquiry.
>
> (Goody 1992: 146)

This history of projects is also evident as one examines the Annual Reports for Taita Taveta County as well as the District Development plans. In reviewing these reports from 1970 to the 1990s, it becomes clear that there is a long-standing relationship with donors in this area. This relationship has informed people's knowledge of 'what works' and 'what does not work' in health and development projects. As an appendix to the annual reports, there is a list of those who visited the area in official capacity. Since 1970, a plethora of representatives from international development agencies have visited the area. Many represented United Nations system agencies such as the United Nations Development Program, Food and Agriculture Organisation and the United Nations Children's Fund. Other organisations listed include the Danish International Development Agency, the Swedish International Development Agency, and organisations such as CARE International in Kenya, Plan International and the Kenya Red Cross. While the annual reports do not contain information on the exact nature of the visits, other documents outline the role these organisations have played in local development. The District Development Reports for 1994–1996 and 1997–2001, for instance, contain tables that list the planned development projects, as well as the funder, whether government or donor. In some cases the donors are mentioned specifically (see Figure 4.2) while other cases may only list the funder as 'donor' (Ministry of Planning and Development 1994).

HEALTH PROJECT AND PROGRAMME PRIORITIES FOR THE 1994–96 PLAN PERIOD

A. Ongoing Project

Project name Location/Division	Description of activities
1. Tausa Dispensary Mbololo Location Voi Division	Completion of the dispensary block, staff house, drainage and fencing Funding source: Government of Kenya
2. Wundanyi Health Centre	Construction of maternity block, laboratory, offices kitchen and laundry Funding souce: Plan International
3. Nyache Health Centre Wumingu Location Wundanyi Division	Construction of laboratory block, offices and VIP latrines Funding source: Plan International
4. Mrugua Dispensary Bura Location Mwatate Division	Construction of consultation block and construction of type 'E' twin staff house Funding source: Plan International
5. Preventative maintenance of rural health facilities (District wide)	Minor repairs to existing facilities Funding source: Government of Kenya
6. Anti-malarial drain Bura Town Mwatate Division	Construction of permanent malarial control drains Funding source: Plan International
7. Screening of school children on malaria, worms and bilharzia Mwatate Location Mwatate Division	Screening of school children to gauge the morbidity rate in communities Funding source: Plan International

Figure 4.2 Excerpt from the 1994–1996 District Development Plan for Taita Taveta
Source: Ministry of Planning and Development 1994.

While there have certainly been health projects in Taita Taveta County prior to the maternal, newborn and child health project, they seem to have been smaller in scale or funded by the Government of Kenya. Furthermore, previous health programmes were overshadowed by a larger number of internationally funded projects that focused on agriculture, wildlife and forestry. Social and economic development projects (such as the support of local tradespeople and women's groups) have also received support from foreign donor agencies. This has important implications for a project that incorporates both health and agriculture as few projects before had brought the two sectors of development together along with the different knowledge and experience of local staff members.

The greater number of projects devoted to agriculture can be explained by the long history of periodic famine and crop failure in Taita Taveta, a reality that was evident in the annual reports for the county. Annual reports contained lists of the famine relief foods distributed in Taita Taveta, documenting the numbers of bags of *ugali* (maize flour) and other foodstuffs.

This history of food aid is relevant to the monitoring of the maternal, newborn and child health project in two ways, by shedding light on factors affecting the uptake of project activities. First, people in the area were familiar with one system of receiving food aid – that of 'blanket' relief food given to everyone in need. This was the frame of reference for many of the local people targeted by the maternal, newborn and child health project. However, the project model, which aimed to 'empower' people to produce their own food from start-up materials offered by the project, did not fit easily within this frame of reference. The project's food security field officers experienced this mismatch in expectations as a major obstacle to recruiting and retaining people for the intervention. They often characterised local people's current expectations around food security as part of a 'dependency culture' wherein individuals were unwilling (from their perspective) to 'do something' (such as build the chicken coops or rabbit houses) to improve their own situation.

Second, the maternal, newborn and child health project only selected a subset of beneficiaries who met specified criteria for the food security component; this inadvertently led to some suspicion in the community. In the past, project staff were told by community members that the Canadian International Development Agency gave everyone food – why was food only given to a carefully selected group of individuals now? From the perspective of local inhabitants, the new project was incongruent with their previous experiences with food aid project funding. Despite careful negotiations to explain why the current project deviated from previous projects, the discomfort over this discrepancy expressed by local communities re-surfaced during the project evaluation process. Community members again told enumerators who led the data collection that only some individuals in their communities received the agricultural inputs because, they believed, project staff (particularly community health volunteers) were pocketing the remainder of the project resources. This suspicion posed a challenge for the volunteers the first author spoke to who had to visit these households on a regular basis for project activities and monitoring purposes. Indeed, tensions such as these could have been addressed earlier if the monitoring system had attended to the local history of development in the region.

Local knowledges

During the project evaluation, enumerators hired to conduct the household survey attended three days of training before heading to their respective sub-locations for data collection. Topics covered during the training included a project overview, introduction to research ethics, sampling and an overview of the different sections of the survey tool. As the group went around the room and read and discussed the survey questions, the project supervisors placed emphasis on making sure that the enumerators understood what the project team hoped to learn from each section. Any questions people may have had about the questionnaire were addressed during these sessions. Enumerators were advised not to attempt to explain the survey questions but to administer them as they were stated in the instrument. They were also told to record responses that did not fit into the given response options as 'other, please specify' and to record any information they thought may be helpful in interpreting results in the comment section on the profile page of the tool. On the final day of training, all enumerators were instructed to go to a village to conduct a practice survey. Upon their return to the conference venue (where the training had been conducted) any challenges and questions were discussed before the teams departed for their respective sub-counties and seven days of data collection.

Although the focus of the training sessions was not on educating enumerators around maternal, newborn and child health issues, some basic knowledge on these issues was conveyed to ensure that enumerators properly understood the questions they would be asking. While discussing a section on breastfeeding, for instance, the facilitator began the session by asking enumerators about any breastfeeding myths with which they were familiar. The training group then discussed these myths, as the project's health and nutrition field officers endeavoured to dispel them. Similarly, enumerators were provided with basic information on antenatal care, nutrition, food insecurity and how to take measurements of children to determine their nutritional status (including height, weight and mid upper arm circumference).

The first author served as supervisor for a team of four enumerators in one sub-location during data collection. Members of the technical team based in Nairobi and Manitoba had selected the sample from a list of villages within the intervention sub-locations based on population size (probability proportional to population). The first author travelled to the selected communities and reviewed household questionnaires for completeness before recording information about the location and the respondents on a master list. In examining the questionnaires, she noticed that some enumerators had composed handwritten comments on the survey tool itself. In some cases these comments followed the instructions received during training and provided information that could be helpful in interpreting results of the project activities. In other cases, however, the information recorded in the margins or at the bottom of the page reflected enumerators' reluctance to fit the information received into given survey response options. A question about the barriers to attending antenatal care (see Figure 4.3) elicited one such comment from an enumerator. Instead of checking a given response option the enumerator wrote that the respondent said she had not gone to receive antenatal care because she was 'not yet six months pregnant'. Another supervisor had checked the specific questionnaire and admonished the enumerator for writing a comment, telling her to just tick 'too early' in the provided list of responses. In a later discussion, the other supervisor told the first author that the enumerator was still too unfamiliar with the tool, which is why she was writing notes. However, in informal conversations with the enumerator the first author realised that it was not a lack of knowledge or confidence that underlay the enumerator's comments but rather a sensitivity to the production of knowledge taking place in the survey process. She was attempting to capture something more complex than whether the respondent had attended antenatal care or not: she was attempting to document the conflict in knowledge systems she was experiencing. While the female respondent may have thought six months was too early for antenatal care, the enumerator – based on the training she had received for

What are the reasons that you did not see someone for antenatal care? CHOOSE ALL THAT APPLY.	☐ 1 No healthcare provider available
	☐ 2 Could not afford
	☐ 3 Distance too far
	☐ 4 Lack of transportations
	☐ 5 Poor road conditions
	☐ 6 Husband/partner would not permit
	☐ 7 Afraid of doctor, nurse, or other provider
	☐ 8 Have never used doctor, nurse before
	☐ 9 Not treated well previously
	☐ 10 Embarassed or ashamed
	☐ 11 Too early in pregnancy
	☐ 12 Not enough time
	☐ 77 Other (specify)
	☐ 99 Refused

Figure 4.3 Question in survey tool eliciting reasons for not attending an antenatal clinic

this project – was aware that the current scientific, biomedical standard held that women should attend their first antenatal care during the first trimester (prior to four months) (WHO 2007). Therefore, the response of 'six months' did not fit in the response option 'too early'.

What is vital to note here is that the astute thinking of the local enumerator will not be captured during the data entry and data cleaning process as the response will most likely be entered as 'too early'. This in many ways parallels the work of anthropologist Crystal Biruk (2012) in Malawi in which she describes the social production of the numbers recorded on survey pages through messy negotiations. Through this process we find the 'transformation of complexity into simplicity. Stories become marks in a survey box, people become data points, and households become dots on a map' (Biruk 2012: 352). It was exactly this complexity our enumerator was trying to highlight. In this way, the primacy of the quantitative logic of standardisation effectively erases local knowledge as it purifies the information collected, thus constituting legitimate knowledge as only that which can fit the predetermined response options, categories that are themselves circumscribed by the scientists who devised the survey and the supervisors who reinforce this logic.

At the same time, the intent of local enumerators, as they drew upon their knowledge and experience, should not be understood as aiming to denigrate quantitative research. Such hand-written comments on the surveys do not merely exemplify a lack of concern for the integrity of the monitoring and evaluation procedures. In fact, the enumerator was driven by a concern for precision. While attending the enumerator training it became clear that the trainees were well versed in quantitative survey design and research methodology. The enumerators, who were predominantly young people from Voi, had been recruited through the Kenya Bureau of Statistics. Many of them had previous experience with conducting surveys, including the Kenya Demographic Health Survey. One enumerator said it was the third survey he had conducted – the most recent having been an evaluation for World Vision. Conducted in late 2014, he said, it had been very similar to the tool we were using in the maternal, newborn and child health project. Moreover, the enumerators' familiarity with conducting surveys was evident in discussions during the training when the trainees took up the need to define the word 'household'. After some discussion they agreed that three criteria needed to be satisfied for a group of people to be considered a household: they had to live together, eat together, and recognise one household head. The discussion and conclusion highlighted that the enumerators understood that a standardised definition was necessary for conducting effective quantitative research. Other issues initiated by the group of enumerators during the training related to whether responses should be circled or checked, and whether the 'skip patterns' should be followed or re-worked in certain sections (i.e. whether a question needed to be asked based on the response to a previous question). This highlights their attention to the conventions of quantitative research as well as the effect that historical experience has on monitoring and evaluation practices at any particular time.

At the closing of the enumerator training, the director of the local partner organisation told a story about a survey they had previously conducted as part of their on-going food aid activities. The survey instrument asked people to recall the meals they had eaten in the last 24-hour period. The director explained that the results from this question suggested that people were eating well; they were often eating multiple meals a day, even up to six meals in some instances. As an organisation, therefore, they had to contend with questions from the funder who, based on the survey results, was concerned that the project was targeting the wrong community, and not reaching those most in need of food aid. But, the director said, in the opinion of those who had conducted the survey, this simply was not a true reflection of the need for food aid in the area. Those conducting the survey, and who lived in the area, insisted that there was a set of local moral implications around discussing issues related to hunger and household food insecurity that influenced the knowledge that was 'captured' by the survey. From first-hand experience they knew that the communities experienced hunger, but they were also keenly aware that people were misrepresenting their food intake to avoid publically admitting their hunger to others as this would also indicate that they could not provide for their families.

By recounting his experience, the director was imploring the enumerators to use their understanding of their communities and the local environment to 'probe carefully' when asking their questions (which likely contributed to the practice of hand-written notes made on the questionnaires). Similar to the enumerator's comments written on the questionnaire, the director's anecdote demonstrates an understanding of the unavoidable complexities and epistemological ambiguities of using questions derived from standardised survey tools in local settings. These examples also highlight the fact that expert and local knowledge systems are neither mutually exclusive nor static, but are actually mutually constitutive. Community members, project staff and academics are not bound by a singular knowledge system – rather, we concur with Jordan (1997: 56) that 'equally legitimate parallel knowledge systems exist and people move easily between them, using them sequentially or in parallel fashion for particular purposes'. In recording the woman's response, the enumerator was caught between two understandings of what 'too early' for antenatal care meant – one imparted to her during training and that she, as enumerator was expected to follow, and an understanding that was born from her being a mother from that community.

Conclusion

Applicable to both monitoring and evaluation practices, the above examples of the way in which enumerators and project staff accessed different knowledge systems and struggled to make sense of opposing understandings of concepts such as antenatal care is reflective of the process of negotiation that took place during the course of the project. In implementing project activities, staff negotiated shared meanings and moved between different knowledge systems to negotiate appropriate implementation strategies. These negotiations are crucial to understanding the complexities around how a project is actually implemented; but these complexities are generally elided beneath the way standardised, quantitative monitoring tools are deployed. The information collected in the maternal, newborn and child health project's monitoring tool was focused on predetermined project indicators derived from the current global scientific knowledge of what indicates improvement in this health area. Through a reliance on quantitative checklists, local knowledge about maternal, newborn and child health is subjugated, rendered invisible in the official monitoring system and project documents.

However, at the same time, discounting local knowledge systems and the role they actually do play in the implementation and success of interventions ignores a crucial part of why an intervention may be successful or a failure, and how it can be replicated; it misses important lessons that could inform eventual scale-up. While some of this may be noted in process evaluation, integrating ethnographic methods into monitoring and evaluation systems could highlight how conflicting epistemological systems interact and thus allow project staff to address these tensions before they derail project activities.

References

Adams, V. (2013) 'Evidence-based global health: subjects, profits, erasures', in J. Biehl and A. Patryna (eds) *When People Come First: Critical studies in global health*, Princeton, NJ: Princeton University Press, pp. 54–90.

Bhushan, A. (2014) *The Muskoka Iniative and Global Health Financing: North–South Institute*. Available at: www.nsi-ins.ca/wp-content/uploads/2014/05/Muskoka-Final.pdf (accessed 6 February 2015).

Biruk, C. (2012) 'Seeing like a research project: producing "high-quality data" in AIDS research in Malawi', *Medical Anthropology*, 31(4): 347–366.

Emerson, R.M., Fretz, R.I. and Shaw, L.L. (2011) *Writing Ethnographic Fieldnotes*, Chicago, IL: University of Chicago Press.

Erikson, S.L. (2012) 'Global health business: the production and performativity of statistics in Sierra Leone and Germany', *Medical Anthropology*, 31(4): 367–384.

Evans, C. and Lambert, H. (2008) 'Implementing community interventions for HIV prevention: insights from project ethnography', *Social Science & Medicine*, 66: 467–78.

Good, M.J. (1992) 'Local knowledge: research capacity building in international health', *Social Science & Medicine*, 35: 1359–1367.

Goody, J. (1992) 'Local knowledge and knowledge of locality: the desirability of frames', *The Yale Journal of Criticism*, 5: 137–147.

Horton, R. (2008) 'Maternal and child undernutrition: an urgent opportunity', *Lancet*, 371(9608): 179.

IDRC (2014) *Global Health Research Initiative: Innovating for maternal and child health*. Available at: www.idrc.ca/EN/Programs/Global_Health_Policy/Global_Health_Research_Initiative/Pages/Innovating-for-Maternal-and-Child-Health.aspx (accessed 3 June 2014).

Jordan, B. (1997) 'Authoritative knowledge and its construction', in R. Davis-Floyd and C.F. Sargent (eds) *Childbirth and Authoritative Knowledge: Cross-cultural perspectives*, Berkeley, CA: University of California Press, pp. 55–79.

Lewis, D., Bebbington, A.J., Batterbury, S.P., Shah, A., Olson, E., Siddiqi, M.S. and Duvall, S. (2003) 'Practice, power and meaning: frameworks for studying organizational culture in multi-agency rural development projects', *Journal of International Development*, 15: 541–557.

Maina, S.B. (2014) 'Experts raise alarm over high maternal deaths in childbirth', *Daily Nation*. Available at: www.nation.co.ke/news/Maternal-Mortality-Health-Report-Kenya/-/1056/2521710/-/nsy0naz/-/index.html (accessed 15 November 2014).

Markowitz, L. (2001) 'Finding the field: notes on the ethnography of NGOs', *Human Organization*, 60: 40–46.

Maternal and Child Nutrition Study group (2013) 'Executive summary of the Lancet maternal health and nutrition series', *Lancet*. Available at: www.thelancet.com/series/maternal-and-child-nutrition (accessed 1 November 2013).

Ministry of Planning and Development (1994) *Taita–Taveta District Development Plan: 1994–1996*, Nairobi: Government Printer.

Mosse, D. (2004) 'Is good policy implementable? Reflections on the ethnography of aid policy and practice', *Development and Change*, 35: 641–644.

Mykhalovskiy, E. and McCoy, L. (2002) 'Troubling ruling discourses of health: using institutional ethnography in community-based research', *Critical Public Health*, 12: 17–37.

Republic of Kenya (2013) *A Strategic Framework for Engagement of the First Lady in HIV Control and Promotion of Maternal, Newborn and Child Health in Kenya*. Available at: www.emtct-iatt.org/wp-content/uploads/2013/12/Strategic-Framework-for-Engagement-of-the-First-Lady-in-HIV-Control-and-Promotion-of-MNCH-in-Kenya.pdf (accessed 2 October 2014).

Rugene, N. (2015) 'County gets new maternity units', *Daily Nation*. Available at: http://mobile.nation.co.ke/counties/Taita-taveta-County-gets-new-maternity-units/-/1950480/2589276/-/format/xhtml/-/u3ncs9z/-/index.html (accessed 1 March 2015).

Smith, D.E. (2001) *Institutional Ethnography: A sociology for people*, Lanham, MD: AltaMira Press.

Steckler, A.B. and Linnan, L. (2002) *Process Evaluation for Public Health Interventions and Research*, San Francisco, CA: Jossey-Bass.

Taita Taveta County Government (2014) *Supporting Quality Life for the People of Taita Taveta: The first Taita Taveta County integrated development plan, 2013–2017*. Available at: http://ke.boell.org/sites/default/files/uploads/2014/05/revised_draft_cidp_30_april_2014_2.pdf (accessed 1 March 2015).

Taita Taveta County Government (2015) *County Government Sign MOU with University of Maryland Baltimore (UMB)*. Available at: http://taitataveta.go.ke/mou%20with%20UMB# (accessed 1 March 2015).

UNAIDS (2014) *New "Beyond Zero Campaign" to Improve Maternal and Child Health Outcomes in Kenya*. Available at: www.unaids.org/en/resources/presscentre/featurestories/2014/january/20140130beyondzerocampaign (accessed 7 March 2015).

WHO (2005) *The World Health Report 2005: Make every mother and child count*. Available at: www.who.int/whr/2005/en (accessed 20 February 2015).

WHO (2007) *Provision of Effective Antenatal Care*. Available at: www.who.int/reproductivehealth/publications/maternal_perinatal_health/effective_antenatal_care.pdf?ua=1 (accessed 1 March 2015).

Part II

Programme design

5

Permissions, vacations and periods of self-regulation

Using consumer insight to improve HIV treatment adherence in four Central American countries

Kim Longfield, Isolda Fortin, Jennifer Wheeler and Dana Sievers

Introduction

Population Services International (PSI) is a global health organisation that has implemented social marketing programmes for more than 40 years. Social marketing is typically defined as the use of marketing principles to target audience behaviour in ways that benefit both the individual and society (Lee and Kotler 2011). PSI uses these principles to make it easier for people in developing countries to lead healthier lives and plan the families they desire by marketing affordable products and services.

PSI routinely conducts qualitative studies to understand consumer behaviour and inform programme design. Consumer focus is the basis of social marketing. Researchers and marketers work together to identify appropriate areas of inquiry and refine research questions in order to gather consumer insight, which helps shape and tailor marketing messages for different audience segments, and create a 'brand'. The brand message is then used to promote a product, service or behaviour. Consumer insight supported by 'thick description' (Geertz 1973: 3) of the target audience is central to creating campaigns that are emotionally engaging, relevant to the consumer and effective for changing behaviour (Lee and Kotler 2011: 45). This chapter focuses on a Central American case study where a member of PSI's global network, the Pan American Social Marketing Organisation, used ethnographic research to gather consumer insight to shape the marketing planning process and programme design for a campaign to improve adherence to HIV treatment.

Barriers to HIV treatment in Central America

Costa Rica, El Salvador, Nicaragua and Panama have concentrated HIV epidemics, whereby prevalence among the general population is low (0.3–0.7 per cent), but is much higher in key populations at risk (UNAIDS 2013). For example, rates of HIV infection are highest among men who have sex with men. Prevalence estimates in this group range from 6.6 per cent in Nicaragua, to nearly 11 per cent in

Costa Rica. Recent estimates of HIV prevalence among female sex workers also illustrate a disproportionate burden compared to the general population: from 1.8 per cent in Nicaragua (Morales Miranda 2010) to 5.7 per cent in El Salvador (Programa Nacional de ITS/VIH/SIDA 2010: 78).

In these four Central American countries, an estimated 61,400 people are currently living with HIV. More than one third of them live in El Salvador (UNAIDS 2013). Eligibility for antiretroviral therapy differs by country and is dependent upon CD4 count. As of July 2013, in line with the World Health Organisation's (WHO) 2010 guidelines, people with CD4 counts of 350 or less were eligible to receive treatment in El Salvador and Panama. In 2014, policies in Costa Rica and Nicaragua were in line with the most recent WHO 2013 guidelines, which state that people with CD4 counts of 500 or less are eligible for treatment (WHO 2013: 25). Exceptions to these criteria – including people living with HIV who are diagnosed with tuberculosis or hepatitis B, who are pregnant, or serodiscordant couples – are often eligible for antiretroviral therapy regardless of their CD4 count. For all others, tests are required to determine CD4 counts to assess eligibility (UNAIDS 2013: 51).

Under these conditions, of the 61,400 diagnosed people living with HIV in the four countries, approximately 56,000 are eligible for antiretroviral therapy. Coverage is less than optimal among the adult population eligible for treatment: Costa Rica (76 per cent), El Salvador (50 per cent), Nicaragua (72 per cent) and Panama (76 per cent) (UNAIDS 2013: A83–97). Once eligible people with HIV obtain treatment, adherence is critical to ensure suppression of viral load. Adherence is also important when antiretroviral therapy is used to decrease risk of HIV transmission, through treatment as prevention (UNAIDS 2012: 4). However, adherence figures bring the total number of people receiving appropriate medication down even further. Figures are not available for all countries, but among treatment recipients in El Salvador and Nicaragua, only 87 per cent and 74 per cent remain on antiretroviral therapy 12 months after initiation, respectively (UNAIDS 2013: A79).

Data from Nicaragua provide an illustration of the progressive decline between eligibility for treatment, and adherence. In 2012, when eligibility criteria corresponded to the 2010 WHO guidelines, 3,053 people were living with HIV, 2,190 were eligible for treatment, 1,613 remained on treatment after 12 months, and 1,051 had an undetectable viral load. Therefore, only one third of people living with HIV benefitted from consistent and effective antiretroviral therapy (PAHO 2013: 39).

A number of factors influence access to treatment and treatment adherence. For example, social and structural factors inhibit people's access to HIV services along the treatment cascade and impede their ability to receive effective HIV care. In a concentrated epidemic, it is common for people living with HIV to experience multiple levels of stigma and discrimination due to their HIV-positive status, their sexual identity, or their status as sex workers. At health facilities, health workers' homophobic attitudes and the criminalisation of sex work can impede the ability of men who have sex with men, transgender women and female sex workers to access antiretroviral therapy (UNAIDS 2013). When people internalise stigma and discrimination, it can cause psychological distress and can prevent them from accessing healthcare services and seeking social support (Caceres 2002). Time since diagnosis can also influence adherence. High levels of stress immediately after diagnosis due to frustration about a lack of immediate benefit from treatment caused some recently diagnosed HIV-positive people in Mexico to give up on their regimen soon after starting treatment (Piña López et al. 2009, 2011). However, the same studies found that people who had lived with their diagnosis for more than 55 months were more motivated to adhere to treatment despite setbacks, due to a better understanding of the nature of their illness.

A combination prevention programme for HIV

In 2010, the Pan American Social Marketing Organisation and partners started a five-year USAID combination prevention programme for HIV in Central America and Mexico. Using behavioural, biomedical and structural prevention strategies, combination prevention programmes aim to meet the specific needs of populations at risk of HIV by addressing structural and psychosocial barriers to seeking treatment and treatment adherence (UNAIDS 2010). This combination prevention programme targeted vulnerable groups, including men who have sex with men, transgender women, female sex workers, and other men at risk (including those who spent long periods of time away from their family and had multiple sex partners, such as migrant workers, uniformed men, and truckers). It also included women from the general population who were infected by their male partners.

The programme offered an intervention package for each target population. For people living with HIV, the minimum package included: behaviour change communication interventions; referral to screening and treatment of sexually transmitted infections, treatment for opportunistic infections, and access to antiretroviral therapy; and referrals to complementary services (e.g. family planning, support groups, legal support, treatment for alcohol and drug use). In this chapter we focus on the antiretroviral therapy treatment component of the programme and highlight how consumer insight was used to design a programme that would increase people's ability to access and adhere to antiretroviral therapy.

The need for consumer insight

In 2012, the Pan American Social Marketing Organisation's social marketing team needed insight into the experience of people living with HIV, and a consumer profile that could be used to shape the programme's communication strategy to increase treatment adherence. Consumer profiles are a common tool in marketing and are used to inform decisions about the 4Ps (product, price, position and place). They aim to provide rich descriptions of the target audience and typically contain information about current behaviour, socio-demographic characteristics, lifestyles and competing factors that get in the way of the desired behaviour.

This process helps social marketers segment target audiences into more manageable subgroups of consumers to effectively target behaviour change communication. A typical approach would involve dividing the population of interest into subgroups of men who have sex with men, transgender women and female sex workers. In this case, the team segmented members into different stages along the treatment continuum – diagnosis, treatment initiation and treatment adherence – regardless of subgroup. This approach helped the team move their work with providers from a clinical perspective on adherence to the more human experience of treatment successes and challenges over time. The team also focused on the psychological changes that typically occurred after diagnosis through the adoption of treatment and adherence. Doing so allowed them to explore adherence within the context of living with a chronic illness, rather than an acute health issue.

Methodology

Data were collected using two qualitative methods: in-depth interviews utilising a life history approach, and focus group discussions. Life history research collects personal narratives about a person's experiences throughout a life course (Atkinson 2002). In this study, life histories encouraged participants to describe their treatment experiences and share their memories and values, which shaped their current attitudes and behaviours. The research team used life histories to identify key moments in the treatment continuum when adherence was compromised, and explored the meaning that participants attached to those moments. Focus group discussions were used to generate consensus from people living with HIV regarding what they believed to be key elements of the adherence process. The combination of life history interviews and focus group discussions helped identify perspectives on adherence as well as the multiple meanings people brought to their treatment experiences.

The study was conducted in Costa Rica, El Salvador, Nicaragua and Panama. Two cities were sampled in each country: the capital city, and another city selected on the basis of HIV prevalence and programming priorities. Study participants were included in the research if they were 25 years or older, HIV positive and identified as belonging to one of the combination prevention programme's target groups (i.e. men who have sex with men, transgender women, female sex workers, men at risk and HIV positive women from the general population). The team used their personal and professional contacts with partner organisations, other non-governmental organisations, support groups, and hospitals to purposively sample HIV-positive people for inclusion in the study.

Study participants were initially recruited for in-depth interviews according to time since diagnosis. Based on earlier work by Piña López et al. (2009), they established 55 months as a threshold and tried to recruit an equal number of participants who had been diagnosed for 55 months or longer, and those who had received a more recent diagnosis. This strategy proved problematic since some people living with HIV, especially those who experienced psychological distress when diagnosed, were unable to recall exactly when they were diagnosed and had only a vague recollection of the time period. Others had lost track of the time since diagnosis because it happened so long ago. Some people, however, could remember their diagnosis date and experience quite vividly. The team found that people who had been diagnosed for 55 months or longer were more willing to participate and were able to provide more complete life histories than those with a more recent diagnosis. Consequently, there were more participants in life history interviews with a diagnosis of 55 months or longer (n=36) than those with a more recent diagnosis (n=25). Diagnosis dates were not recorded for participants in focus groups.

Data collection took place between June and November 2013. A total of 61 life history interviews (six in Costa Rica, 24 in El Salvador, 19 in Nicaragua and 12 in Panama) and 20 focus groups (eight in Costa Rica, four in El Salvador, five in Nicaragua and three in Panama) were conducted. Study participants were interviewed only once: they either gave life histories or participated in focus groups.

Semi-structured discussion guides were used. Life history interviews generated narratives focusing on a person's life and how it changed after diagnosis and along the treatment continuum. Probes helped elicit accounts of the doctor–patient relationship, experience with support groups, and short- and long-term expectations for treatment. Focus group discussions also included personal accounts and identified common emotions experienced before, during and after diagnosis. Focus group participants shared their knowledge about HIV, living with a positive diagnosis, expectations for the future, experience with antiretroviral therapy, and sources of support.

PSI's Research Ethics Board approved the study, and the Pan American Social Marketing Organisation team secured authorisation to collect data from the Ministry of Health in each country. Participation in the study was voluntary and anonymous. All participants were informed about the study details and the risk of participation through a verbal informed consent process.

All interviews and focus groups were audiotaped and transcribed. Data were coded by hand using an inductive approach to identify emergent themes, particularly themes not already covered in the literature. Common themes were identified in the study transcripts and then categorised along the treatment continuum: diagnosis, treatment initiation and adherence. Data analysis was iterative and happened throughout fieldwork – researchers discussed, revised and validated findings with the marketing team after completing sets of interviews and focus group discussions.

Findings

Study findings indicated that there was no specific pattern of adherence that could be generalised to all people living with HIV. Living with HIV was defined by constant fluctuations and changes in emotional and physical well-being.

While such ups and downs may be a common experience, they were particularly significant in people living with HIV because of the threat of suffering, stigma and discrimination, and even death.

> It goes up and down ... sometimes I feel very happy, very optimistic and then, all of a sudden, sad again. [It happens] perhaps every three months, but it doesn't last but a day or a week. When I'm like this, I go to my brothers' or my friends'.
> (Woman living with HIV, >55 months, Nicaragua)

> I feel like I have my ups and downs. They still happen on occasion, when, for example, I have a partner and I tell him that I'm HIV positive and then he distances himself from me ... I feel bad, but I try to overcome it. I understand. Perhaps I would do the same.
> (Man who has sex with men, >55 months, Nicaragua)

Key moments along the treatment continuum at which there were setbacks or challenges in adherence were identified that could be targeted with tailored messages. These moments, which are portrayed in the New Framework for Treatment Adherence (Figure 5.1), were linked to programmatic implications and informed the communications strategy developed for the combination prevention programme.

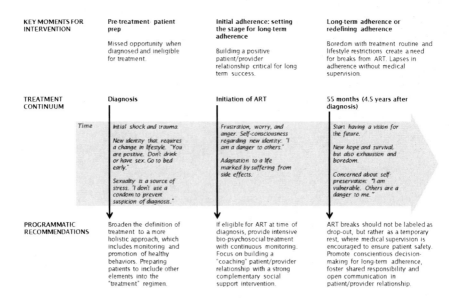

Figure 5.1 A new framework for treatment adherence for people living with HIV

HIV diagnosis

The quality and experience of HIV testing and diagnosis varied greatly across the four countries and individuals. The period immediately following diagnosis and post-test counselling was critical, as it influenced people's process of coping, and coming to terms, with a positive diagnosis. Participants' narratives demonstrated that the identity assumed by those diagnosed with HIV is not static, rather, it is situational and dynamic and only one of many that a person may adopt over time.

> At first I thought it would be more difficult. With time, I realised that most days I don't remember that I'm HIV positive. I forget. It's there, and maybe it's the treatment that reminds me, but sometimes when I'm running around, working, studying, traveling, and doing the activities that I do, I take my medicines as if they were acetaminophen, as if my head hurt. I've already forgotten that I'm HIV positive, and sometimes I have to be reminded.
> (Man who has sex with men, <55 months, Costa Rica)

The specific experiences of coping with a diagnosis varied between individuals. However, common patterns were identified within participants' narratives. They included an overlay of emotional well-being against a backdrop of physical health that were both sensitive to phases of trauma, denial, anger, acceptance, recovery, depression and other life events.

People's understandings of what it meant to be diagnosed with HIV also changed over time. Among newly diagnosed participants, initial self-perception was often dominated by feelings of guilt, and being a danger and infectious to others. Conversely, some people who had lived with an HIV-positive diagnosis for a longer period of time perceived themselves as vulnerable and had transitioned to the belief that HIV is a chronic condition.

> I didn't take care of myself, I infected myself. I didn't think 'who was it [that infected me]?' but 'who have I infected?'
> (Man who has sex with men, <55 months, Panama)

> The virus mutates ... and can become immune to the medications. Those of us who are carriers must be much more careful than others. We can infect other people, but we must also take care of ourselves.
> (Man who has sex with men, >55 months, Panama)

Participants who experienced a negative interaction with the health system at the moment of diagnosis tended to delay or refuse to seek care. Lack of social support, follow-up or reliable sources of information during the diagnosis period were reported as curtailing some participants' engagement and access to treatment.

And [the doctor] said to me, 'you already know that you have AIDS and there's no cure. Those are the consequences of sleeping around. How many [men] have you slept with?' I remember that I didn't say anything, and the tears just fell. I felt the impact of it and I felt like I wanted the earth to swallow me. That was the first and only time I went to [that hospital], I've never been back.

(Woman living with HIV, <55 months, El Salvador)

In contrast, other participants reported on more positive experiences, and appreciated how 'lucky' they were to have received good treatment from their providers.

[My doctor] is considered one of the most humane clinical infectologists that works on the patient care side. There are many complaints about the care that infectologists provide: they simply prescribe medication. They never ask patients how they feel, how things are going, what's happening. With this doctor, I've felt really good. His recommendations have been excellent. He always asks how I'm doing.

(Man who has sex with men, <55 months, Costa Rica)

Treatment initiation and adherence

A time lapse between diagnosis and the initiation of treatment created a missed opportunity to engage newly diagnosed patients in managing their health and building an early and positive patient/provider relationship. Not all the individuals in the study were immediately eligible for antiretroviral therapy at the time of diagnosis. The time between diagnosis and treatment initiation could have been used to engage them in support groups, nutrition counselling or psychotherapy, which may have improved their future engagement with the health system and adherence to antiretroviral therapy.

I spent the first nine years without regular [medical] visits. I'm not doing that until now. What I needed back then was emotional support.

(Man at risk, >55 months, Nicaragua)

Factors such as time constraints, overworked health staff and mistrust between healthcare providers and patients created a negative environment between some participants and health service providers, both in terms of communication and care.

She didn't know that I had had hepatitis ... she just said 'very well, fill out the form, see you later'. Perhaps we need an examination that is a little more thorough. Sometimes [doctors] don't even get out of the chair. Sometimes it's just file, pen, chair, prescription and 'see you later'.

(Man who has sex with men, >55 months, Costa Rica)

Overall, the relationship between providers and patients tended to be hierarchical. The doctor prescribed medications and the patient assumed responsibility for starting treatment, and trying to adhere to the medication regimes. The volume of information provided at the time of diagnosis and/or treatment initiation, and service providers' expectation for immediate behaviour change, was overwhelming to participants. It created a relationship of tension, resentment and fear of failure that interfered with successful treatment adherence in the short, medium and longer term.

> In the health system, they saturate you with information when recently diagnosed ... The day you start therapy they tell you what you should and shouldn't eat, interactions between some of the medications, that you can't drink [alcohol] ... It's too much information on a single day ... The rest [of the treatment] is just appointments, so the process fails.
> (Man who has sex with men, >55 months, Panama)

In addition to taking antiretroviral therapy correctly, doctors prescribed lifestyle changes that could be overwhelming for study participants. In interviews and focus groups, they discussed the challenges involved in modifying their diet, eliminating alcohol and cigarettes, increasing physical activity, adopting healthier sleeping schedules, and disassociating from social circles and activities that could lead to unhealthy behaviours.

> [Doctors] are so strict ... they tell us 'you must take [the medications] at a certain hour', and we must adapt to that schedule strictly. Everything that deviates from that norm is bad ... to the point that you can't do anything else ... you can't be ... truly happy with your therapy ... Because they take everything away, including things that we enjoy eating or things that we enjoy doing ... And little by little, we stop enjoying things that all humans enjoy, including our social life.
> (Man who has sex with men, >55 months, Panama)

In cases where interactions between providers and patients were infrequent and distant, participants spoke of wanting more from treatment, and of being dissatisfied with the very sporadic engagement and lack of continuity they experienced.

> Yes, I ask questions. [The doctor] sees my lab results. In fact, she says since I'm undetectable, there is no 'risk'. I said, 'Doctor, excuse me, but don't you think that it's too long [between visits]? I should have follow up, be monitored.' But she says, 'no, you're fine'. I'd rather my appointments not be so far apart.
> (Man at risk, >55 months, Costa Rica)

Participants who had a strong relationship with their health provider discussed how important a more holistic approach – including social and emotional support – was for adherence. Those who felt that their providers were more engaged in their care, and interested in them as people, were more motivated to be adherent, and more likely to have an honest and positive relationship with their provider.

> The virus is under control. My immune defences are always on the rise. [My doctor] congratulates me and motivates me. You can see it in his face that he's happy to see that one of his [patients] is following the plan exactly. For me, seeing his face, and that he's happy with me, motivates me. He asks me about my life, whether I've been drinking and smoking. I try to be honest … because at first I wasn't honest [with him].
> (Man who has sex with men, >55 months, El Salvador)

People living with HIV for many years displayed a greater understanding of the challenges associated with adherence, and recognised that psychosocial factors such as self-esteem, individual and collective empowerment, and mental health play a critical role. Periods of instability were red flags for non-adherence. In absence of holistic care and regular follow-up, there was no support to patients during bouts of depression and no intervention to reduce the risk of non-adherence.

> But if I fall into depression, it's a lie that I'll be adherent, because I'll become so depressed that I don't even want [the medicines]. It's happened to me. There are moments when I say: 'why should I take them? It's not worth it.' And I have stopped taking them.
> (Man at risk, >55 months, El Salvador)

Client approaches to 'treatment adherence'

Newly diagnosed participants used biomedical terms when speaking about antiretroviral therapy and their understanding of treatment adherence. Those who had been diagnosed for some time described their evolving needs, changing expectations for treatment, and strategies for adapting treatment to fit into their lives. People adopted those strategies, which usually had unknown implications for their long-term health, in response to a medical system they perceived to be overly strict and inflexible. Even though they adopted alternatives, participants did not consider themselves non-adherent. Five different kinds of alternatives were identified during the study.

The first occurred when people were conscious of the need to take antiretroviral therapy, but had difficulty adhering because they forgot or struggled to establish a routine. This usually occurred at treatment initiation, when taking medication according to a schedule was not yet habitual. Participants aspired to be adherent, and described a range of strategies they used to remind themselves to help adhere to treatment.

> When you begin, you have these small lapses of forgetfulness ... so I would turn on the alarm on my phone ... That's how I started getting closer [to adherence] ... until the moment when, thank God, I was adherent.
> (Woman living with HIV, <55 months, El Salvador)

The second strategy took the form of 'abandonment', when people decided to stop taking treatment definitively. Abandonment typically occurred when participants were unable to cope with the side effects of medication, were depressed, or felt a loss of control. Abandonment was seen as a way to regain control over their lives.

> Those nightmares were terrible. I would always have the same dream ... I was stabbing a man ... When I left the hospital, I would stop taking [my medication] ... I was afraid that one day I'd wake up and find that I'd stabbed my children! [The dreams] were so real! So that's how I left things.
> (Woman living with HIV, >55 months, Panama)

The third consisted of a strategy whereby people who were usually adherent gave themselves permission to stop taking treatment during short and discrete periods of time. These permissions were usually motivated by a specific event that involved alcohol consumption, such as attending a wedding, party or graduation. Participants indicated that they would never request permission from their doctor in such situations, but instead took short breaks which they felt 'liberated' them from the restrictions of medication. People still considered themselves adherent and even viewed the decision as responsible, especially when they avoided combining medication and alcohol.

> Since I know that [my viral load] is undetectable, sometimes I go out and have a few drinks, to be able to have some fun, get out of the routine ... but I don't do it all of the time. In my case, I get bored and tired and I say, 'today I'll rest' and I don't take [my medication]. But the next day, I say, 'today I'll take them!'
> (Woman living with HIV, Panama)

> I usually take [my medications]. I remind myself that they're the motor that keeps me going ... I don't take them when I know that I'm going out over the weekend. Some of my friends take [their medications] with a swig of beer. Not me. I respect that ... If I know that I'm going out at night, I take one pill in the morning at 9am like normal, but I won't combine the pills with liquor. I try to follow the instructions exactly.
> (Man who has sex with men, Costa Rica)

The fourth strategy consisted of people deliberately stopping taking their medications for a defined period of time, based on a need to be free from the treatment routine. While the third strategy was usually associated with a specific event, the fourth was born out of treatment fatigue, with no reference to a specific event to justify a lapse. Patients adopting this strategy explained that treatment 'vacations' gave people a chance to feel 'normal' for a while. After such vacations, people felt more able to continue with treatment.

> It's been 13 years of taking so many pills, and you get tired and say, 'no, I'm going to give myself a vacation.' I said once, 'I'm taking a vacation' and I stopped taking [my medication] for a month.
> (Woman living with HIV, Costa Rica)

Finally, participants described a process of self-regulating their medication, modifying their dosage or administration schedule to better fit within their lives or to decrease side effects. They felt that such a strategy gave them some control over treatment, without completely abandoning it or feeling non-adherent.

> I've never had a lapse, and I hope not to have one. So I'm always on time [taking my medication] and I try to, every day of the week up to Friday. Because when Friday comes around it's party time! And I forget about the pills until Sunday. On Monday I start taking them again. It's just Friday and Saturday that I take my days off.
> (Woman living with HIV, Panama)

Hierarchical and distant relationships between providers and patients fostered a lack of communication and prevented honest discussion about patient-initiated treatment breaks.

> I've never sat down with a doctor to discuss whether or not it's good to take a break from the medication because I don't have the confidence to ask. On the other hand, it could be the system itself: the routine, the lack of resources, the environment. [Ideally], I think the key would be to ask the doctor.
> (Woman living with HIV, >55 months, Nicaragua)

While most participants knew that adherence was important, they found justifications for disrupting treatment. Some cited scientific debate about whether taking a break would cause specific effects. Others talked about a lack of antiretroviral therapy availability in the health system, or used their personal experiences with lapses in treatment without health consequences to defend their actions.

> It's proven that we can take vacations. In December, there's no medication [at the hospital] and I am so happy. So, unconsciously it's scientifically proven that we can take vacations, because when [the] health [sector] doesn't have money, and they don't buy it and they don't supply it, then it doesn't get to the user.
> (Woman living with HIV, Panama)

Design implications

Study results and data from life histories provided insight into people's lived experiences with treatment and services, their motivations and concerns, the social context within which events unfold, and the challenges and successes they experienced along the treatment continuum. A wide range of programme strategies were developed from this data, and integrated into the annual USAID combination prevention work plan for 2015. For illustrative purposes, we focus here on opportunities along the treatment continuum most critical for targeted communications.

Immediately after receiving an HIV-positive diagnosis, people are enrolled into the programme, which prepares them for treatment initiation and case management, and supports and motivates them to make healthy lifestyle changes. In this way, each country programme now targets people living with HIV before they become eligible for treatment.

For clients already enrolled in comprehensive care, a diary-based tool will be used to document and track health status and progress along the treatment continuum. The diary functions as a logbook, but also serves as an information resource on nutrition, medications and side effects, emotional support and medical appointments. Diary keeping aims to improve people's engagement in their own care by increasing their knowledge and ability to track viral load and providing guidance for effective personal treatment management.

Mobile technology and social media are also important programme components. For clients who have access to mobile technology in El Salvador, a pilot mobile phone application and SMS messaging, designed to complement the diary, could serve as a resource to remind clients about medical appointments and treatment adherence, and provide motivational messages about nutrition and self-esteem.

The combination prevention programme updated its current social media strategy and online platform (www.yahoraque.info) – which is designed for people living with HIV and their family members, friends and partners – to include a private, confidential discussion forum. Forum topics will be aligned with key study findings and include healthy lifestyles, self-esteem, nutrition, antiretroviral therapy, adherence, stigma and discrimination, and human rights.

To improve psychosocial support, the Pan American Social Marketing Organisation's partner REDCA+ (Central American Network of People Living with HIV) is responsible for implementing a support group strategy. This strategy is flexible and adaptable to the contexts of people living with HIV, catering for the diversity of needs according to time of diagnosis and issues specific to men who have sex with men, transgender women and female sex workers. REDCA+ has developed an interactive, game-based model entitled *Porque soy capaz, yo actuo* ('because I can, I act'), which covers emotion management among programme recipients. During an eight-week regional training course, forum group facilitators are trained in skills to manage groups, support recipients, and help mitigate risks for non-adherence.

At the health provider level, a new intervention will engage medical staff to improve treatment and care for people living with HIV. The intervention will include job aids, such as a newly formatted chart for patient health records to improve follow-up and expand the data collected beyond medication administration to include contextual information that will capture patients' experiences and challenges with adherence.

Using consumer insight to influence national HIV treatment policy

The topic of adherence is not new, but is increasingly relevant within the context of universal access to treatment, especially given the potential of treatment as prevention as a strategy to curtail the HIV epidemic. The Ministries of Health in Costa Rica, El Salvador, Nicaragua and Panama have expressed interest in better understanding the phenomenon of adherence. They see achieving a high level of treatment adherence as a marker of effective and efficient treatment intervention. Improved adherence also indicates improved service quality, which will be reflected in the health and wellbeing of people living with HIV.

In Nicaragua, the Pan American Social Marketing Organisation team has recently conducted a workshop, in collaboration with the US President's Emergency Plan for AIDS Relief. Participants included 30 individuals from different sectors, including non-governmental organisations, donors, USAID Combination Prevention Program personnel, and psychologists. Participants used study findings, along with the field experience of implementing NGOs, to identify actions that existing support groups could adopt to assist people in overcoming setbacks to adherence. Study findings were also used during a forum in Nicaragua in 2014 to revise intervention and care protocols for treatment adherence for people living with HIV. Protocol revisions included improving care for people living with HIV, redefining treatment to reflect a broader definition of care, and better coordinating with other sectors such as peer support groups, that offer services and can contribute to more holistic treatment regimens.

Conclusions

This case study illustrates how ethnographic methods can significantly improve programme design. The team gathered insight into the lived experience of people living with HIV and developed an adherence framework that could be used to shape the combination prevention programme's communication strategy to increase treatment adherence. This permitted a better understanding of people's realities, motivations, concerns and behaviours, and the successes and setbacks they experience along the treatment continuum. As a result, the team was able to identify the most critical moments for targeted communications and intervention. However, study findings also influenced policy, especially advancing the dialogue on universal access and treatment as prevention in the four countries under study.

The team's use of stages of treatment as a segmentation strategy was something of a departure from typical marketing approaches that more typically focus on subgroups of consumers. Examining adherence along the treatment continuum helped move from a clinical perspective on adherence to the more human experience of treatment successes and setbacks over time. Findings challenged the programme to support people within the context of a chronic condition, and acknowledge that treatment is dynamic and multiple factors compete with adherence.

Linking programme development strategy to high quality ethnographic research, through careful analytical processes located in the reality of people's daily lives, results in more successful social marketing programmes. Such approaches challenge social marketers to appeal to consumers on an emotional level and target them at the most relevant moments for intervention.

References

Atkinson, R. (2002) 'The life story interview', in J.F. Gubrium and J.A. Holstein, J.A. (eds) *Handbook of Interview Research: Context and method*, Thousand Oaks, CA: SAGE, pp. 121–140.

Caceres, C.R. (2002) 'HIV among gay and other men who have sex with men in Latin America and the Caribbean: a hidden epidemic?' *AIDS*, 16(Suppl. 3): S23–S33.

Geertz, C. (1973) *The Interpretation of Cultures*, New York: Basic Books.

Lee, N. and Kotler, P. (2011) *Social Marketing: Influencing behaviors for good*, Thousand Oaks, CA: SAGE.

Morales Miranda, S. (2010) *Encuesta Centroamericana de Vigilancia de Comportamiento Sexual y Prevalencia de VIH e ITS Comportamiento Sexual y Prevalencia de VIH e ITS en poblaciones vulnerables ECVC Nicaragua 2009: Principales Resultados en la población de trabajadoras sexuales*, Managua: conference presentation.

PAHO (2013) *Tratamiento antirretroviral bajo la lupa: un análisis de salud pública en Latinoamérica y el Caribe*, Washington, DC: PAHO.

Piña López, J.A., Davila Tapia, M., Sanchez Sosa, J.J., Cazares Robles, O., Togawa, C. and Corrales Rascon, A.E. (2009) 'Efectos del tiempo de infección sobre predictors de adherencia en personas con VIH', *International Journal of Psychology and Psychological Therapy*, 9(1): 67–78.

Piña Lopez, J.A., Sanchez Sosa, J.J., Fierros, L.E., Ybarra, J.L. and Cazares, O. (2011) 'Psychological variables and adherence among HIV persons: evaluation based on length of infection', *Terapia Psicologica*, 29(2): 149–157.

Programa Nacional de ITS/VIH/SIDA (2010) *Encuesta Centroamericana de Vigilancia de Comportamiento Sexual y Prevalencia de VIH/ITS en Poblaciones Vulnerables*, San Salvador: Ministerio de Salud de El Salvador.

UNAIDS (2010) *Combination HIV Prevention: Tailoring and coordinating biomedical, behavioural, and structural strategies to reduce new HIV infections*, Geneva: UNAIDS.

UNAIDS (2012) *Treatment 2015*, Geneva: UNAIDS.

UNAIDS (2013) *Global Report: UNAIDS report on the global AIDS epidemic 2013*, Geneva: UNAIDS.

WHO (2013) *Consolidated Guidelines on the Use of Antiretroviral Drugs for Treating and Preventing HIV Infection: Recommendations for a public health approach*, Geneva: WHO.

6

Generating local knowledge

A role for ethnography in evidence-based programme design for social development

Ruth Edmonds

Introduction

This chapter discusses how the generation of 'local knowledge' (Geertz 1983) using an ethnographic approach can be used in social development to ensure that programming is meaningful, impactful and responsible towards programme beneficiaries or service users. It draws on empirical research experiences in Rwanda aimed at understanding girls' emotional, rational and practical realities to inform the design of girl empowerment programmes. Using the case study, the chapter demonstrates how an understanding of important cultural concepts can help make sense of findings about girls' daily lives. It shows how this local knowledge has the potential to make the difference between programme success and failure in terms of making programmes locally effective and meaningful.

Evidence-based programming: a role for 'local knowledge'

In the fields of health and social development, much attention is paid to evidence-based programming, stemming from demands for greater levels of efficiency and effectiveness within the public and not-for-profit sectors where there is pressure to justify expenditures and activities (Miller and Rudnick 2012). In social development contexts in particular, the term 'evidence-based programming' is increasingly popular: programming, in itself, is no longer considered a legitimate and worthwhile exercise unless it is somehow evidence based. Moreover, engaging in evidence-based programming has become synonymous with achieving effective programme approaches with high levels of impact and desired results. Despite this, it is pertinent to ask: what has really changed, in practice, about the way evidence is generated and used in the design of social development programmes?

A typical approach to social development programming involves six stages, although these vary in their manifestation from one organisation to another (Edmonds and Cook 2014). They include: (1) the identification of needs and problems at community, regional or state level; (2) insight research or needs assessment, typically involving assessments and surveys, to reveal information about the problem and develop indicators upon which programme effectiveness can subsequently be evaluated; (3) programme planning, usually drawing on existing programme models and typologies as well as the information gathered; (4) programme delivery, involving the 'rolling out' of activities; (5) programme evaluation, in which research is conducted to assess programme 'effectiveness' measured against predetermined indicators; and (6) the documentation of 'best practice', which serves as a basis for future models and from which programme approaches can be scaled up (see Figure 6.1).

Current problems with evidence-based programming

Despite the promise of an evidence-based approach, programme decisions are still often made based on the result of political negotiation and a combination of the opinion and experiences of programme staff (Miller and Rudnick 2012, Miller et al. 2010). While these are important, they do not constitute a rigorous basis for programme design. The distinction between 'planning' programmes and 'designing' them is useful here. While there is talk of programme design in social development, the process by which knowledge is moved into action rarely constitutes an actual design process (Miller and Rudnick 2010, Miller et al. 2010). Political negotiation and experience are more commonly applied within an expedient 'plug and play' process in which development problems are addressed in formulaic ways through the application of tried and tested programme models (Edmonds and Cook 2014). Knowledge is used to adapt existing models for different target areas and audiences rather than to design new ways of doing things and, in many cases, programme models are applied with little attention to local social and cultural specificity (Edmonds and Cook 2014).

There are three problems with the use of the term 'evidence-based' in programming for social development. First, there remains insufficient interrogation about the type and quality of evidence used. This is partly due to a lack of information and expertise among programme staff to assess the quality of evidence. This requires deep attention to research design where research aims and questions are clearly defined and are used to shape the methodological approach. In

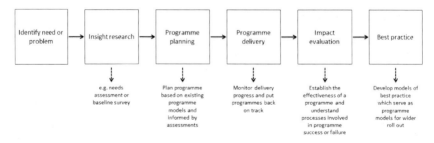

Figure 6.1 Key stages of a typical programme cycle in social development contexts

practice, a 'method-led' approach is common where limited knowledge of available research methods drives methodological decisions. This is demonstrated by the large number of tenders for research that present almost identical methodologies (e.g. questionnaires, focus groups, surveys) for a vast range of research questions and concerns. Quality assessment also requires attention to the design of an appropriate analytical approach to make the responsible moves between data, interpretation and 'claim' that are needed to generate 'evidence'. Analysis is something that is often overlooked or viewed as of secondary importance, despite the fact that, without it, we are acting on the basis of 'information' rather than 'evidence' (Miller and Rudnick 2012).

Second, programming is more often inspired by evidence rather than systematically informed by it (Miller and Rudnick 2011, 2012, 2014). In other words, evidence is not used in a rigorous process to verify and falsify programme ideas that are developed on the back of research (Miller and Rudnick 2011). Rather, these are based more loosely on recommendations for practice, although some attempts to repackage such knowledge in practical and accessible ways are laudable (e.g. RAPIDS, Overseas Development Institute). Service design approaches that aim to move knowledge into action through a process of co-design to develop ideas to solve social development problems (e.g. IDEO's Human Centred Design approach) also hinge on 'inspiring' rather than 'informing'. Co-design uses insight for 'idea generation' – the development of prototyped ideas for services or policy solutions that are subsequently tested in practice with stakeholders. Insight is used to sense-check ideas (i.e. can we see a connection to the evidence in this idea?) rather than to systematically identify pieces of evidence to falsify or verify the prototyped solutions (Miller and Rudnick 2014).

Finally, evidence used to determine programme success is problematic because it involves assessment against indicators that are largely upwardly accountable to donors and policy makers. This means that programme assumptions do not necessarily align with the perspectives of programme beneficiaries (Mosse 2001). As empirical material from Rwanda will demonstrate, goals and approaches can be in direct contradiction with beneficiary perspectives and their sociocultural realities. Consequently, research to inform programme approaches (from which programme indicators are developed) frequently reflect measures of success from donor and implementing organisations' perspectives rather than what constitutes success from a local point of view.

A role for local knowledge

Attention to generating local knowledge can help overcome some of these problems with evidence-based programming. The term 'local knowledge' was coined by the anthropologist, Clifford Geertz, who described it as 'understanding of understandings not our own' (Geertz 1983: 5). Simply put, local knowledge refers to knowledge *of* a place, people or practice, as understood by community members within their own social and cultural frame of references (Miller *et al.* 2010).

It is useful to distinguish this from 'local-level knowledge', which refers to knowledge *about* a place, people or practice, and might include the knowledge that programme staff have about social development problems in local communities (Miller et al. 2010). This distinction is important: even the most participatory research processes can result in a reflection of local power rather than accessing real voices of community members (Mosse 2001). Project staff are not passive recipients of knowledge but are often the owners of research tools, topics and modes of recording data, and extract information according to their own project criteria or relevance. Consequently, their local-level knowledge can become synonymous with the local knowledge of community members. Moreover, community members themselves have become expert research participants, manipulating local knowledge so that it becomes compatible with bureaucratic planning (Mosse 2001: 32).

Approaches that enable the generation of local knowledge are vital for evidence-based programming. These processes reveal the understandings of programme beneficiaries that are relevant for developing programme activities that are locally situated, meaningful and effective (Miller and Rudnick 2010). Taking an ethnographic approach to the generation of local knowledge enables learning about cultural systems and the symbols, meanings and practices that articulate daily life for a group of people (Hammersley and Atkinson 2007).

Using an ethnographic approach to generate 'local knowledge'

Ethnography is an approach to understanding people, cultures and societies from the 'inside out', from the vantage point of those who are being studied (Wolcott 1999, Herbert 2000, Hammersley and Atkinson 2007). In this sense it is an emic rather than etic approach (Hammersley and Atkinson 2007). It involves understanding the systems of meanings and practices that animate daily life for the people we study, and privileges the categories, explanations and interpretations of those we study rather than viewing these things from our own frames of reference (Hammersley and Atkinson 2007). Traditionally, ethnography was the choice approach for anthropologists who often spent long periods of time living with those being researched, to engage in their daily lives and experience it with them. It is now used (and abused) by a range of people and organisations from different disciplines and fields of practice. This has led to some confusion of what can be termed truly ethnographic, with a number of new types of ethnography emerging – such as 'design ethnography', 'visual ethnography' and 'digital ethnography' – in new journal publications and university curricula. In some cases, ethnography has become synonymous with conducting in-depth qualitative research. Indeed, while many new forms of ethnography view it as a set of methods and tools (e.g. case studies, participant observation, in-depth interviewing, life and family histories, focus group discussions) which can be used to generate insights, ethnography is actually an approach to research, underpinned by some key principles that inform how certain choice methods and tools are employed (see Cook 1997, Kees van Donge 2006). Some of these principles include: participation, observation, listening, reflexivity, and taking an iterative approach to research. In an ethnographic approach, research is recognised to be subjective and positioned but still valid and valuable, provided that analytic moves are made in responsible ways to safeguard the subjective point of view, and frame it in references that are relevant and meaningful to the data. It is these analytic moves that are frequently missing from some of the newer, emerging forms of ethnography. For example, design ethnography uses methods from social science to generate information about user experiences, but not to analyse or interpret such information (Leighter *et al.* 2013).

An ethnographic approach is useful for evidence-based programming because it can illuminate how programme stakeholders construct and interpret the programme and its effects in light of their own social and cultural realities and meaning systems (Dorr Bremme 1985, Miller and Rudnick 2010, Bell and Aggleton 2012). Such insights are vital when designing programmes that are effective and successful from the perspective of recipients, rather than donors, policy makers and programme implementers with their external frameworks for making sense of what will and will not work.

Research to generate local knowledge in Rwanda

The rest of this chapter focuses on empirical ethnographic research in Rwanda that was commissioned to inform the design of girl empowerment programmes and communication campaigns. The aim of the research was to better understand what girls think, feel and believe, to design interventions that were effective in terms of being meaningful to girls themselves. Knowledge generated would be used to develop initiatives and communications that could positively change girls' behaviours in line with a number of programme goals that aimed to give girls more control over their lives. These included, for example, enabling girls to finish school, marry, have children later, look after their own health and take control of their own finances.

The girl-led research approach drew on a range of research theories and methodologies, including youth and child-led research (Johnson *et al.* 2014), ethnography (Hammersley and Atkinson 2007), peer-to-peer methods (Price and Hawkins 2002) and participatory techniques (Cook 1997, Kees van Donge 2006). Thirty girls, aged between 16 and 18 years, who were either 'in' or 'out' of school, were involved as researchers. The research project was located in three contrasting locations – Kigali, a provincial town and a rural community – to involve girls with different life experiences and access to different opportunities. Girls were recruited from different geographic areas within each research location to ensure that the research reached a wide range of social networks and reflected the diversity of cultural, social and economic backgrounds. Local partner organisations provided access to research communities, made introductions to key stakeholders, recruited girl researchers, provided logistical support and acted as a referral point for the research team and girl researchers.

Girls were involved in the research as co-researchers, key informants, co-designers and co-analysts. They led the research, making decisions about research themes and questions, and shaping the methodological and ethical approach so it was locally appropriate. They conducted six in-depth interviews each, including with two younger girls (12–15 years), two same age girls (16–18 years) and two adults (one male, one female), resulting in a total of 178 interviews across the three locations. Interviewees encompassed a mix of girls in and out of school, as well as a diverse range of personal experiences, including girls who worked as house maids and girls who had personally experienced rape, abortion, domestic violence, forced marriage or early pregnancy.

The research process was based around three stages: training, supported fieldwork and analysis. The training was highly interactive and focused on building girls' confidence and self-esteem as researchers to ensure they had the capability and confidence to lead the research process and understood their ethical responsibilities. During fieldwork, girls were mentored through weekly one-to-one support and group meetings. These meetings continued to build girls' research capacities by hearing feedback about interview experiences and conducting group problem-solving activities to address challenges. They also ensured that detail from interviews was captured. Following fieldwork, a period of dedicated analysis saw the researchers making sense of their data, drawing on their own experiences to support interpretation. This involved girls reporting back in detail on their findings and organising data on each research topic according to age group, school attendance and gender of interviewees. Areas of overlap and difference, points of contention and particular interest were then explored in more detail through discussion. Girls were also engaged in the co-design of evidence-based principles for interventions based on key messages from the research.

The research process produced the following data sets: field diaries kept by the research team; field notes from workshop and mentoring sessions, including notes from focus groups and accounts of the conversational interviews; and field notes from weekly in-depth interviews with research assistants. Data analysis was ongoing, involving the researchers alongside local research assistants, to encourage iterative learning, and ensure the process of making sense of data was immersed in local interpretation. In particular, two analytic tools or processes that are central to an ethnographic approach were used to generate local knowledge with girls in Rwanda. The first was 'thematic analysis', a favoured analytic tool for analysing ethnographic data to ensure a central focus on participants' values, interpretations and meanings. Thematic analysis of data ensures that programme design is rooted in local explanation, as well as researchers' observations and interactions. The research process is iterative, beginning with generative questions that serve as a guide to the research but are neither static nor confining. Thematic analysis involves searching for themes in the data that emerge as important to the description of phenomenon and are meaningful by virtue of being recognisable and holding some degree of importance to the community in which the data was generated (Schutz 1967, Rice and Ezzy 1999).

The second analytic tool used was 'discourse analysis', drawn from the theoretical orientations of the Ethnography of Communication (Carbaugh 2007). We drew on Cultural Discourse Analysis (Carbaugh 2007) to treat communication as a socially situated practice. This involved listening for local terms and treating them as cultural symbols through a cluster analysis around significant terms that explored how the term is manifested through people's practices and what forms and meanings they attached to these. While this did not constitute a comprehensive use of the Cultural Discourse Analysis method, it allowed us to understand how key local concepts are recognised in cultural life, in turn, providing a lens through which to interpret the data.

The importance of local knowledge in programme design

This section demonstrates how local knowledge generated from this research had important implications for designing girl empowerment programmes that are more meaningful from the girls' perspectives. It provides a discussion of a local term (*agaciro*) and its significance to young women in relation to programme activities connected with delaying marriage and pregnancy. It shows how, without local knowledge, research data is cast in a different light and not sufficiently based in the cultural logic of girls involved in this research.

Agaciro: a local lens for understanding girls' daily lives

In Rwanda, girls negotiate a complicated terrain of cultural and social expectations, emotions and practical realities (McLean Hilker 2014). This delicate negotiation is encapsulated in one local Kinyarwandan term that effectively served as a lens for understanding girls' lives: *agaciro*. Literally translated, *agaciro* means 'value'. *Agaciro* is closely connected with the notion of respect (*kwiyubaha*) and is something that is attached to individuals and can be both given and received. It can also be given by an individual to themselves ('you are always valued if you value yourself'). *Agaciro* is inherently connected to the way a girl handles herself – her decisions and actions, attitudes and behaviours that lead to gain and loss of value. As girls explained: 'you start respecting yourself and then you get it.'

Girls described how there is a 'correct' way to behave that allows them to gain *agaciro* from family and wider society. This narrative of girlhood broadly involves: following the advice of parents; having respect for yourself (e.g. 'looking after your body') and treating others with respect (especially elders); avoiding 'bad' behaviour (e.g. sexual relationships before marriage); getting married at the time specified and to the person chosen by parents; having money (through 'honest' work); having children; and getting an education (although this was not universally viewed as a requirement for being a person who has *agaciro*).

Girls contrasted this narrative of girlhood with another in which attitudes and behaviours are in stark contrast to what is expected of them and that, ultimately, leads to losing value. This narrative was described by girls as 'getting all the consequences' and involved a chain of events in which girls are depicted as becoming 'delinquent' either because they do not follow, or receive, advice. Girls presented this in terms of a worst case scenario involving sexual relationships with boys, getting pregnant outside marriage, contracting sexually transmitted infections and HIV, being abandoned by relatives who are ashamed of their association with them, and engaging themselves in prostitution to earn a living.

In reality, girls' lives do not play out neatly according to one of these narratives. Neither do these narratives paint a true picture of the emotional rationale driving the decisions they make, the opportunities available to them and the constraints facing them. Life for girls in Rwanda is full of tensions and contradictions in terms of what is expected of them by their families, communities and wider society, what they want themselves, and the way they negotiate and shape pathways available to them. Girls overcome many obstacles to fulfil societal and personal expectations. They seek to conform to the socially and culturally accepted narrative of girlhood but are not passive recipients of this. Rather, they make rational choices that do not consistently conform to either mainstream expectations or discourses promoted by non-governmental organisations and international development agencies (see also De Boeck and Honwana 2005, Payne 2012). Understanding what drives girls' behaviours, especially when this contradicts accepted narratives, especially those of social development programmes, is important to ensure interventions are meaningful to girls and will be accepted by them.

During the research, it was important to explore the differences between what girls *can* and *want* to do in terms of their agency to make and enact decisions about their lives, and the social and cultural contexts that influence their abilities to do so in positive and negative ways. This is because, in many cases, girls' perspectives on gaining *agaciro* were in direct contrast with programme goals for empowering girls. Table 6.1 illustrates how girls' goals differed, sometimes very subtly, from those of organisations designing girl empowerment programmes.

In only one of the themes (school) did the organisational and girls' goals match. In all the others, there were subtle differences between them. Marriage and pregnancy are two examples of contrasting programme goals. These illustrate the importance of understanding local knowledge when designing programmes that resonate with girls' own values and ambitions. For both marriage and pregnancy, girls were not concerned with the age at which these things happened, only that they happened in a particular order – marriage first, then pregnancy – to ensure they gained *agaciro*. Consequently, while programme goals included empowering girls by helping them delay marriage, girls were actually more concerned with having greater control over who they married and their sexual lives. This helped to prevent unwanted pregnancies that might either end in marriage to a man they did not want to marry, or detrimentally affect their ability to form a respectable marriage in the future. The following sections elaborate on these issues in the context of local knowledge about *agaciro*.

Table 6.1 Comparing and contrasting programme goals and girls' goals

Empowerment theme	Organisational goal	Girls' goals
Girlhood	I enjoy being a girl	I want more control over my life
School	I want to finish secondary school, and I can	I want to finish school, and I can
Marriage	I want to marry later, and I can	I want to choose who I marry
Pregnancy	I want to have babies later, and I can	I want to have babies once I am married
Health	I want to look after my own health, and I can	I want to be more informed about my health to address problems better
Money	I want to look after my own money, and I can	I want to be 'self-sufficient' (being self-sufficient is a concept that does not easily translate into a singular term in either English or Kinyarwanda. In Kinyarwanda, girls used phrases such as 'kuba wishoboye', referring to a situation in which a person is able to financially support both themselves and any dependents and not be dependent on any external support)
Ambition	I can do what I want with my life	I want to succeed in life

Local knowledge about marriage

Girls' reasons for wanting to get married were focused around the *agaciro* that being married affords a girl. They included having children and the expectation to have children within marriage rather than outside of it; being financially supported through marriage; escaping from unhappiness at home; being emotionally supported and advised; being in love; and gaining the respect of family members and the wider community, connected to dominant sociocultural norms and values that dictate that parents should give daughters away respectfully by arranging their marriage to a suitable man:

> The family will feel proud to give the girl away when she gets married. It's a respectful thing when a girl gets married ... It's a good thing when you invite people to the wedding. At a wedding they say congratulations to the parents because you gave the children away respectfully.
>
> (Woman, Kigali)

The research highlighted a number of barriers faced by girls in terms of their choices about getting married, providing important knowledge for programmes that aim to support girls to meet their marriage expectations. Parents were one barrier because they want girls to marry boys from families of which they approve. This usually means families from the same ethnic group, who are also respectable, and able to financially support their daughter:

> Sometimes our parents want to control us and who we should marry. Parents want boyfriends to have some money. They want to know he can take care of you, especially when you come from a rich family. [When you come from a rich family] you can't marry someone poor.
> (Girl, Kigali, 12–18yrs)

A second barrier is getting pregnant outside marriage, which results in losing *agaciro*. When this happens girls feel they have no choice but to marry the father of their child, and are often forced into doing so by parents rather than burdening the family for support. Girls who are unable to marry the father of their child sometimes try to earn their own money through petty business or prostitution, or have abortions. In addition, they often find their opportunities for getting married to a person of their choice are limited because they have lost *agaciro* due to the stigma associated with having sex outside marriage:

> Girls want to be 'on the market' but if you get pregnant you are off the market …. Once you are not a virgin, you are used, you are scrap. But if you have a baby you are scrap times ten. If you have a baby [out of marriage] the community treats you as a whore. Boys will say 'ah she had a baby with so and so, let me go and help myself'. They treat you like a ball they can bounce around.
> (Girl, rural area, 12–18yrs)

In reality, girls' reasons for getting married often lie in complete contradiction to the programme goal that specified the idea of getting married later. Where girls' reasoning may often be hidden from public conversation, this has important implications for programme success in terms of ensuring girls buy into what organisations are trying to achieve. In particular, the complexities surrounding the concept of *agaciro* and how it is applied in the context of girls' relationships and marital choices are important. For example, empowerment programmes that encourage a link between choice and losing value will alienate girls. In contrast, programmes that encourage and enable girls to 'wait until they are sure' would achieve both programme goals for delayed marriage and girls' own desires for more choice over marriage, while avoiding suggestions that choice equals losing value.

Local knowledge about pregnancy

Programme goals specified increasing the age of girls at first pregnancy as empowering. However, girls' primary concern was to get pregnant after marriage, and they generally interpreted 'early pregnancy' as referring to pregnancy outside marriage rather than pregnancy at a young biological age. Girls in Kigali explained that for the *Abanyamurenge* (a pastoralist ethnic group in the Eastern Democratic Republic of Congo) it was 'okay' for girls to have babies when they were young because girls in this particular ethnic group usually married at an early age. Early pregnancy, as defined by girls themselves, was viewed as problematic:

> If girls and boys are not careful, it brings about pregnancy but it's the girl's responsibility. Boys don't have this – the girls get all the consequences.
> (Girl, rural area, 12–18yrs)

Girls' reasons for wanting to get pregnant within marriage were essentially connected to keeping *agaciro*. A girl who becomes pregnant before marriage loses *agaciro* from family and wider society because she has not adhered to social norms and values. However, this varied according to the different research locations. In rural areas it is considered particularly taboo for a girl to become pregnant outside marriage compared to in the city where it is frowned upon but often accepted as part and parcel of daily life. There was some disagreement over whether it is worse for younger or older girls to get pregnant outside marriage. If a young girl becomes pregnant, girls felt people will either blame the parents or assume she has been raped so she might be relinquished of responsibility for the pregnancy. However, if an older girl becomes pregnant, people will think she 'should have known better', shaming her more for her 'mistake'. Girls who become pregnant are often prevented from socialising with non-pregnant girls because of the bad influence they pose and because they are perceived to be on a 'different level':

> Parents will tell their daughters not to socialise with the girl who got pregnant because they are worried that their daughters will also get pregnant.
> (Girl, provincial town, 12–18yrs)

Despite a strong desire to have babies within marriage, girls often struggle to achieve this for several reasons. Girls experience considerable pressure from friends to have boyfriends and begin sexual relationships. In turn, they are pressured for sex from boyfriends and sugar daddies and feel unable to control these encounters, either in terms of saying 'no' or ensuring that boys use protection. Girls described this as 'being deceived' because they felt obliged to have sex with boyfriends and sugar daddies who gave them gifts and money:

> A sugar daddy can ask for sex and a girl doesn't say no … When you don't say no he can think you are saying yes. When they give you materials and ask for sex, you will not say 'no' or 'yes'. You think he might take back the things.
> (Girl, provincial town, 12–18yrs)

Girls were keen to point out that they want to have sexual relationships, even if this means engaging in sex outside marriage and in spite of the risks of getting pregnant:

> Girls and boys talk about sex when they are in relationships. They talk about it and they do it. It's all about sex. You can start meeting in lodges. You will be doing that thing always – that's what it's all about.
>
> (Girl, Kigali, 12–18yrs)

Parents can be instrumental in encouraging girls to have relationships with boyfriends and sugar daddies in an attempt to secure financial support, which leads to girls becoming pregnant outside marriage:

> Sometimes, when parents don't have the means, they allow girls to get a sugar daddy because he will also support the family. Sugar daddies and boyfriends are encouraged by some parents because they bring money into the home.
>
> (Girl, provincial town, 12–18yrs)

Girls often defended sugar daddies, and described deliberately seeking their company to fulfil needs for money, material items and sex. Their defence was that while such behaviour means they lose *agaciro* from wider society, money obtained through relationships with sugar daddies can be used for school fees and to support parents, thus increasing a girl's *agaciro* in other ways, by fulfilling expectations to get an education and support family.

Being fertile gives a girl *agaciro* because she is able to fulfil sociocultural expectations around giving birth and raising a family. Consequently, girls feel pressurised by boyfriends to prove they are fertile, or feel that, by demonstrating this, boyfriends will be encouraged to marry them:

> Some girls love to get pregnant before marriage. It's proof that the girl is not barren.
>
> (Woman, Kigali)

Consequently, despite a strong desire to get pregnant within marriage, girls often struggle to achieve this.

The concept of *agaciro* is an important lens for understanding the impact pregnancy outside marriage has on a girl's life, especially in terms of her opportunities for marriage and getting an education. Pregnancy outside marriage can also be responsible for creating stigma between girls that put them on 'different levels', creating challenges to empowerment programming that aims to be inclusive of all girls.

Empowerment programmes will benefit from working with the concept of *agaciro* while recognising the tensions that exist in girls' daily realities. For example, programmes might emphasise the *agaciro* a girl gains from having babies within marriage while recognising the necessary role risky sexual relationships play in enabling girls to get things they need. Cultural and social pressures on girls to prove their fertility pose challenges for empowerment programmes that aim to delay pregnancy, in terms of not exacerbating assumptions that girls who do not marry or produce children early are more likely to be infertile.

Conclusion

This chapter has highlighted the problems with current styles of evidence-based programming, and the role that generating local knowledge can play in making programmes more sensitive to people's own values and sociocultural realities. It shows how local perspectives about what are potentially empowering courses of action in the context of marriage and pregnancy with girls in Rwanda can subtly, but significantly, contrast with the goals and approaches of empowerment programmes. Without an understanding of the concept of *agaciro* and how it is articulated in empowerment themes of marriage and pregnancy, programmes are unlikely to be meaningful to girls themselves. They might also promote messages that inadvertently lead to experiences of disempowerment.

The concept of *agaciro* and understanding about how it manifests in different aspects of girls' lives can, therefore, be used to enhance empowerment programming so that it is grounded in the cultural logic of girls in Rwanda and aligns with their frame of reference for living their lives. An understanding of the role *agaciro* plays in girls' lives, the complex ways in which they want and can act to gain *agaciro*, and the practical realities that cause them to lose *agaciro* are important for evidence-based programming. This would result in locally situated programme designs that have greater potential for impact and more appropriate measures of success based on the perspectives of beneficiaries themselves. By contrast, if programme goals and designs are externally driven and determined, they can contrast so much with young people's own realities that they will never succeed.

References

Bell, S.A. and Aggleton P. (2012) 'Integrating ethnographic principles in NGO monitoring and impact evaluation', *Journal of International Development*, 24: 795–807.

Carbaugh, D. (2007) 'Cultural discourse analysis: communication practices and intercultural encounters', *Journal of Intercultural Communication Research*, 36: 167–182.

Cook, I. (1997) 'Participant observation', in R. Flowerdew and D. Martin (eds) *Methods in Human Geography: A guide for students doing a research project*, Harlow: Longman, pp. 127–149.

De Boeck, F. and Honwana, A. (2005) *Makers and Breakers: Children and youth in postcolonial Africa*, Oxford: James Currey.

Dorr-Bremme, D.W. (1985) 'Ethnographic evaluation: a theory and method', *Educational Evaluation and Policy Analysis*, 7(1): 65–83.

Edmonds, R.E.D. and Cook, M.R. (2014) 'Starting a Conversation: the need for and application of Service Design in International Development' Conference proceedings, ServDes 2014, Lancaster. Available at: www.servdes.org/conference-2014-lancaster (accessed 16 March 2015).

Geertz, C. (1983) *Local Knowledge: Further essays in interpretive anthropology*, New York: Basic Books.

Hammersley, M. and Atkinson, P. (2007) *Ethnography: Principles in practice*, Abingdon: Routledge.

Herbert, S. (2000) 'For ethnography', *Progress in Human Geography*, 24(4): 550–568.

Johnson, V., Hart, R. and Colwell, J. (2014) *Steps to Engaging Children in Research*, Brighton: University of Brighton. Available at: www.bernardvanleer.org/steps-to-engaging-young-children-in-research (accessed 16 March 2015).

Kees van Donge, J. (2006) 'Ethnography and participant observation', in V. Desai and R.B. Potter (eds) *Doing Development Research*, London: SAGE, pp. 180–188.

Leighter, J.L., Rudnick, L. and Edmonds, T.J. (2013) 'How the ethnography of communication provides resources for design', *Journal of Applied Communication Research*, 41(2): 181–187.

McLean Hilker, L. (2014) 'Navigating adolescence and young adulthood in Rwanda during and after genocide: intersections of ethnicity, gender and age', *Children's Geographies*, 12(3): 354–368.

Miller, D. and Rudnick, L. (2010) 'The case for situated theory on modern peacebuilding practice', *Journal of Peacebuilding & Development*, 5(2): 62–74.

Miller, D. and Rudnick, L. (2011) 'Trying it on for size: design and international public policy', *Design Issues*, 27(2): 6–16.

Miller, D. and Rudnick, L. (2012) *A Framework Document for Evidence-Based Programme Design on Reintegration*. Available at: www.unidir.org/files/publications/pdfs/a-framework-document-for-evidence-based-programme-design-on-reintegration-396.pdf (accessed 16 March 2015).

Miller, D. B. and Rudnick, L. (2014) *A Prototype for Evidence based Programme Design for Reintegration*. Available at: www.unidir.org/files/publications/pdfs/a-prototype-for-evidence-based-programme-design-for-reintegration-en-610.pdf (accessed 16 March 2015).

Miller, D., Rudnick, L., and Kimball, L. (2010) 'Designing programmes in contexts of peace and security', *SEE Bulletin*, 4: 3–7.

Mosse, P. (2001) '"People's knowledge", participation and patronage: operations and representations in rural development', in B. Cook and U. Kothari (eds) *Participation: The new tyranny?* London: Zed Press, pp. 16–35.

Payne, R.E.D. (2012) 'Extraordinary survivors or ordinary lives? Embracing "everyday agency" in social interventions with child-headed households in Zambia', *Children's Geographies*, 10(4): 399–411.

Price, N. and Hawkins, K. (2002) 'Researching sex and reproductive behaviour: a peer ethnographic approach', *Social Science & Medicine*, 55: 1325–1336.

Rice, P., and Ezzy, D. (1999) *Qualitative Research Methods: A health focus*, Melbourne: Oxford University Press.

Schutz, A. (1967) *The Phenomenology of the Social World*, Evanston, IL: North Western University Press.

Wolcott, H.F. (1999) *Ethnography as a Way of Seeing*, London: SAGE.

7

Interpretation, context and time

An ethnographically inspired approach to strategy development for tuberculosis control in Odisha, India

Jens Seeberg and Tushar Kanti Ray

Introduction

'Bausenpali'[1] is situated more than one hour's drive from the nearest primary healthcare centre on a small metal road. When we arrive, it takes around 20 minutes for people to gather to talk with us in the central square of the village. They tell us that there are 73 households in the village. Two or three households are from the robe makers' caste, two or three are blacksmiths, two or three are *Dalit*, occupying the lowest position in the caste system, but most households belong to the *Khonda* scheduled tribe. Asked about their daily life, the villagers tell us that they go to the forest in the early morning at 5–6am and return around 9am due to the heat. The people in the house nearest to the meeting place are not present. They have some land where they grow turmeric, and they also have a place there to stay. Turmeric is a major crop here. They also collect *bidi* [local cigarettes] leaves from the *saal* tree [*shorea robusta*], and leaves used to make cups and plates that are sold to the restaurants in Nuagaon [nearest town]. From the *saal* tree, they also get seeds that are used to produce oil to the shops in the town market. All families are involved in this. In a good year the yield will ensure survival for three months, but this year is not good. There is no water now, so they cannot grow anything in the fields. They cannot do much about the problem. It's too dry. There is seasonal variation of income. In summer they can only sell those leaves, and in the rainy season they cultivate rice, maize, pulses, turmeric and oil seeds, and they sell this in the winter season and keep some of it.

(Fieldnotes, Bausenpali village, Kandhamal District, Odisha, India)

The evaluation team of four 'experts' arrived after a long drive between villages and small towns in mountainous parts of Gajapati and Kandhamal districts in the Indian state of Odisha. The objective was to generate primary data that would feed into the development of a strategy for enhancing tuberculosis (TB) diagnostic and treatment services in difficult-to-reach areas of the state. At the time of independence, the fathers of the Indian constitution had developed the concepts of 'scheduled castes' and 'scheduled tribes' to refer to some of the poorest and most marginalised groups in a caste-based Indian society. Despite the measures designed to uplift such groups into the mainstream of society through reservation policies in the educational and political systems, many remained living in villages like this. Because of this, the political framing of ethnicity, caste and class forms part of the context that we deem necessary to understand how access to health services may fail or succeed in any Indian state.

An interpretive approach is valuable in any endeavour that seeks to elicit local perceptions and knowledge, since the processes by which we describe peoples and events, and how we analyse meanings, are necessarily interpretive. By 'local' we indicate that there is some kind of nexus between place, people and social practice (Leach 2006) that can be defined as a 'field' of inquiry, or as a site for fieldwork. Our visit to Bausenpali village was one of several activities designed to develop a Tribal Action Strategy for the state of Odisha in order to increase access to TB diagnostic and treatment services, improve public awareness of TB and improve health seeking behaviour among tribal communities. In this chapter, we focus in on the notion of context as a core element of an interpretive approach to evaluation and public health strategy development.

TB control in 'tribal districts' in India

When the World Health Organisation (WHO) developed the Directly Observed Treatment, Short-course (DOTS) strategy for TB control in the 1990s, India contained approximately 40 per cent of the world's notified TB cases (WHO Tuberculosis Programme 1993). DOTS was in many ways a complex health intervention (Gericke et al. 2005), requiring simultaneous actions at different levels of the health system. The aim of DOTS was to achieve a minimum case detection rate of 70 per cent of all actual cases, and a minimum cure rate of 85 per cent. Patients were given a combination therapy with four different types of antibiotics during an intensive phase of two months, followed by a continuation phase of an additional four months. For treatment to be directly observed, it required the patient to be put in contact with a so-called DOT provider, with the patient visiting this provider three times a week (during intermittent treatment) and taking the medicine in front of the provider.

In India, the DOTS strategy was implemented by the Revised National Tuberculosis Control Programme. In addition to a locally available DOT Provider, DOTS required patient visits to a diagnostic centre. This involved the detailed monitoring of each individual patient, and the transmission of patient data from village level through a communication chain resulting in aggregate data at the national level. However, this complex programme was implemented through the existing health system and, because of this, the programme proved more difficult to implement in contexts where there was poor infrastructure, a large distance between healthcare delivery points, and locally competing systems of belief about health and the determinants of illness. As illustrated in our field notes, such configurations are typical of the so-called tribal districts:

The *Anganwadi* worker [local health worker with special focus on child health and related issues] in the village gives medicine for malaria and if it's serious they'll go to the hospital. Apart from malaria she can also treat diarrhoea. If some patients don't feel better she sends them to Nuagaon Primary Health Centre [PHC]. They have to walk or go by bicycle. It's 12km. It takes two and a half hours to walk. … Nobody has been to the hospital recently. *(Here, the* Panchayat *[village council] Secretary explains the situation on behalf of his village.)* The villagers believe in witchcraft and the work of the gunia [shaman]. *(The* Panchayat *Secretary is dressed in trousers and shirt, unlike all the others who wear* lungi *[loincloth].)* There are two types of healers. One is *boidya* who gives herbal medicine. Another is *gunia*, who provides ritual services. … Only after the disease gets serious they [the villagers] go to the *gunia*. After rituals, if they are cured, fine, if not they go to *boidya*. The *boidya* sometimes refers to the hospital and says he's unable to handle the case. For other diseases he provides medicines. He provides only roots and herbs and explains how to use them. The cost for the *gunia*, when he enters the village, is one bottle of alcohol, costing INR 20 [GBP0.25]. Then the *gunia* checks the patient physically. They say it is evil spirits or somebody has put something on the body. … For cough they go directly to hospital if there is blood in the sputum. They say it means TB. Two people are currently taking medicine for TB *(they are not present)*. The villagers don't know the duration of the treatment, except for the panchayat secretary who says six months. He has learned this from seeing one of the patient's treatment cards at the PHC. If they discontinue treatment, it's increased to eight months. Till now, that patient has not completed the course. He felt well after three months. Also, his wife told him to discontinue. He took his medicines for one month, two months, like that. They do not know that the medicine is free. They will ask the patient's wife, then they will know. They do not suffer from TB. That is why they do not know whether the treatment is free.

(Field notes, Bausenpali village, Kandhamal District, Odisha, India)

The challenges of geographical distance to the nearest health hospital and the coexistence of competing medical systems are clearly present in the above account. The field notes paint a picture of a rural Indian village setting in which the workings of medical pluralism involved a number of local specialists who were consulted on the basis of suspected causes of disease. Most health problems were managed (though not always successfully) through a network that included ritual specialists, entrepreneurs and volunteers, whose training depended on access to educational activities offered by public health programmes with specific focus areas such as mother and child health, malaria control or TB control. The same excerpt illustrates that TB was most usually diagnosed (if at all) at a late stage when haemoptysis occurred, and that even the most basic government healthcare facilities were only accessed when the disease was considered very serious. There was no general understanding that TB diagnosis and treatment should be available free of charge, even though this had long been a key message in health communication regarding TB in the state. It also seems that at least one patient was taking medicine irregularly, and likely without knowing the associated risk of drug resistance, although we could not confirm this.

The Tribal Action Plan

To address the needs of 'tribal'[2] communities for TB detection and treatment, the Government of India developed a Tribal Action Plan (Central TB Division 2005). This plan was a requirement defined by the World Bank as one of a number of conditions in relation to its financial support for the second phase of the DOTS programme in India. The Tribal Action Plan was based on limited secondary research and consisted of a long list of bullet points that were not explicitly related to one another. Hence, there was a need for a strategy for implementation in states such as Odisha with a large Scheduled Tribe population.

The Tribal Action Plan constituted a point of departure for the development of this strategy. However, the document was somewhat generic, and offered an insufficient knowledge base on which to build the strategy. Instead, we had to treat the Tribal Action Plan as secondary data in need of analysis rather than as a given. We undertook a thematic content analysis of the Tribal Action Plan to try to make sense of, and organise, the various problems, challenges and proposed solutions within it. The core problem identified by the plan was the inadequate utilisation of Revised National TB Control Programme services in tribal areas. Four areas pointed to challenges contributing to this overarching problem, including a weak primary healthcare infrastructure (distant location of services, poor access to services, inappropriate clinic timings, diagnostic facilities not available, information education and communication activities not undertaken, lack of integration of TB services within health system); inadequately supported health providers (e.g. lack of supervision and monitoring, vacant posts, communication and cultural barriers); and challenges associated with local communities (lack of local confidence in the health system, little or no community participation, traditional healers working in parallel). Grouping the specific challenges raised in the Tribal Action Plan in this way provided an initial indication of the scope of the research, and the design of potential interventions. The plan also provided a list of suggestions for interventions intended to improve the situation, including, for example, a tribal area allowance for supervisors, monetary incentives for patients, community engagement, training of staff and filling of vacant posts. However, it was not clear which interventions were supposed to address which issues.

Our analysis pointed to two issues that were of strategic importance yet unclear. First, many of the identified problems and proposed interventions were not specific either to tribal populations (as opposed to other marginalised groups) or to TB services (as opposed to healthcare services in general). They were general in nature and reflected the fact that the TB control programme would only function well if the general health services functioned well. Therefore, certain interventions that would be important for TB control needed to address general barriers to marginalised people's access to the health system. Second, in spite of its status as a national strategy document, and despite significant variation across different states of India, the Tribal Action Plan did not contain any efforts to prioritise problems and interventions.

To establish a basis for development of a draft strategy, we had to redefine the task at hand. The Tribal Action Plan was a policy document that was supposed to provide a rationale for the strategy. But our analysis of the plan demonstrated a need to test the problems identified in it against local realities in Odisha, to identify additional problems that had not been included in the Tribal Action Plan but were important in Odisha, and to prioritise among problems and interventions. This called for a more grounded approach based on rapid ethnographic research, paying attention to the important issue of understanding context. The analysis of the Tribal Action Plan had also transformed the context of this work, since the assumptions that were built into the plan were no longer treated as a given but were themselves potentially open to challenge as a possible outcome of the empirical study.

An ethnographic approach to developing a tuberculosis control strategy

Ethnography is commonly associated with anthropology where it often constitutes the primary approach to creation of data. In its classical form, ethnography implies that an ethnographer lives in the community under study for a prolonged period of time, engages with interlocutors and participates in daily chores and activities. Data is created through participant observation and interviews that may range from informal conversation to structured questioning. Field notes are developed to capture observations, based on the insight that there is no simple relationship between what people say they do and what they actually do (Bernard 1994). Qualitative techniques are often supplemented with other research methods, such as surveys, mapping and use of local secondary data sources (such as newspaper photos, and in our case, the Tribal Action Plan), and the analysis and interpretation of such materials transforms them into ethnographic data (LeCompte and Schensul 1999).

While the ethnographer will, inevitably, have preconceived ideas and assumptions about the field prior to fieldwork, it is a virtue of good ethnography to be able to bracket these and focus on the perspectives that emerge in the field and from the interlocutors (Bernard 1994). The relevance of ethnographic analysis rests on its alignment with what is important in the lives of people inhabiting the field under study. This does not necessarily mean that the ethnographer has to agree with the views of the interlocutors (Farmer 1992). A good ethnographer should be able to represent these topics of importance in such a way that it becomes possible to understand how they are perceived and practised locally, and how such perceptions and practices are embedded in the local political economy as well as in broader social and cultural contexts (cf. Scheper-Hughes 1992).

Ethnography does not only involve the application of ethnographic tools, even if these form an important part of the ethnographer's research practice (LeCompte and Schensul 1999). Ethnography is also an analytical activity that strives towards a situation in which little is taken for granted. The ethnographer has to be open to the constant challenges that ongoing dialogue and interaction with interlocutors pose for the assumptions that are brought to the field in the form of research protocols, terms of reference and interview guides, and that may result in changing assumptions and the development of new questions (Agar 1986). This analytical activity is frequently embedded in a theoretical understanding of concepts such as context, interpretation, reflexivity and positionality.

We distinguish three interconnected levels in ethnographic methodology: methods, analysis and theory. The term 'methods' refers to the toolbox of data collection techniques mentioned already. Analysis refers to the ongoing interpretive practice that takes place before, during and after fieldwork. Examples include instances when, during an interview, the interlocutor provides information that needs to be analysed immediately in order to frame the next question. Analysis also refers to the interpretive practices of coding the data (i.e. identifying themes and topics that are discussed by interlocutors). The development of such codes depends on the analytical framework and the interpretive process. For example, narrative analysis might emphasise details within a person's life story, whereas comparative analysis might examine similarities and differences between different settings. Finally, the analytic framework is based on theory. Theory refers the position of the research vis-à-vis the larger body of anthropological (or other) theory and knowledge that is relevant to the research problem. Theory also requires that assumptions are made explicit regarding the scientific status of the data that emerge during fieldwork and it frames how findings and interpretations may (or may not) be generalised.

In this chapter, we focus primarily on the analytical level, especially in relation to the framing of context. Context is not easily defined since it is potentially limitless (Dilley 1999). Context can be understood as 'that which environs the object of interest and helps by its relevance to explain it' and being 'temporal, geographical, cultural, cognitive, emotional – or any sort at all' (Scharfstein 1991: 1). Relevance is the key word here. In our case, relevance is defined by the problem of access to TB services for people defined as tribal in the state of Odisha.

Time is important in any qualitative study, and ethnographic fieldwork is arguably one of the most time-consuming and labour-intensive form of data collection in the social sciences. For this reason, but also because of its resistance to premature analytical closure, ethnography is not always considered as a suitable approach to evaluation. Evaluations often share two characteristics that are antithetical to more traditional forms of ethnography. The first is time: those who need an evaluation may want results quickly, which may pose challenges for high quality research. The second is the confusion between methodology and methods. Ignoring the value of a clearly defined analytical framework, approaches are often reduced to qualitative and quantitative methods, or mixed methods if both are used. Findings may derive from results from questionnaires and/or qualitative interviewing with little or no triangulation. Instead of interpretive analysis, a descriptive summary of interviewees' statements may be provided. An industry has developed around the use of this standard approach; if the evaluation questions are sufficiently simple – as opposed to complex and context-dependent – this, it is claimed, can produce useful results. In more complex circumstances, such as developing a strategy for TB diagnosis and treatment for indigenous peoples in rural areas, the issues under study are highly context-dependent, suggesting the need for a more ethnographically informed approach.

Methods

Due to the short period of time that was allocated for fieldwork within the available budget, purposive sampling (Atkinson and Pugsley 2005) was used to select two districts with large Scheduled Tribe populations, namely Gajapati and Kandamal districts in Odisha. Neighbouring districts were chosen to save travel time. In each district, two blocks (sub-district administrative units) were selected. In each block, a health institution was selected in an area considered geographically inaccessible. In each, the Medical Officer in-charge (if present) and other staff were interviewed about the functioning of the TB control programme in general and TB services to tribal people in particular, using an open-ended interview guide. A total of six villages from within the catchment area of the health institutions and with TB patients registered at the clinic were selected. Care was taken to ensure that remote villages with poor road infrastructure were included. Upon arrival in the village, a group discussion was conducted with all available villagers. Ten to 30 villagers participated in each group discussion. No effort was made to select specific subgroups within villages from the outset, since this initial meeting was intended to provide an overview of the social landscape and health problems as perceived by the villagers. After an initial open group discussion, smaller and more focused group discussions were undertaken with woman's groups and families with TB patients. Observation of service provider practices at the health institutions was also undertaken, and additional interviews were conducted with health volunteers, individual patients and one private practitioner who practised western biomedicine without any formal qualifications.

Time, team and the importance of context

In addition to five days for literature review and report writing for the first author, five days had been dedicated for fieldwork in Odisha. This was a rather modest investment of time and resources. At a general level, this reflects a tension between contractors' interests in getting a job done at the smallest possible cost versus the time needed for high quality output. This tension often translates into necessary compromises in choice of methods, giving preference to rapid appraisal tools and descriptive (rather than interpretive) analysis, with less emphasis given to context. As illustrated by Ferguson in his classical critique of de-politicised development, the consultant may not be expected to know anything about context and yet be supposed to provide solutions to local problems:

> What, I asked, did this consultant know about Zimbabwe's agriculture that they, the local agricultural officers, did not? To my surprise, I was told that the individual in question knew virtually nothing about Zimbabwe, and worked mostly in India. "But," I was assured, "he *knows development.*" It is precisely this expertise, free-floating and untied to any specific context, that is so easily generalised, and so easily inserted into any given situation.
> (Ferguson 1994: 258–259)

Ferguson (1994) suggests that such an approach is part of a global development industry, and for people who have been involved in development projects it is surely a recognisable phenomenon, irrespective of the value and quality of the contribution of 'global' expert consultants. The global consultant may compare the situation in one country with that in another country, and use this comparison as a context across societies. This implies that emphasis is placed on those phenomena that can be compared across different scenarios. In our case, the team of four people (including the authors) all had substantial work experience on access to TB services among Scheduled Tribes and Castes in Odisha. Hence, we had the advantage of being able to compare what we found during this mission with other work that we had either been directly involved in or had intimate knowledge about within the context of TB control in the state. We felt that building the team around such knowledge was a precondition for a meaningful work process, given the tight time frame of the project. Importantly, none of us currently worked in the TB control programme in Odisha, and we had no direct stakes in the outcome of the study. We felt we were equipped to identify relevant questions without being biased towards politically 'desirable' results, and we were not expecting to be involved in the implementation of the resulting strategy, should it be accepted.

Tension between pressure of time and the importance of context is common in policy-related consultancies. Put differently, the composition of the team should consider time available to work with contextual matters during a project versus the experience brought into a project by team members who have previously worked on core issues in the same context. Our team consisted of one former health systems research advisor, one former project advisor, and two former health communication officers, all of whom had worked on the Danida-funded 'Danish assistance to the Revised National Tuberculosis Control Programme in India' project in Odisha until it was closed down at the end of 2005.

Clearly, one could point to both pros and cons of a team with prior insider knowledge of the programme and each other. Disadvantages might include cultural blindness (Lykkeslet and Gjengedal 2007), whereby researchers take too much for granted rather than creating the necessary analytical distance during and after data collection. Another potential disadvantage could include having been involved in shaping the programme that was under review. Such issues are important and should be considered seriously, and prior identification and discussion of key assumptions that are broad to the field (e.g. normative views about how TB control ought to work, or stereotypes about Scheduled Tribes) can help in addressing these.

However, in this particular case, we felt that the advantages outweighed the disadvantages. We had knowledge about the distribution and variation of Scheduled Tribes and Castes in the districts that we selected for the study. We felt that purposeful sampling of districts and health institutions with focus on those placed in 'inaccessible' areas was more appropriate than random sampling, and we were able to perform this selection ourselves, thereby eliminating any risk that better health institutions were selected for us. Villages were only selected when we reached the health institution responsible for treatment, since we wanted to ensure that TB patients under treatment lived in the villages we visited. More important than sampling issues, we were able to draw on contextual knowledge about health politics and policies in Odisha, the social dynamics that regulate the lives of people classified as Scheduled Tribes and Castes, earlier interventions that had been undertaken to achieve what the Tribal Action Plan tried to accomplish, and our understanding of the somewhat marginal position of this plan in relation to the mainstream plans of the TB control programme in India. Important contextual knowledge also included the healthcare reform named the National Rural Health Mission that had been implemented in India prior to our field visit. It was important to see the extent to which this reform – with its emphasis on free medicines and strengthening of peripheral health services – had reached these remote areas, and if so, how it interacted with the Revised National TB Control Programme.

From tribal action plan to empirically grounded strategy

Interpretation as an analytical practice is, by definition, the process of developing meaning in context (Wilden 1972). Context may be delineated at many levels. One approach to defining levels is by scale, ranging from a local micro-level to a global systems level (Baer *et al.* 2003). Above we have considered context at meso-level, understood as larger patterns of social life (e.g. the marginal existence in Odisha of most people defined as Scheduled Tribes) and of policies at state and national levels (e.g. the governance structures embedded in the Revised National TB Control Programme). Interpretation must also be grounded in the daily local social and political realities of the people whose input is requested. Analytical development of a contextual understanding at the micro-level of social interaction among villagers and in clinical settings was also part of the research, since many of the problems that the strategy was expected to address played out at this level. Every evening, interviews and observation notes from that day were transcribed and coded, and the analysis informed the following day's data collection. Coding implied the identification of themes that appeared in the interviews and field notes and that were important to the interlocutors. If a theme was new to us, it would be added to the list of issues that we would take up during subsequent data collection.

Using the second extract from field notes presented above as an example, an on-the-spot analysis pointed us to some expected issues that had been identified in the Tribal Action Plan. These included problems related to distance to primary health services ("It takes them two and a half hours to walk"), and access to relevant information (only the *Panchayat* Secretary had information about TB, and only rudimentary), including when to react to early symptoms (postponing a visit to the Primary Health Centre till haemoptysis occurs). But we also made observations of new issues. One such example involved the behaviour of the *Panchayat* Secretary. His eagerness to speak for the group could be seen as asserting his status as the village leader. But it could also indicate that his language skills in the official state language of Odisha, *Oriya*, were superior to those of the villagers. As we later discovered, his enthusiasm resulted from a combination of the two. However, when directly exploring the issue in smaller groups and individually, we found that among middle-aged and elderly, and very frequently among women, people only spoke their native language. In the case of the *Khunda* inhabitants of Bausenpali, their language was *Kuvi*. Yet, healthcare programmes and clinical interaction were carried out in Odisha based on the assumption that everybody speaks *Oriya*. In some cases the doctor would speak *Oriya* without discovering that the patient did not understand the language. This observation was confirmed in other villages. One health worker, who was able to speak the local *Adivasi* language, said that she did not use that language for health information because, in her experience, when her performance was assessed, the person doing so would only be able to communicate in *Oriya*. Assessment would only check whether the target community was able to reproduce her standard messages in *Oriya*. To protect herself from poor outcomes in performance assessments, she used *Oriya* for communication even if many did not understand it, as long as they could reproduce the slogans.

Another example of exploratory analysis during data collection that was visible in the above field notes was the uncertainty about payment. At face value, not knowing whether TB treatment is free can be seen as an indication of lack of information, especially in connection with the language problem. Above, we saw that direct treatment costs for local healers were comparatively small, even if any monetary cost can be insurmountable in a very poor community. But we were also told that one man had visited the hospital last year:

> He had joint pain in knees and hands. First he went to the *gunia*. He spent INR40–50 [GBP0.5–0.6]. Then *gunia* referred him to hospital. If he had been cured, he would not have gone (*an agitated discussion evolves about the role of the* gunia *versus the 'modern' hospital, lead by* Panchayat Secretary). At the hospital, the doctor saw his convulsions and gave him medicines and injections. He did not understand what the doctor explained. The doctor told

him that he had to go and buy drugs in the market. The cost was INR800 [GBP10]. He is happy that he was cured.
> (Fieldnotes, Bausenpali village, Kandhamal District, Odisha, India)

We know very little about this particular patient's actual diagnosis or treatment, but we understand that the cost of treatment was very high for village standards and that, for this reason, it is important and fortunate for the patient that the treatment was effective. We pursued the question of costs of treatment irrespective of diagnosis, both when talking to villagers and health staff and when observing prescription practices in the clinics and hospitals that we visited.

As mentioned above, the National Rural Health Mission had led to an increase in availability of free drugs for a wide range of conditions at the primary health centres. Such drugs were widely dispensed, and in no cases did we find that money was charged for them. Yet, invariably patients had to pay out-of-pocket for free treatment provided at the government health institutions. This paradox arose because doctors in all the cases we observed added drugs to the prescription that were not available within the range of free drugs provided. Therefore, the patient had to go to one of the local chemists that thrived in the immediate neighbourhood of the hospital and buy these additional drugs. Often, the medical officer, when asked directly, found it difficult to justify the use of such medicines medically; instead it was suggested that patients wanted such drugs, including syrup versions of drugs available at the hospital, in tablet form. In all cases, the patient was instructed to return from the chemist and show the purchased drugs.

Local chemists informed us of daily aggregate sales around INR 2–3,000 (GBP25–38), largely based on such prescriptions. All medical officers were observed to use prescription pads from a local chemist. In addition, medical officers in remote villages were being targeted by the pharmaceutical industry. Posters, stickers, calendars and gift items were visible at the primary health centres. When asked, one medical officer estimated that patients were provided with 60 per cent of their drugs from the free government stock and had to buy 40 per cent from the chemist. It was striking that while medical officers recognised that abject poverty was the main cause of patients' health problems, at the same time they did nothing to minimise their treatment costs but seemingly created unnecessary expenses for treatment.

We found no evidence during the study that doctors benefited financially from informal agreements with chemists. However, the extent of these prescription practices was a cause for concern. Irrespective of the nature of the health problem, the patients learned that treatment at the government hospital was not free. They had to pay, even if the point of payment was located outside the hospital. This had an overall negative impact on the image of government facilities among the communities and also influenced perceptions of the TB control programme. Villagers may find it difficult to believe that TB treatment under the Revised National TB Control Programme was free when their general experience was that it was rarely, if ever, free of cost to visit the hospital. We believe that this is why, when directly asked, villagers did not know whether TB drugs were available for free. We observed that this question could only be clarified by TB patients who had actually received treatment. The answer had to be embedded in lived experience on a case-by-case basis. These two examples illustrate how on-going analysis of the data is central to an ethnographically informed approach that can open up subsequent exploration of unforeseen questions.

Designing the local TB control strategy

While the Tribal Action Plan had a tendency to focus more on perceived tribal issues, overall we found that a much stronger focus on health service providers and infrastructure was required to deliver the Tribal Action Plan in practice. Our analysis suggested a focus on the issues presented in Figure 7.1. Hence, the analysis pointed to a need to expand the attention from the four areas described in the Tribal Action Plan as related to healthcare providers (Figure 7.1) to a new set of focus areas.

This led the development of a Tribal Action Strategy in two directions. First was the identification of local preconditions for the Revised National TB

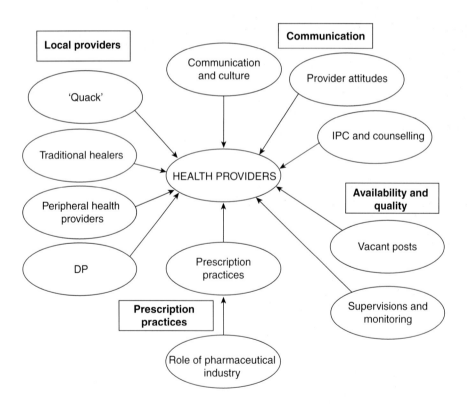

Figure 7.1 Issues related to health providers

Control Programme to function. This included a healthcare system that needed further strengthening, and a better understanding of the target tribal populations. The plural form is important here, given substantial ethnic and language variation among peoples classified as Scheduled Tribes. Second, as presented in Figure 7.2, a number of specific problems could be grouped under three main areas – transport, cost and communication. Together, these provided a higher-level framework to think about the kinds of change required, and point to the need for policy-level collaboration across government departments to ensure that access to services for marginalised population groups is effectively addressed.

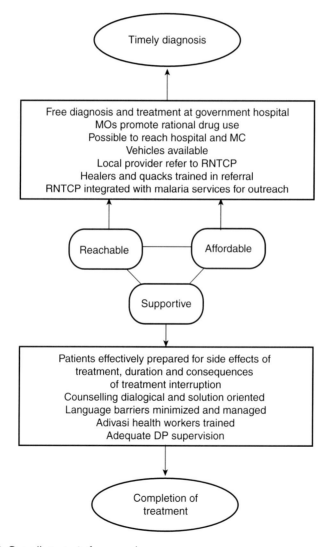

Figure 7.2 Overall strategic framework

Figure 7.2 illustrates the centrality of these three areas in relation to the diagnostic process (i.e. barriers leading to diagnosis) and the treatment process (i.e. barriers leading to interruption of treatment schedules).

Conclusion

In this chapter, we have discussed the development of a strategy for implementation of TB services in 'inaccessible' areas of the state of Odisha in India. We have suggested that while limited time may often preclude standard forms of ethnography as an evaluation approach, as was certainly the case here, ethnography may inspire the analytic strategy used during fieldwork. In the case described here, the deconstruction and contextual analysis of the Tribal Action Plan allowed us to pursue questions in the field that were important to attaining the objectives of this plan, yet invisible in its understanding of the issues. This allowed us to move beyond some of the implicit assumptions in the plan about Scheduled Tribes and about TB services as seen in isolation from the larger system, and include living conditions of the target group as well as impediments and shortcomings of the healthcare system that was supposed to serve them.

An understanding of context can be developed during fieldwork through an iterative research process (Spradley 1980) that opens up new questions to be included in the continued data collection. Time constraints may sometimes inhibit the possibility of taking an ethnographically informed approach. However, this may, to some extent, be countered by the inclusion of team members with prior context-specific knowledge that is grounded in long-term engagement with the communities and society in question.

Grounding the development of a strategy for the implementation of TB services in tribal districts of Odisha made it clear that the social and political marginalisation of this target group could neither be ignored nor satisfactorily addressed within the limited scope of the Revised National TB Control Programme. The political will to more whole-heartedly address the underlying reasons for social exclusion of villagers like those we visited has historically been limited. The resulting draft strategy was well received by the International Union Against Tuberculosis and Lung Disease, who commissioned the consultancy, and by the Government of Odisha. Hopefully, steps will be taken in the future to address the social exclusion that Scheduled Tribes of Odisha face in their daily lives, of which their relative lack of access to TB treatment is but a symptom.

Notes

1 The name of the village and all other names that could be used to identify specific persons have been altered.
2 While we are concerned with the use of the label 'tribal' due to its problematic ideological and historical content, it is retained as an important administrative category in India. As such, we use the term throughout this chapter.

References

Agar, M.H. (1986) *Speaking of Ethnography*, Newbury Park, CA: SAGE.
Atkinson, P. and Pugsley, L. (2005) 'Making sense of ethnography and medical education', *Medical Education*, 39: 228–234.
Baer, H.A., Singer, M. and Susser, I. (2003) *Medical Anthropology and the World System*, Westport, CT: Praeger Publishers.
Bernard, H.R. (1994) *Research Methods in Anthropology*, London: SAGE.
Central TB Division (2005) *Tribal Action Plan for RNTCP II*, India: Government of India.
Dilley, R. (1999) *The Problem of Context*, New York: Berghahn Books.
Farmer, P. (1992) 'New disorder old dilemmas: AIDS and anthropology in Haiti', in G. Herdt and S. Lindenbaum (eds) *The Time of AIDS: Social analysis, theory, and method*, Newbury Park, CA: SAGE, pp. 287–318.
Ferguson, J. (1994) *The Anti-Politics Machine: "Development," depoliticization and bureaucratic power in Lesotho*, Minneapolis, MN: University of Minnesota Press.
Gericke, C.A., Kurowski, C., Ranson, M.K. and Mills, A. (2005) 'Intervention complexity: a conceptual framework to inform priority-setting in health', *Bulletin of the World Health Organization*, 83: 285–293.
Leach, J. (2006) 'Out of proportion? Anthropological description of power, regeneration and scale on the Rai Coast of Papua New Guinea', in S. Coleman and P. Collins (eds) *Locating the Field: Space, place and context in anthropology*, Oxford: Berg, pp. 149–162.
Lecompte, M.D. and Schensul, J.J. (1999) *Analyzing and Interpreting Ethnographic Data*, Walnut Creek, CA: AltaMira Press.
Lykkeslet, E. and Gjengedal, E. (2007) 'Methodological problems associated with practice-close research', *Qualitative Health Research*, 17: 699–704.
Scharfstein, B.A. (1991) *The Dilemma of Context*, New York: New York University Press.
Scheper-Hughes, N. (1992) *Death without Weeping: The violence of everyday life in Brazil*, Berkeley, CA: University of California Press.
Spradley, J. (1980) *Participant Observation*, New York: Holt, Reinhart & Winston.
WHO Tuberculosis Programme (1993) *Tuberculosis Notification Update*, Geneva: WHO.
Wilden, A. (1972) *System and Structure*, London: Tavistock Publications.

8
Designing health and leadership programmes for vulnerable young women using participatory ethnographic research in Freetown, Sierra Leone

Naana Otoo-Oyortey, Elizabeth Gezahegn King and Kate Norman

Introduction

Development practitioners are increasingly recognising the value of investing in girls and young women, especially those who live in vulnerable communities whose needs are often invisible in development interventions. Securing girls' rights is vital if young women are to realise their full potential (UNFPA 2013). However, many girls in developing countries continue to face multiple challenges that hamper their development and full participation in society. These include poverty, discriminatory social norms, early sexual initiation, gender based violence and inadequate laws (FORWARD and IPPF 2012). The ability to respond adequately to these challenges is hampered by insufficient disaggregated data to help track progress on the situation of girls in marginalised communities (The Chicago Council on Global Affairs 2011), as well as difficulties accessing young women during their everyday lives to gather in-depth insight needed to design transformative interventions. A report on adolescence by the United Nations Children's Fund (UNICEF 2011) reiterates the urgent need for international agencies and governments to collaborate and invest in data collection and analysis to improve existing knowledge on young people that will help inform the design of programmes and policies. The report also reiterated recommendations from the Committee on the Rights of the Child to governments to ensure young people are included in data collection, stating, 'where appropriate, adolescents should participate in the analysis to ensure that the information is understood and utilised in an adolescent-sensitive way' (UNICEF 2011: 64).

The Foundation for Women's Health Research and Development (FORWARD), a UK-based women's not-for-profit organisation that works to eliminate harmful practices, has learned over the years to value the role of insider knowledge in our programmes. Access to community perspectives and norms has helped to inform our campaign and support work. We work to improve the sexual and reproductive health and rights of African women and girls, focusing on the sensitive issues of female genital mutilation, child marriage and related health issues including maternal health and obstetric fistula. Over the last ten years the foundation's work has focused on 'girls left behind', a term we adopted in direct response to the invisibility of the needs of girls and young women in rural and slum areas in development programming. Young women in these contexts tend to be disproportionately affected by the triple burden of gender, social and physical environment, and age (Chicago Council on Global Affairs 2011). The beneficiaries of our programmes include child mothers, pregnant girls, child brides and those at risk of multiple forms of abuse and gender inequality, many of whom lack control over decisions in relation to their sexual lives and bodies. In this chapter, we share our experience using participatory and ethnographic research to inform and shape a girls' health and leadership programme in Sierra Leone.

Young women at risk in Sierra Leone

The long civil war in Sierra Leone had devastating effects on the social and economic development of the country and adversely affected the attainment of the Millennium Development Goals (Government of Sierra Leone 2010). Sierra Leone was ranked at 183 out of 187 countries in the Human Development Index in 2013, and 73 per cent of the population lived below the poverty line, while more than 55 per cent of these were on less than a dollar a day (UNDP 2014). According to the Government's Poverty Reduction Strategy Paper 2013–2018 (Government of Sierra Leone 2013a), the highest levels of poverty and unemployment are found among young people, women and other vulnerable groups.

Girls and young women living in resource poor environments often experience tremendous pressure to initiate sex early, putting them at increased risk of early pregnancy, early motherhood, and sexually transmitted infections, including HIV (FORWARD and IPPF 2011). Teenage pregnancy and early motherhood are perceived as critical development challenges in Sierra Leone, which occur primarily due to early sexual initiation and high rates of child marriage (Government of Sierra Leone 2013a). The Sierra Leone's Child Right Act, 2007 (Government of Sierra Leone 2007) makes marriage below 18 years illegal, yet in the country, 30 per cent of girls aged 15–19 are married (Population Council 2010). In 2008, over 34 per cent of all pregnancies occurred among teenage mothers, and 26 per cent of young women aged 15–19 years already had a baby (Government of Sierra Leone 2013b). A study conducted in 24 communities in four regions in Sierra Leone found a high level of risky sexual activity and unwanted pregnancies among girls aged 12–20 years (Coinco 2010). Younger girls who become pregnant are often withdrawn from school; early pregnancy is cited as the third most common reason for girls dropping out of school in Sierra Leone (Government of Sierra Leone 2013b).

In 2010, we began to implement a 14-month pilot project with financial support from the International Planned Parenthood Federation. The project, called

'Empowering Girls at Risk', was part of a broader IPPF initiative called 'Girls Decide' that aimed to address young women's sexuality and pregnancy-related matters. In Sierra Leone, the project was implemented with the Sierra Leone Family Planning Association, and aimed to involve girls and young women living in poverty and affected by teenage pregnancy in the poorest areas of Freetown. The project goal was to improve the lives of young mothers and girls at risk, by enabling them to claim their entitlements and increase their knowledge of sexual and reproductive health and rights. Programme activities included education sessions to increase knowledge of sexual and reproductive health and rights issues and develop self-expression and confidence, the creation of a platform for young women to raise their voice and claim their entitlements, and the establishment of social support networks for girls and young mothers. Ethnographically informed participatory research was undertaken with young women to inform the design of this project.

An ethnographic approach to programme design

In order to design an effective programme, it was important to conduct research with young women in order to strengthen understanding of young women's experiences of sex, teenage pregnancy and early motherhood, as well as the root causes of these, the impact these had on their lives, and the contexts within which these occurred. The data collection methodology used in this study was based on a peer ethnographic method developed by Price and Hawkins (2002). In this method, members of the target community are selected as peer researchers who are trained to carry out in-depth conversational interviews with individuals they know from their own social networks, 'based on the premise that what people say about social life and behaviour changes according to the level of familiarity and trust established between the researcher and the researched' (Price and Hawkins 2002: 1328). The method aims to tap into the existing established relationship of trust with the individuals who peers interview. Importantly, the method uses 'third person' interviewing techniques, whereby respondents are asked about people like themselves in their communities, rather than about their own personal experiences and opinions. In doing so, it can yield rich narrative data to help understand health and risk perceptions and behaviours from an insider's point of view, generate detailed understanding of the context in which these behaviours occur, and provide a more intimate engagement with the realities of young women's lives (Price and Hawkins 2002).

Given the project's aim of empowering young women to speak out about their needs, this method was also chosen as it has been documented as having a transformational effect on peer researchers (Price and Hawkins 2002). This was perceived as important, given the programmatic aim of establishing a platform for young women's action, and social support networks.

Recruitment and training

The research was led by two programme staff members and a lead researcher. Each had prior experience using the research method and expertise in adolescent sexual reproductive health issues. A further five research supervisors – who had previous knowledge of peer education and sexual and reproductive health issues – were recruited by the Family Planning Association of Sierra Leone to assist with the research. Their main role was to support the data collection process, communicate regularly with young people involved in the research to ensure the research process was running smoothly, and to ensure accurate recording of the data collected.

Fifteen young women aged 15–20 years living in poorer areas of Freetown – including Brookfields, Grey Bush, Waterloo and Red Pump – were selected as volunteer peer researchers. Half of them had experienced teenage pregnancy, and the majority had dropped out of school. These peer researchers were recruited using 'snowball sampling' techniques through girls who were working with the Family Planning Association of Sierra Leone as peer educators, or were part of their ongoing youth programmes. These young women took part in a four-day participatory training workshop in Freetown. The aim of this was to train peer researchers in conversational research skills, and build confidence to enable them to discuss sensitive research topics. Training was conducted in Creole, the *lingua franca* spoken widely throughout Sierra Leone. During training, the supervisors and peer researchers worked together to agree the overarching research questions – why are girls living in poor communities in Freetown at risk of teenage pregnancy? What is the impact of teenage pregnancy and early motherhood on the lives of these girls? What do girls say about the availability of appropriate services and information and what change do they want? They also developed six to seven questions as prompts to use for each of the three themes.

Data collection

Over a four-week period, peer researchers carried out three interviews with three friends on each of the three themes, resulting in nine interviews each, and 135 interviews in total. Interviewees were encouraged to share stories or examples of events they had heard about. Interviews were carried out in the third person, and no names were used:

> [A]ll interviews are conducted in the third person, in an attempt to elicit narrative accounts of how interviewees conceptualise the social behaviour of 'others' in their networks, not accounts of their own behaviour or normative statements about how they 'ought' to behave.
>
> (Price and Hawkins 2002: 1329)

Peer researchers were asked to make brief notes on the key issues, words used and events described immediately after interviewing their friends, to enable them to capture the stories and themes. The supervisors' role was to meet the peer researchers every week to make sure the data was being collected on the themes, to collect their findings, and make detailed notes on challenges and issues that resulted from the interviews. During these meetings, peer researchers and supervisors reviewed the content of the interviews and addressed any issues raised during the week. The supervisors then sent all collated data to the lead researcher.

Once all data under each theme was collected, the lead researcher organised in-depth interviews with each peer researcher and a focus group discussion to explore issues that needed further clarification. The focus group discussion helped to validate the data, and the in-depth interviews enabled the research team to probe further and obtain additional explanations to aid interpretation of the data. Both methods enabled the peer researchers to reflect on their own experiences as well as their discussions with their interviewees.

Finally, a full day debriefing workshop with the supervisors and peer researchers was undertaken in order to develop and discuss the main findings, and articulate possible short and long term programmatic solutions. This workshop also provided the opportunity to thank everyone for taking part in the process and to distribute completion certificates.

Data analysis

Data were analysed under the three themes by the lead researcher. A process of thematic coding was undertaken, whereby recurrent findings were assigned codes and clustered together under the three themes of the research. In practice, the data were divided into text units made up of paragraphs, quotes and stories and arranged under the cluster of codes. In each cluster, data were then re-read, and a proportion of quotations were selected to capture the essence of each code.

Stakeholder consultation

A stakeholder consultation meeting was organised to create a platform for peer researchers to engage in dialogue with government officials and other decision makers and agencies at local level. The consultation was designed as a participatory forum with girls taking part in panel discussions to share their experiences of the process, their findings and recommendations. The participating stakeholders – including representatives from government ministries and development agencies working on sexual and reproductive health issues, as well as community leaders and programme staff from the Sierra Leone Family Planning Association – were asked to read some quotes from the study to put themselves in the girls' shoes. This provided a platform for disseminating the results of the study to wider audiences and decision makers.

Designing health and leadership programmes 115

In their own words: findings from formative research

The research documented rich stories of vulnerability and risk taking, as well as the heavy toll of teenage pregnancy and early motherhood on girls' lives. These findings informed the development of the young women's health and leadership programme.

The causes of teenage pregnancy and early motherhood

Interviews highlighted a number of factors that enhanced the vulnerability of girls at high risk of teenage pregnancy. These included poverty and social pressure from families for young women to earn an income; peer pressure; lack of opportunities to access education and health services within their communities; and the separation of families arising from the long years of civil war. Young women also described a lack of basic information on sexual matters, sexual exploitation and abuse of girls by older men, and low use of contraception.

Girls also shared stories of the daily struggle of families to provide them with food and other basic items, such as school fees. Many parents were unemployed or worked long hours for little pay, working as manual labourers and petty traders in the market. Parents were away from home for long periods of time and struggled to provide adequate parental care. Unable to obtain financial support from their parents, many girls were forced to support themselves by looking for ways to earn money to buy their basic necessities often through transactional sex, and sometimes relying on multiple sexual partners.

> High teenage pregnancy is because of no home attention. Single parents definitely find it harder. They are always at work and not around to discipline their children.
> (Young woman from Freetown)

> You ask your mum for something and when she can't give it to you, you ask one of your boyfriends, but he definitely won't give it to you unless you sleep with him. Nothing for nothing!
> (Young woman from Freetown)

> It is best for a girl to have as many boyfriends and sugar daddies as possible. We say 'John buy di trousers, peter go buy di top' [John buys the trousers, Peter buys the top] and we say 'one close, not di full up box' [One cloth will not fill up the suitcase, meaning you require different men to fill your wardrobe].
> (Young woman from Freetown)

> Girls say there is unemployment for them in the community so that is the reason why they turn to prostitution so that they can be able to feed themselves.
>
> (Young woman from Freetown)

Some girls also shared stories of family pressure to earn money to support their family. Many parents did not question their daughters about where their income came from, whilst other parents encouraged their daughters to attract support from men.

> If you are beautiful in a poor family your parent will pressure you. They will say there are lot of men coming your way, why can't you make provision for the family? The family will force you, even if you don't want it. Use what you have to get what you want. This happens in poor families all over, especially poor families and single parent families. If the man proposes to a beautiful young girl to have sex with him, even if she says no he may go and discuss it with her mother. Even if that girl go out late at night and never come home, they will never question her because she is the one bringing the money.
>
> (Young woman from Freetown)

Girls growing up in poor communities in Freetown often have very limited job options, which is problematic for girls who drop out of school due to becoming pregnant. Interviewees explained that dropping out of school early is common for girls, as many mentioned that parents do not value girls' education and put pressure on girls to marry (see also Government of Sierra Leone 2013b). This was reported as such a common occurrence that interviewees explained that many young women view pregnancy and early motherhood as their only future.

> Parents do not care much about girls' education, they say school is not for girls it is for boys. It is common for girls to drop out of school early, but not the boys, boys are more important to finish. Girls get pregnant and drop out. Boys cannot get pregnant.
>
> (Young woman from Freetown)

Although it was evident that some girls lacked correct information on prevention of pregnancy, this was more common for those who had recently moved to the city from the rural areas. Many of the girls involved in the study were aware of modern family planning methods to prevent pregnancy, and knew that condoms protected against sexually transmitted infections.

> Most girls in Freetown our age now know about sex and how to prevent pregnancy and HIV. But most people say that HIV is not existing here. It is not around.
>
> (Young woman from Freetown)

However, there was a significant gap between this knowledge and girls' actual behaviour. Youthful naivety, common myths and beliefs, traditions, religious beliefs and gender roles, all weave together to explain this disparity between what girls – for the most part at least – know, and what they do when it comes to protection. Young women knew that contraception helped to prevent pregnancy and sexually transmitted infections, but they did not appear to think that they needed to use contraception themselves. Some interviewees indicated that some girls use pregnancy as a strategy to keep their boyfriends.

> As a girl if you carry condoms the men will think you are a prostitute. Some girls are ashamed to buy condoms because when they go to where it is being sold they are being judged as wrong.
> (Young woman from Freetown)

> Women don't use condoms to show their boyfriends how much they love them.
> (Young woman from Freetown)

> Some girls want to get pregnant at an early age because they do not want to lose their boyfriends.
> (Young woman from Freetown)

Girls' stories made frequent mention of sexual exploitation, incest and rape, often by older men in positions of power, including teachers, relatives and guardians. In these circumstances, girls reported being unable to protect themselves or have the confidence to report this abuse. Stigma associated with rape was reported as being common, and some interviewees explained that young women tend to be blamed for being raped.

> Rape cases are still high around here. Some men even rape their own children. 'If you prepare the soup, you should be the first to taste it.' In other words she is my daughter; I should be the first to have sex with her.
> (Young woman from Freetown)

Peer pressure affected girls in different ways. For example, interviewees reported that girls with low self-esteem want acceptance and praise from their peers. In some instances, these young women might follow a crowd of peers who influence them to seek men to obtain support, in the form of material items such as gold chains, clothes, earrings and slippers. Some young women join such a peer group because their parents cannot provide for them.

> They say pressure from friends is bad because they pressure them to engage in premature sexual activities.
> (Young woman from Freetown)

The impact of pregnancy and motherhood on young women's lives

The findings indicate that girls were very much aware of the huge impact of pregnancy and early motherhood on their lives. Narratives indicated that early pregnancy created many new hardships. These included being shunned by friends and rejected from their homes due to family shame, having to drop out of school due to school policy or being too embarrassed to continue with their education, boyfriends denying parental responsibility, and struggling to provide for their babies' upkeep when they themselves depend on their poor families.

> As soon as I find out I am pregnant I leave school because I feel shame – I drop out of school, I don't want the teacher or other people to know about it.
> (Young woman from Freetown)

> When I am pregnant my community are laughing at me and calling me names. They laugh at you and point finger on you.
> (Young woman from Freetown)

> The consequences that girls face are that their parents drive them out from their houses and they find it very difficult to take care of their babies.
> (Young woman from Freetown)

In order to avoid stigmatisation and the burden of caring for a baby, some young women described vivid narratives of unsafe forms of abortion, using dangerous chemicals or backstreet practitioners. Abortion is legally restricted in Sierra Leone (United Nations n.d.), so young women are often unable to access safe abortion services. Girls shared numerous accounts of their own and others' dreadful experiences – many of which ended with death, or with long term damage or disability.

> Most girls try to take something to abort. Some are using traditional medicine; some are using ampiclox (antibiotics). I myself took ampiclox with coke and stood up on a mortar and jumped to get rid of the baby. It didn't work. Some are taking blue – a chemical for washing cloth. You mix with water and drink it.
> (Young woman from Freetown)

> When they want to make an abortion, girls use a medical instrument or some even go to fake doctors. It causes infertility in young girls and women, cause internal bleeding which leads to death or destruction of the womb.
> (Young woman from Freetown)

Even when young women give birth, maternal and child morbidity and mortality remain a major risk, due to the girls' young and often underdeveloped and malnourished bodies not 'being ready' for childbirth. Anecdotes indicated that some of those who made it through delivery often did not have the necessary skills to nurture and take proper care of the baby. Interviewees reported that young women in these situations face a life of poverty, especially those who drop out of school and are unable to return due to punitive school policies.

> Teenage pregnancy destroys their future plan and makes them unable to be useful to the community.
> (Young woman from Freetown)

> Girls are not happy about their teenage pregnancy. They can become uncaring mothers and in regard to that, their babies suffer a lot and that can lead to infant mortality.
> (Young woman from Freetown)

> Young mothers and their babies find it very difficult to live because they hardly have their daily bread. Young mothers or babies can find it so hard – they are often the ones who get into prostitution as the only way of supporting [their child].
> (Young woman from Freetown)

> Girls want to be a very useful person in their community and country as a whole but so many get teenage pregnancy for difficult reasons, they are now drop-outs and they think that's the end of their future. When some are now pregnant they think that's the end of their world.
> (Young woman from Freetown)

Young women's views on access to information, health and support services

One of the key findings from the interviews concerned the limited sources of information available to young women on matters such as sexual development, sexual behaviour and sexual and reproductive health. The majority of peer interviews indicated that young women had received some form of sex education at school (although information was perceived as inadequate, especially for younger girls), as well as at healthcare settings (e.g. hospitals, clinics) and drug stores, or by hearing or seeing educational messages on the radio or television (although relatively few households had their own television). While the media may help raise awareness on sexual matters, most of these messages fail to provide girls with the skills to negotiate safe sex. Few interviews reported that girls had discussions with parents about sexual matters.

> Girls around here get their information about sex and reproductive health from the hospitals, clinics, drug stores and even from public outlets such as

the radio, television and movies. They sometimes get their information from their friends and parents.

(Young woman from Freetown)

Sometimes you will hear on the radio or television – but let's be honest, if we hear a health programme we will change the channel to hear the music or watch the Nigerian movie instead.

(Peer researcher, focus group discussion, Freetown)

Sex education is limited. They don't have any in primary school and yet there are girls up to the age of 14 even in primary school, plenty of them are already having sex.

(Young woman from Freetown)

Sex was not often openly discussed in the home, although some mentioned conversations with grandmothers or other older people as being helpful. However, this tended to refer to information obtained by girls from grandmothers during the female genital mutilation rites which is widespread in Sierra Leone, and noted by girls as important for relationships with partners and husbands. Other communication about sexual issues at home was rather incomplete.

It is very rare for parents to do a good job at telling children about sex. One woman told her daughter 'do not let a man lie on top of you – if you do you will become pregnant and disgrace the family'. When the girl became pregnant she said she told her mother that she climbed on top of the man. The mother later said I should have told her the whole truth.

(Peer researcher, focus group discussion, Freetown)

Despite there being a number of potential channels for accurate information on sexual matters, girls on the whole agreed that the information they received was 'not enough', and that sex was still considered a taboo topic that was rarely openly discussed. Peer researchers readily acknowledged that they wanted and needed the right information on sexual matters. Many girls had to rely on their friends for information – be it right or wrong – about sex.

In terms of specific sexual and reproductive health services available, the peer supervisors involved with the local branch of the Family Planning Association of Sierra Leone talked positively about the youth friendly services available in the clinics. The majority of interviewees, however, indicated that girls tended not to use these services – many were not aware of them, while others knew about the clinics but lived too far away to access them. Where young women reported using modern forms of contraception, narratives indicated that they tended to access services in a range of settings – from local hospitals and clinics (not specific to sexual and reproductive health) to pharmacies, to buying from 'men who roam around our community selling drugs at a cheaper price'. Data collected indicated that girls generally felt that the essential youth friendly services were not available or were too few in number. Poor signposting of services was also flagged up as an issue by a number of girls.

> Some girls say that they don't even know whether there are services available, while others said that there are services of course but they don't know too much about it so they don't know what to say about them.
> (Young woman from Freetown)

> Some girls around here say support services for pregnant teenagers and young mothers are not available and that they need more. Some girls say that there are no supporting services for girls and this just leaves the girls to be vulnerable to all kinds of problems.
> (Young woman from Freetown)

> Some girls say that there are no support services for teenagers or young mothers so you will have to struggle on your own if you don't have people to care for you.
> (Young woman from Freetown)

Young women shared stories of the varied traditional and alternative methods used to prevent pregnancy. Many believed strongly that these worked and continued to use them, while others cautioned that these only worked under specific conditions. Some girls said that their mothers arranged for them to access these traditional methods from traditional herbalists. Other contraceptive methods included drinking salt water after unprotected sex, as well as washing immediately after intercourse.

> You can use traditional rope and tie it around your waist and it will stop you getting pregnant. The female traditional healers give you the rope, you pay for it and say how long you don't want to be pregnant for. And to be honest it works – all the people believe it. We do know some people who got pregnant with the rope but that is because some people are not the real traditional people, they are selling you the wrong rope.
> (Peer researcher, focus group discussion, Freetown)

The shame associated with accessing adult health services was illustrated in stories that described the poor treatment of teenage girls by government health workers. Stories of being judged and abused when seeking advice about family planning or pregnancy, and specifically when giving birth, were common among young girls in the study.

> Some nurses treat you badly – as if you are not a human being because you don't have money. Even they will beat you up while you are supposed to be delivering your baby – they will beat you mercilessly, they hit you and say

'hurry up I have other things to do. I was not the one who told you to go and spread your legs in the first place.'

(Young woman from Freetown)

Transitioning from research to the girls' programme

As illustrated, research findings highlighted a number of challenges experienced by young pregnant women, those at risk of becoming pregnant, and young mothers living in poor and marginalised communities in Freetown. With support of the peer researchers, recommendations forming the basis of the programme were made. These included the provision of a supportive environment and skills for young mothers; supporting girls to continue their education; and the provision of safe youth friendly spaces to access information and support.

> I want a place where girls will be happy. Somewhere that will help us to prevent teenage pregnancy, show us how to have a good life.
> (Peer researcher, focus group discussion, Freetown)

> We need microfinance support – along with training on how to do business, how to save money etc.
> (Peer researcher, focus group discussion, Freetown)

> Girls want to go back to school; after they have the baby they leave but they realise what they are missing. They want a second chance.
> (Peer researcher, focus group discussion, Freetown)

> We want somewhere only for young people. We don't want to meet up with our mother there. There is no privacy and we don't feel free to say what we want. We want to speak to someone who we have confidence in, not some old person asking us a lot of questions and embarrassing us.
> (Peer researcher, focus group discussion, Freetown)

Three of the supervisors and two peer researchers who had shown an interest in taking action in their community were included in four days of training about confidence building and working with girls. This was organised in Freetown for staff and youth volunteers of the Family Planning Association of Sierra Leone. Interactive training used group discussions, films, photo stories and presentations to show how best to empower girls to become leaders, develop communication and assertiveness skills, and tackle gender-based violence. The training also explored strategies for running a girls' empowerment programme and developing action plans to meet young women's needs. This capacity building training resulted in the five representatives developing an action plan to work with girls from their community following on from the research.

With FORWARD's support, each of the five representatives established a girls' club in their local area, and recruited girls to join these clubs. Efforts were made to continue to build the capacity of these five individuals, which included funding a study visit to Ghana to meet a young women's organisation that was implementing a girls' network. During this visit to Ghana, these five young women decided to set up what is now called the Girl2Girl Empowerment Movement. Funding was secured to recruit a part time coordinator for this Movement in 2013, and it has since been registered as a community-based organisation with the Government of Sierra Leone. A resource centre was set up in the office, providing a meeting place for the leaders to plan their programmes and organise joint meetings of the girls' clubs. There are currently six clubs being run in six areas in Freetown, involving 100 girls so far. These clubs provide leadership training, sexual and reproductive health information and sign posting to health services, as well as income generation training activities. The girls are trained as peer educators and supported to undertake outreach in their local areas on teenage pregnancy and rights of girls to be free from practices such as female genital mutilation and gender-based violence.

Reflections and conclusion

We adopted a peer ethnographic methodology to improve understanding on the situation of girls at risk of, and experiencing, pregnancy and early motherhood living in poor areas of Freetown. The research revealed new and fresh insights into the experiences and lives of girls at risk. The study provided rich stories of vulnerability experienced by young women and young mothers in their daily lives.

Importantly, the study was led by girls from the local community, who were trained to become peer researchers. Participation in, and confidence developed from, each of the different aspects of the research led to some of the young women involved – as peer researchers and research supervisors – becoming activists and agents of change, using research findings to lead change in their communities. These girls and young women became experts in the issues affecting their own lives.

The research findings informed the design of a girls' empowerment programme, called the Girl2Girl Empowerment Movement, which is now working with girls in four communities in Freetown. The transformation and confidence that the peer researchers developed over the course of the peer study and the transition into a new girls' intervention was remarkable, clearly showing the added value of listening to young women's voices and supporting their participation in shaping and designing programmes for girls in similar difficult situations to themselves.

References

Chicago Council on Global Affairs (2011) *Girls Grow: A vital force in rural economies. A girls count report on adolescent girls*. Available at: www.ungei.org/resources/files/GirlsGrowReportFinal.pdf (accessed 25 May 2015).

Coinco, E. (2010) *A Glimpse into the World of Teenage Pregnancy in Sierra Leone*, Freetown: UNICEF.

FORWARD and IPPF (2011) *'In Their Own Words': Girls from Sierra Leone on Sexuality, Pregnancy and Services*, London: FORWARD.

FORWARD and IPPF (2012) *'In Their Own Words': Girls from Liberia on Sexuality, Pregnancy and Services*. Available at: www.forwarduk.org.uk/wp-content/uploads/2014/12/Girls-from-Liberia-on-Sexuality-Pregnancy-and-Services.pdf (accessed 25 May 2015).

Government of Sierra Leone (2007) *The Child Right Act, 2007*. Available at: www.sierra-leone.org/Laws/2007–7p.pdf (accessed 25 May 2015).

Government of Sierra Leone (2010) *Millennium Development Goals Progress Report 2010*. Available at: www.sl.undp.org/content/dam/sierraleone/docs/MDGdocs/undp_sle_mdgreport2010.pdf (accessed 25 May 2015).

Government of Sierra Leone (2013a) *The Agenda for Prosperity, Road to middle income status. Sierra Leone's Third Generation Poverty Reduction Strategy Paper 2013–2018*. Available at: www.undp.org/content/dam/sierraleone/docs/projectdocuments/povreduction/undp_sle_The%20Agenda%20for%20Prosperity%20.pdf (accessed 25 May 2015).

Government of Sierra Leone (2013b) *Let Girls be Girls, Not Mothers. National Strategy for the Reduction of Teenage Pregnancy, 2013–201*. Available at: http://hivhealthclearinghouse.unesco.org/sites/default/files/resources/Sierra_Leone_National_Strategy_for_the_Reduction_of_Teenage_Pregnancy.pdf (accessed 5 June 2015).

Population Council (2010) *The Adolescent Experience In-Depth: Using Data to Identify and Reach the Most Vulnerable Young People: Sierra Leone 2008*, New York: Population Council.

Price, N. and Hawkins, K. (2002) 'Researching sexual and reproductive behaviour: a peer ethnographic approach', *Social Science & Medicine*, 55: 1325–1336.

UNDP (2014) *Human Development Report 2014*, New York: UNDP.

UNFPA (2013) *Motherhood in Childhood: Facing the challenge of adolescent pregnancy*, New York: UNFPA.

UNICEF (2011) *State of the World's Children 2011: Adolescent, an age of opportunity*, New York, New York: UNICEF.

United Nations (n.d.) *Sierra Leone Abortion Policy*. Available at: www.un.org/esa/population/publications/abortion/doc/sierraleone.doc (accessed 25 May 2015).

Part III

Monitoring processes

Using social mapping techniques to guide programme redesign in the Tingim Laip HIV prevention and care project in Papua New Guinea

Lou McCallum, Jennifer Miller, Scott Berry and Christopher Hershey

Introduction

Papua New Guinea (PNG) occupies the eastern half of the island of New Guinea and is geographically the largest country of the Pacific region. It is one of the world's most ethnically diverse countries, with over 850 indigenous languages, and its population in 2011 was estimated at 7.5 million. Demographically, PNG is a young country: 76 per cent of people are under 35 years of age and 40 per cent are under the age of 15 years; 85 per cent of the population live in rural areas and 75 per cent of households depend on subsistence agriculture (UNDP 2014). Despite intensive development in recent years through the sale of natural resources, significant challenges exist in raising health, education and employment levels. Law and order problems persist.

PNG has an HIV epidemic that has followed different patterns in all four of its geographical regions. National projections conducted in March 2014 estimated the overall prevalence of HIV in PNG at 0.65 per cent and the number of people living with HIV in 2013 was estimated at 31,945. Only the National Capital District and the Highlands provinces of Enga, Jiwaka and Western Highlands are estimated to have an HIV prevalence greater than 1 per cent (PNG Department of Health 2014). The prevalence of sexually transmitted infections across PNG is among the highest in the world, with the majority of cases reported from the Highlands Region (PNG National AIDS Council 2011).

The potential for sexual transmission of HIV is heightened by a range of factors including early sexual debut, often in situations of coercion and abuse; multiple and concurrent sexual partnerships, including polygyny, extramarital sexual partnerships and inter-generational sex; the widespread exchange of sex for cash, goods and security, and family disruption; low and inconsistent condom use; high levels of sexual violence and rape; mobility; and the use of penile inserts and modifications (PNG National AIDS Council 2011).

This chapter focuses on a research study that was conducted early in the second phase of PNG's largest HIV prevention project, after an independent evaluation of the first phase of the project concluded that the project appeared to have 'lost its conceptual focus' (AusAID 2007: 11). A 'social mapping' exercise was conducted by the new managers of the second phase of the project. It was designed to identify the key populations affected by HIV in PNG and, more particularly, to update information on the particular context of HIV risk and impact in different parts of the country and in different environments.

Tingim Laip

Tingim Laip is PNG's largest community-based HIV prevention and care project. Tingim Laip means loosely 'value life' in Tok Pisin, one of the country's three national languages (AusAID 2010). It is a project of the PNG National AIDS Council and is funded by the Australian Government. Tingim Laip emerged in 2006 from the High Risk Setting Strategy, which was part of the AusAID-funded National HIV/AIDS Support Project – NHASP (PNG National AIDS Council 2006). At the end of the NHASP project in late 2006, AusAID changed the name of the High Risk Settings Strategy to Tingim Laip, and the first phase of the Tingim Laip project commenced.

The conceptual framework for the first phase of Tingim Laip was driven by a social mapping study conducted in 19 of PNG's 20 provinces in 2005. This was an extensive study – over 200 field interviewers were trained and mobilised and over 2,000 people were interviewed (NHASP 2005). The four pillars that guided work done in the first project phase came from an analysis of the data collected in this study. These were access to condoms; access to sexually transmitted infection testing and treatment facilities; access to user-friendly voluntary counselling and testing; and access to care and support for people living with HIV (AusAID 2010).

An independent mid-term evaluation of the first phase of Tingim Laip in 2007 identified a number of issues with the project's conceptual focus. It argued that the project was too concerned with condom distribution and had lost focus on its other three key pillars. The review identified the project's volunteer workforce as its key strength, but expressed concerns about an 'incoherent conceptual framework' and a 'sub-optimal communication between the implementing partners' (AusAID 2007: 11). Subsequent to this evaluation, AusAID commissioned a project design for a new phase of Tingim Laip in 2008, and in 2010 a second five year phase of Tingim Laip commenced (AusAID 2010). Its official goal, set out by the funder, was 'to contribute to the reduction of HIV prevalence in the general population, to improve care and support for those infected and minimise the social and economic impact of the HIV and AIDS epidemic on individuals, families and communities' (AusAID 2010: 26).

The purpose of the second phase of Tingim Laip was defined as 'effective prevention at sites where there is a convergence (coming together) of risk behaviour and vulnerability through community centred and interpersonal approaches' (AusAID 2010: 27). The second phase project design document called for a repeat of the 2005 social mapping study in order to ensure that the project implementers had up to date contextual information about HIV risk in and impact on the key populations affected by HIV in PNG (AusAID 2010: 14).

The social mapping methodology

The use of ethnography in health service programming is relatively new, reflecting the historic dominance of quantitative methods in medicine and public health assessment, planning and evaluation (Al-Busaidi 2008). These latter methods have been criticised for largely ignoring the everyday lives of the people they study (Al-Busaidi 2008). Much has been written about the social construction of reality (Burr 1995; Anderson 2006), and how views about morality and social norms are not static, but are constantly in flux and vary widely within social groups (Herzfeld 2005). Ethnographic research, which is sensitive to understanding these local subjectivities (Liamputtong 2007), prioritises research participants' needs and voices during monitoring and evaluation research.

Social and anthropological research on HIV and sex conducted in PNG since the first Tingim Laip Social Mapping study (conducted in 2005) pointed to the need to move away from a research focus on people's knowledge, attitudes and behaviours (Kelly 2009). Instead, it was recommended that the focus be on methodologies that would provide policy makers and programme designers with more information about the social elements that shape people's ability to act on the basis of what they know (Kelly et al. 2011). These elements include personal power; gender norms and practices; dependence on others for money, shelter and safety; intimate-partner, clan and community violence; and alcohol and other drug use (Hammar 2007). In response to this suggestion, the second phase of Tingim Laip sought out specific information on contexts of HIV-related risk and impact that went well beyond descriptions of behaviour. Furthermore, the populations (e.g. sex workers, men who have sex with other men) we sought to access were often marginalised in PNG communities because of the illegality or social undesirability of their behaviour. For these reasons, we chose a methodology for the social mapping study that would allow us to work closely with these populations, and gain specific, personal information that many of the participants might feel disinclined to share immediately with people they do not know or trust (Stewart 2014).

An ethnographic approach was adopted in this social mapping methodology, in the form of participant observation and interviewing, in order to reveal something of the 'insider' experiences of research participants (Adler 2004, Liamputtong 2010). For the Tingim Laip interventions to be available to the people who most needed them and relevant to their lives, it was necessary for the methodology to provide us with specific information about the context of the lives of people most affected by HIV. How was information about HIV incorporated into the thinking and behaviour? What power did they have to act? Who and what influenced their decisions or had power over their lives? How might these power relations be shifted?

Thematic focus

We started developing the methodology by identifying a set of 'domains of interest' for the study. These included mobility; power; gender; risk settings and factors; populations most-at-risk; money and poverty; employment; violence, including sexual violence; alcohol and other drug use; gambling; and local culture and religion. Our enquiry was not limited to these domains, and the mapping teams were encouraged to follow leads that took them beyond these. Analysing power relations is an essential part of responding to HIV. Promoting simple messages such as 'use a condom' or 'visit an STI clinic' does not take into account the power or permission that different people have to seek in order to protect themselves and their partners.

Study locations

Before the existence of a parallel programme in PNG – the Asian Development Bank Enclaves Project – commenced its work in 2006, there had been a particular focus in PNG on finding and mapping 'HIV hot spots'. These included bars, bus terminals, parts of town where sex was bought and sold, where people gathered to drink and have sex, where men were living away from wives and family, and where money flowed freely.

The Enclaves Project had broadened this focus into an interest in environments and industries rather than just physical locations (Asian Development Bank 2006). This broader perspective – that included a focus on the movement of people along a major trading route (e.g. the Highlands Highway), or the impact of a big development project such as a gas mining project on a small town (e.g. Tari, in the Highlands) – provided opportunities to understand how people move in and out of environments, and how power relations within these environments influence people differently. We explicitly engaged with these opportunities as part of work done during the second phase of Tingim Laip.

PNG has few major roads because of the inaccessible nature of its terrain. The Highlands Highway is the busiest and most important transport corridor in the country, stretching from the inland Highlands towns of Tari, Mount Hagen and Goroka, to the north coastal ports of Madang and Lae. Our work focused not just on specific locations, but on who was moving along the Highway, how and why they gather, and who they interact with. In addition to the Highway, several other 'corridors' of risk exist, exemplifying PNG's widespread dislocation of people. For example, the Liquefied Natural Gas pipeline project is a relatively new development project that runs from the Highlands to the coast, and involves the regular movement of goods and people for work, which in turn generates a significant support industry providing lodging, food, alcohol and sex. The Palm Oil industry of the coastal areas supports the seasonal movement of workers, and the housing of seasonal workers in compounds away from families and a significant informal support industry. The military moves mostly men from their homes to more isolated bases such as those in Wewak, Kiunga and Vanimo.

Mapping team selection and training

Two teams, each comprising a coordinator and three mappers, were established to move easily through the populations and settings we wanted to observe. One team focused on the Highlands Highway and Liquefied Natural Gas project, and the other focused on the Palm Oil Industry and the Military. The team leaders were both non-Papua New Guineans who had lived and worked in PNG for considerable periods, were fluent in Tok Pisin, had extensive experience of cultural norms and practices in many parts of PNG, and were well known to civil society groups. This was important to ensure little impact on the settings we were moving through. The remaining mapping team members were PNG nationals, experienced in social research data collection, fluent in several PNG languages and with good basic writing skills. Most were known to people working in the HIV and community sectors, and were comfortable moving around the settings and among the populations we needed to reach.

As in other contexts, people in PNG often behave differently in the presence of an unknown stranger. For example, the perceived opportunity for gain or benefit can lead respondents to say what they think researchers want to hear, or a lack of familiarity and trust can lead to suspicion and reluctance to share thoughts. Trust is essential to engaging with people. A strong *wantok* (one-talk) system, in which immediate and extended family clan lines are the foremost element of social structure, forms the basis for social support, yet at the same time restricts large-scale social mobilisation due to allegiances or demands by the *wantok* systems. Fear of sharing information that might be reported back to a family member or an opposing *wantok* group can also affect responses. This is particularly true when talking about the private aspects of life. Trust can also be built quite quickly in many parts of PNG, if people can build connections and trust, either through a *wantok* connection or the sense of 'genuineness' the research team brings.

The mapping team members participated in a five-day workshop that familiarised them with the research methodology through a series of practical exercises. They interviewed people, practised holding focus groups, documented findings, and held practice 'group talk' meetings to go over what they had observed and heard. Mappers were provided with a toolkit to assist them in documenting observations, interviews and focus groups. This contained an overview of the aims and process; an explanation of the domains of interest; a visit schedule for teams to complete to assist in planning; tips for what to observe at sites; sample questions for individual interviews and focus groups; and detailed templates for recording data.

Data collection, reflection and analysis

Two cycles of field work (consisting of observation and interviews) separated by 'group talk' sessions in Madang, were repeated in each of the four environments (e.g. Highlands Highway, Palm Oil sites, Liquefied Natural Gas pipeline sites and military sites) during the social mapping process. The teams visited a range of sites for field work, and recorded what they found in diaries and through maps or drawings. When they returned to the Tingim Laip national office in Madang, each of the two teams met separately first, and then together in the 'group talk' sessions, to discuss their site-by-site findings. They compared and contrasted their findings, identified gaps in the data and information they had collected and agreed upon common themes across all the sites. The second cycle then followed in each site.

Observation and interviews were focused on particular research participants, chosen based on their relevance to the study, our emerging understandings of risk and impact for HIV at the selected locations and their membership of, or close association with, relevant key populations. Following initial interviews at each site – with Tingim Laip staff, HIV public health officials, doctors and nurses at HIV clinics, non-governmental organisation leaders and local leaders – the teams adopted a targeted sampling process, identifying individuals or groups with characteristics and experiences relevant to the research. Mappers sought out harder-to-reach contacts, such as women involved in transactional sex (including both self-identified sex workers as well as women who exchange sex for safety, goods or favours), their clients, men who have sex with men, and other people moving through these environments.

The mappers observed the sites, and documented what they saw – in the form of text and diagrams – in field diaries throughout the process (Emerson et al. 2011). At the start of each field visit, each team created maps of the sites that reflected the domains of interest, which were revised regularly. At the end of each day, team members worked on their diaries and field notes, frequently meeting to compare observations and information, again informed against the domains. The rationale for this approach was that we were attempting to document large 'maps' across key domains of interest. These maps documented movements of small and large groups of people in and out of, within and around the sites, and also the social influences on actions taken by people at the sites. Once they had completed their work at each site, mapping teams met together with local project staff to describe what they had observed by presenting these diagrams. What project staff saw, heard and felt, and their interpretation of all of this were crucial to accurately recording the trends, movements and issues.

Individual and group interviewing occurred at the places where participants were meeting, working or travelling through (Hood 2007). No voice or video recorders were used in interviews because many were conducted in the open – on streets, along highways, in villages and towns, and in fields. Mappers interviewed participants in pairs, whereby one mapper focused on interviewing the participant and ensuring confidentiality and privacy, while the other mapper focused on taking detailed notes of the interview (Steinar and Svend 2009). Mappers' diaries assisted the teams to accurately recall conversations and observations.

At the end of each day, the team sat down together and shared what they had learned and observed in their interviews, taking particular notice of the similarities and differences on a day-to-day basis. Through this daily reflection, and as they met more people and visited new locations, findings that were either common or different across sites were noted. When they had completed their work at each site, diaries and interview notes were used to produce narratives of the themes identified at each site. We were not attempting to tell detailed stories or histories about the knowledge and experiences of individual respondents. Instead, the exercise aimed to document key themes, patterns and trends that emerged from respondents as they related to different domains of interest.

After each site visit, group talk enabled continuous data analysis throughout the social mapping method (Chamraz 2006). Group talk sessions allowed the teams to come together at the national office several times throughout the data collection process to discuss what they were finding and to modify the methodology to ensure that we were reaching the right people and obtaining the right type of information. For example, a key finding that arose from the first group talk session was that the teams needed to move further into populations, to get past the many gatekeepers and intermediaries, and have detailed conversations with the people that the project most needed to reach. We had deliberately chosen difficult environments, such as the main oval in one town where homeless young women gathered in the evenings to sell sex. Getting access to these young women to have a conversation about their lives meant getting past security guards (sometimes armed) who were guarding the nearby shops at night, but who also protected the women, in exchange for sex or for a share of their takings. In the first round of interviews in this setting, the mapping team had not been able to negotiate enough time or privacy with some respondents in order to obtain information in sufficient detail. This led to the development of strategies to negotiate better in the next round of interviews for the time and privacy we needed.

Group talk sessions also reinforced the need for the teams to document findings each day accurately on site, as, without this, they quickly found that they could not easily recall enough detail in the data analysis meetings. This is important in PNG, where oral culture means that much information is passed on verbally and people may not be in the habit of writing in detail. The group talk sessions encouraged mappers to improve their documentation practice so that they could verify the information they were bringing to the sessions.

Programme changes resulting from the social mapping

The timing of access to the social mapping data was important for the second phase of Tingim Laip. There had been a documented drift away from a focus on key HIV affected populations in the last two years of the first phase of Tingim Laip (AusAID 2012), and at the beginning of the second phase, the new management team set about reviewing and revising the project's policies, guidance and training materials, from the project's previous phase.

This led to the development of a new model of intervention, called the STEPS Model (Figure 9.1). This was designed to expand site-level interventions from awareness raising activities (which most sites were achieving) to include an increasingly broad range of activities relevant to HIV prevention, care and support (Tingim Laip 2012). In addition to reinforcing the need for access to HIV testing, sexually transmitted infection treatment and care and support of people living with HIV, the new model was also designed to address some of the key drivers of the epidemic that contribute to HIV risk and impact, such as alcohol and other drug use, discrimination and intimate-partner violence.

In parallel to the social mapping activity, AusAID commissioned a second independent review of Tingim Laip in 2011. This assessed the fit of the existing implementation model recommended in the project design document (developed three years earlier) to the current HIV epidemic in PNG. This review delivered its recommendations in mid 2012, at the same time that the social mapping data was being analysed. It recommended an immediate shift in focus, from the one-dimensional HIV awareness-raising in the general population that had dominated the latter stages of the first phase of Tingim Laip, to a range of targeted interventions aimed specifically at key HIV-affected populations. It supported the newly designed STEPS Model and recommended its rollout across a smaller number of sites in a more consolidated manner – from 37 sites in the first phase, to 20 sites in the second phase. It also challenged the project to meet a set of prescribed activity targets that included reaching at least 80 per cent of people engaged in transactional sex in each site with prevention messages, condoms and assistance to access sexually transmitted infection and HIV testing (AusAID 2012). The social mapping exercise contributed to the redesign of these activities in between first and second phases of Tingim Laip in several ways.

Clarification of groups and populations to work with

The social mapping data highlighted the inadequacy of the standard key HIV-affected population categories, particularly the category 'sex worker' in the PNG context. While there are a few women in PNG who describe themselves as sex workers and who belong to small local or provincial sex worker groups that are affiliated with the national sex worker organisation, Friends Frangipani, there are significantly more women who trade sex on a regular basis for cash, food, shelter and physical safety. The picture is complex. Some of these women cluster in small groups, living together as single mothers, providing a level of safety, security and support for each other. Many of these women were uncomfortable with the term sex worker, and saw their sexual transactions as a necessary means to an end in a context where there are few opportunities for women to be physically safe and financially independent.

The teams also spoke with a number of women who had several regular sexual partners who travelled through the towns in which they lived and contributed to the cost of housing, school fees and food. There were, of course, also women who

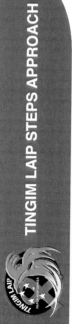
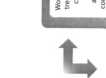

Figure 9.1 The Tingim Laip STEPS Model
Source: Tingim Laip 2013.

had multiple sexual partners, for mutual enjoyment rather than goods or safety. The teams learned that identity as a sex worker did not necessarily mean highest risk. A number of young women who had moved to towns to 'find a husband' reported as much sex and as many partners as women who referred to themselves as sex workers. But these young women were partying, not selling. They accepted drinks from men, and maybe food and physical protection, but saw themselves as quite different from the women they knew who were 'selling' sex.

These examples only serve to highlight some of the complexities of the environments that we worked in, and the inadequacy of an approach that says that a project should only target women who identify as sex workers, and should report contact with sex workers differently from contact with other women whose risk may be similar.

These findings led to spirited but productive debates between the Tingim Laip team, the funding agency, AusAID and the National AIDS Council. There was insistence from some quarters on a 'sex worker only' or 'sex worker first' approach in the second phase of Tingim Laip. These people argued that there were women in many sites who could easily be identified as sex workers, who were selling sex to a number of clients each day and who were mostly cut off from health services. However, in the end a compromise was reached and Tingim Laip adopted the shorthand 'women exchanging sex' in its target setting, reporting and training materials, so that a broader range of women at risk of, and affected by, HIV could be reached. In reality, Tingim Laip's approach was pragmatic. We focused more on the people who move through the environments where sex is transacted and where people are drinking and partying, which are often the same places. Our work connected these people to information, condoms and lubricant, and supported them to access the clinical services, legal aid and welfare services they needed.

Figure 9.2 maps some of the pathways into transactional sex described by women the teams spoke to. Maps like this were used in staff and volunteer training, and in describing our work to external stakeholders. The drawings helped steer conversations away from a focus on simplistic, one-dimensional solutions that were inadequate to address what are complex problems and contexts. They allowed people to better understand some of the realities of the world in which they were expected to work.

The social mapping data also highlighted the need to work not just with women engaged in transactional sex, but also with men who are sexual partners as well as those mediating the transactions. Information on male sexual networks, gender norms and practices, levels of coercion and violence, the role alcohol and other drugs play, and the influence that men have in insecure settings led us to another innovation. Unique within PNG's response, efforts were made during the second phase of Tingim Laip to identify and recruit field staff who could provide outreach and referral services to so-called 'mobile men with money'. For example, Tingim Laip recruited several men as paid peer workers. These men knew their peers though previous employment, and were aware of their movements and the best times to reach them. Some rode with drivers in their trucks

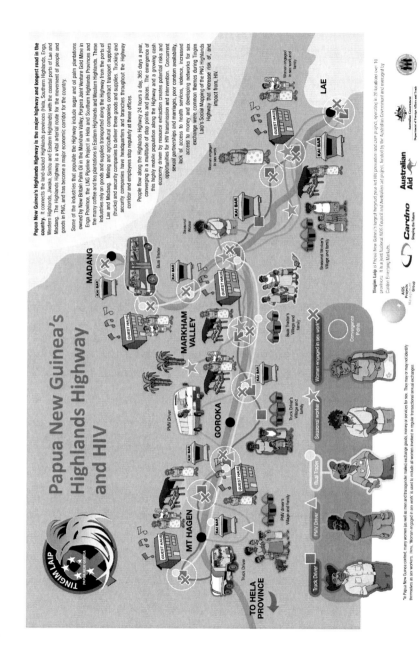

Figure 9.2 Mapping the context of HIV risk and impact along the Highlands Highway in Papua New Guinea

Source: Tingim Laip 2014. © DFAT.

along segments of the Highway and provide information, condoms and access to sexually transmitted infection and HIV testing and treatment. During peer discussions, they sought to challenge norms around sexual violence, alcohol use and the treatment of women. More often, these peer workers reached agreement with their former companies to meet with employees during muster meetings held before and after their shifts.

Environments of risk

Following the social mapping, the second phase of Tingim Laip moved away from hot spot thinking to focus on 'environments of risk'. The previous focus on stand-alone hot spots (including guest houses, bars, clubs, markets) contributed to the one-dimensional awareness raising interventions. Seeing hot spots as part of a connected environment, and understanding population movement through this environment, as well as the factors that lead people into and out of this environment, created greater opportunities for interventions addressing the social and cultural issues contributing to risk, rather than just an individual's behaviour.

Workforce and place of work

It became immediately obvious from the data that there was a mismatch between the experiences and preparedness of volunteer outreach workers from the first phase of Tingim Laip, and the individuals and groups our social mapping identified as being at significant risk of HIV. Many first phase volunteers were committed members of the community who wanted to do something about HIV and who were comfortable raising awareness in schools, workplaces and church groups. Although trained in peer counselling and support, few of them were actually peers of the people we needed to reach in the second phase of Tingim Laip. Men, often community leaders, dominated many of the volunteer committees, while women were meant to be a primary target for interventions. Many of our volunteers felt unsafe going to the places where our new key populations could be accessed, particularly after dark.

We needed to find new outreach workers who were genuine peers – that is, people who had life experiences similar to the people we wanted to work with, giving them legitimacy or permission to move through these environments, and preferably an existing member of their social networks. To provide us with additional information and options, a review of volunteer models in the PNG context was commissioned during the second phase of Tingim Laip. The report found that it would be very difficult to recruit and manage volunteers from a cadre of women who were living in insecure accommodation and trading sex for cash, food and security (van Reyk 2011). This led us to recruit paid part-time casual workers at site level: women involved in transactional sex; transgender people; men who have sex with men; security guards; oil palm estate workers. The effectiveness of this move is evident in the project's 2014 data: casual peer outreach workers spent an average of 2.5 times more hours per week on outreach and registered three times as many peers as volunteers in the same setting. This move has established a highly skilled and experienced network of members from marginalised groups, who are now gaining employment opportunities with other organisations to deliver HIV prevention outreach to key populations.

A greater focus on increasing access to services

Two of the clearest findings of the social mapping exercise were the degree to which people in PNG were on the move, and the difficulties they faced in accessing health and other social services. The study found that the people of PNG are highly mobile, moving between town and home villages for family and cultural commitments, relocating to attend school or find work, moving backwards and forwards to secure and trade goods. However, most clinical services struggle to cater for people who move in this way. One of the main aims of the second phase of Tingim Laip was to connect people to HIV, sexually transmitted infection, maternal and child health, and other services. This is difficult if people are on the move and services have limited service hours. Service providers often expect people will be willing to wait up to eight hours to be seen. Those waiting may lose their place in the queue if they go away to eat. Many respondents also reported that clinic staff in small (and some larger) towns knew who was local and who was just moving through town, and particularly knew which young women were living rough and trading sex, and were openly hostile towards these latter groups.

This led to the need to rethink some of these 'passive' referral strategies, and develop new interventions including the provision of HIV and sexually transmitted infection counselling and testing at non-clinical sites, and at times best suited to reach particular groups. For example, services were established near to a beach where traders dock their boats in the early morning during betel nut season in Oro Province and at a major truck stop late at night on the Highlands Highway. We also supported an HIV and sexually transmitted infection testing service at the early morning mustering point for oil palm workers changing shifts. These initiatives required the cooperation of different people including local clinic staff, and sometimes police to provide security.

It was clear from the social mapping data that we needed to take a longer term interest in health service clients, rather than just giving them information and a condom and expecting them to stay safe and healthy. To support this, we developed a Unique Identified Code system – a code that could be generated from answers to a series of easy-to-remember questions. This meant that no matter how mobile a client was, his or her service needs could be met across multiple sites, and could also be tracked for monitoring purposes.

Many respondents complained of barriers preventing them from accessing clinics. A series of innovations to help clients keep appointments at clinics were developed, including the provision of bus fares for getting to the clinic, and small food and drink packs to ensure that they could stay in the queue and did not have to take medications on an empty stomach. Clinic staff were also trained to reduce stigmatising attitudes and behaviours, and members of the Tingim Laip field workforce were placed in clinics to assist people to navigate the health system, understand test results and decide on their next health care steps. An anonymous card-based referral system gave clients priority to services on particular days – reducing the waiting time and overcoming the stigma they felt in asking for sexually transmitted infection services.

Conclusions

The social mapping study provided Tingim Laip with an opportunity to reconnect with the populations it most needed to serve. The pause in funding and activity between the first and second phases of the project resulted in a significant drift away from these populations. The remaining workforce was not well equipped or supported to go into the environments they most needed to be in, and in many cases did not have enough in common with the people they needed to reach. Taking an ethnographic approach to the social mapping put us in direct contact with the people we needed to be working with, and provided us with a much clearer understanding of the types of interventions that would put them in the best possible position to respond to HIV prevention in their own populations. It also signalled strongly to them that the people in the second phase of Tingim Laip were interested in understanding them and working with them, not just documenting their sexual behaviour.

The information we obtained was directly relevant to the design of the new interventions in the second phase of Tingim Laip, and in particular, laid the groundwork for the hiring of people from key populations as peer educators, condom distributors and field managers. It resulted in a significant improvement in the participation of people from key populations in our work and a significant increase in the number of people we were able to reach in subsequent years.

Although it was time and resource intensive, and presented the project and the research teams with significant logistical challenges, getting this close, both physically and emotionally, to the people we needed to work with led to long-term engagement that has survived throughout the remainder of the project. It brought lasting cultural change in the project, particularly in relation to issues of power and opportunity. The methodology developed has proven to be effective in increasing detailed programme knowledge, as well as in shifting organisational culture relating to the manner in which programmes are designed and put 'back on track' during their implementation.

References

Adler, S.M. (2004) 'Multiple layers of a researcher's identity: uncovering Asian American voices', in K. Mutua and B.B. Swadener (eds) *Decolonizing Research in Cross-Cultural Contexts: Critical personal narratives*. Albany, NY: State University of New York Press, pp. 107–121.

Al-Busaidi, Z.Q. (2008) 'Qualitative research and its uses in health care', *Sultan Qaboos University Medical Journal*, 8(1): 11–19.
Anderson, B. (2006) *Imagined Communities: Reflections on the origins of the nation state*, London: Verso Books.
Asian Development Bank (2006) *Proposed Asian Development Fund Grant Papua New Guinea: HIV/AIDS prevention and control in rural development enclaves project*. Available at: www.adb.org/sites/default/files/project-document/68506/39033-png-rrp.pdf (accessed 23 March 2015).
AusAID (2007) *Independent Evaluation of Tingim Laip: Draft final Report*. Canberra: AusAID. Available at: www.apmglobalhealth.com/tingimlaip (accessed 23 March 2015).
AusAID (2010) *Tingim Laip Phase 2: Value Life – project design document*. Canberra: AusAID.
AusAID (2012) *PNG Tingim Laip Phase 2, Contract 56225, IRM Review Report*. Available at: http://dfat.gov.au/about-us/publications/Documents/png-tingim-laip-phase-2-independent-review-mechanism.pdf (accessed 23 March 2015).
Burr, V. (1995) *An Introduction to Social Constructionism*, London: Routledge.
Chamraz, K. (2006) *Constructing Grounded Theory: A practical guide through qualitative analysis*, London: SAGE.
Emerson, R., Fretz, R. and Shaw, L. (2011) *Writing Ethnographic Fieldnotes*, Chicago, IL: Chicago University Press.
Hammar, L. (2007) 'Epilogue: homegrown in PNG – rural responses to HIV and AIDS', *Oceania*, 77(1): 72–94.
Herzfeld, M. (2005) *Cultural Intimacy: Social poetics in the nation-state*. New York: Routledge.
Hood, J. (2007) 'Orthodoxy vs. power: the defining traits of grounded theory', in A. Bryant and K. Charmaz (eds) *The SAGE Handbook of Grounded Theory*, London: SAGE, pp. 151–164.
Kelly, A. (2009) 'The role of social research in the response efforts to the HIV epidemic in Papua New Guinea', *Papua New Guinea Medical Journal*, 52(1–2): 35–43.
Kelly, A., Kupul, M., Man, W.Y.N., Nosi, S., Lote, N., Rawstorne, P., Halim, G., Ryan, C. and Worth, H. (2011) *Askim na save (Ask and understand): People who sell and/or exchange sex in Port Moresby*, Sydney: Papua New Guinea Institute of Medical Research and UNSW Australia.
Liamputtong, P. (2007) *Researching the Vulnerable: A guide to sensitive research methods*, New York: Cambridge University Press.
Liamputtong, P. (2010) *Performing Qualitative Cross Cultural Research*, New York: Cambridge University Press.
NHASP (2005) *Social Mapping of Nineteen Provinces in Papua New Guinea: Summary report*, Port Moresby: National HIV AIDS Support Project.
PNG Department of Health (2014) *Interim Global AIDS Response Progress & Universal Access Reports Papua New Guinea*. Available at: www.unaids.org/sites/default/files/country/documents//PNG_narrative_report_2014.pdf (accessed 23 March 2015).
PNG National AIDS Council (2006) *High Risk Settings Strategy Report: Moving beyond awareness*, Port Moresby: PNG National AIDS Council.
PNG National AIDS Council (2011) *PNG National HIV and AIDS Strategy 2011–2015*, Port Moresby: PNG National AIDS Council.
Steinar, K. and Svend, B. (2009) *InterViews: Learning the craft of qualitative research interviewing*, Thousand Oaks, CA: SAGE.

Stewart, C. (2014) *Name, Shame and Blame: Criminalising consensual sex in Papua New Guinea*, Canberra: Australian National University Press.

Tingim Laip (2012) *Briefing Note STEPs Model*. Available at: http://apmglobalhealth.com/project/tingim-laip-project-png (accessed 23 March 2015).

UNDP (2014) *About Papua New Guinea*. Available at: www.pg.undp.org/content/papua_new_guinea/en/home/countryinfo (accessed 23 March 2015).

van Reyk, P. (2011) *The Price of Work Sol: A review of Tingim Laip volunteer activity*. Available at: www.apmglobalhealth.com/tingimlaip (accessed 23 March 2015).

10

Pathways to impact

New approaches to monitoring and improving volunteering for sustainable environmental management

Jody Aked

Introduction

The time, energy, wisdom, experience, knowledge and skills that people give to helping one another are often the spontaneous result of human relationships and community life (Halpern 2009), but volunteering is also organised and managed consciously by international development organisations as a means of achieving social development. Arguably, volunteering's contribution as an approach to development has been undervalued in efforts to secure peace, progress and human well-being (United Nations Volunteering 2011), manifest in recent trends to reduce core funding to many long-standing international volunteer cooperation organisations (Lough and Matthew 2013). This has been triggered partly by a culture of auditing and accountability that has made money a central criterion in public decision making, despite recognition that non-monetary impacts (e.g. social and environmental value) are often those that make the biggest difference in people's lives (NEF Consulting 2013). For example, some of the capacities considered crucial for emancipatory social change are the soft and intangible ones (such as identity, confidence and the capacity to establish relationships), which also happen to be the most difficult to identify and develop (Clarke and Oswald 2010). For development programmes working to create change in ways that cannot be easily expressed in monetary or concrete project deliverables (e.g. donations collected, local amenities provided), pressure has been increasing to demonstrate a 'return on investment' for funders (Maxwell et al. 2011).

The indirect, slow and subtle ways in which interventions such as volunteering, as compared with the direct provision of aid or infrastructure projects, work to effect social and political change creates particular challenges for monitoring programme processes and assessing impact. This is especially the case with change processes that are neither wholly technical (The World Bank Institute 2013) nor linear in character (Ramalingam and Jones 2008). End of programme evaluations may provide a snapshot of what has been achieved, but can make it difficult to elicit any insight into *how* change was arrived at in order to attribute contributions to factors such as volunteer effort. Lengthy time lags between the collection and analysis of data, and the application of findings, also make it difficult to use insights to innovate and learn (Marks 2011).

To date, academic research has not been able to offer practitioners much help in these matters, with few studies looking at the links between volunteer activity and development impact (see Lough and Matthew 2013 for overview). To understand volunteering as a force for social change we cannot simply add up all the individual actions people take to explain impact. Rather, we need to find approaches that can explore multiple actions and interactions across a whole system or set of relationships (Burns *et al.* 2012), while also appreciating the contextual nuances and interdependencies of change pathways (Ramalingam and Jones 2008). Global and programmatic theories of change that map the intended relationships between volunteer action and change may be strategically important in communicating with funders, but without on-going monitoring of programme processes it is difficult to verify or adapt the assumptions that underpin them.

This chapter draws on research recently conducted in partnership with Voluntary Services Overseas (VSO) in the Philippines. The research used training in systemic action research to integrate the use of interpretive methods, participatory approaches and systemic thinking into the monitoring of a volunteering programme focusing on the sustainable management of natural resources. It shows how a different approach to monitoring progress, grounded in cycles of action and learning about the realities of practice and experience, can support volunteers to review, adapt and improve the activities they devoted their energies to, while they were still active in the community's development.

The International Citizen Service (ICS) programme

The International Citizen Service (ICS) 2012–2015 is a £60 million programme supported by the UK Government's Department for International Development (DFID) to enable 18–25 year olds to contribute to development through international volunteering. The initiative is expected to have a development impact in the placement community as well as an impact on the volunteer (ITAD 2011). Since October 2012, the ICS programme has been operating via VSO in the Philippines, providing a platform for young people from the Philippines and the UK to work together and make practical contributions to communities facing marginalisation or challenging situations. On the island of Bohol in the Visayas region of the Philippines, multiple cycles of ICS volunteers have worked with local government units, schools, the university and community actors in independent community-based associations called 'people's organisations'. The aim is to achieve the sustainable management of natural resources found within an area of land called the Carood Watershed. Its water system serves rivers, basins and coastal waters that span six municipal boundaries.

Following recruitment, assessment and selection, ten British volunteers are paired with ten Filipino volunteers before they arrive on the island of Bohol.

Pre-departure and in-country training are provided before volunteers settle into their new home and work life for three months. They are supported by two locally based ICS programme supervisors who find host homes for the volunteers and liaise with volunteer placement supervisors to agree work programmes and role descriptions. On arrival, volunteers usually receive briefing by ICS programme supervisors and their volunteer placement supervisors to discuss deliverables. Volunteers usually work in pairs or small teams to influence prevailing social and environmental issues by raising awareness about the watershed and associated risks, affecting behaviour among farmers and residents in relation to the watershed, and building capacity for local youth action and engagement with the management council.

Volunteers are supported to reflect on volunteer outcomes and community outcomes through structured review spaces, usually involving an initial retreat midway through the three-month placement and a second one at the end. This is in addition to one-on-one supervision by ICS programme supervisors themselves. Programme supervisors also meet with all the volunteer placement supervisors at the end of the cycle to collect feedback. The regularity of these review processes almost functions as a continual monitoring process. But there are two notable limitations. First, this learning typically takes place outside of the theory of change and accompanying monitoring and evaluation frameworks that have been introduced by the ICS programme globally, and separate from the annual partnership review between VSO and the local watershed management council. Second, existing review processes tend to focus more on the process of managing volunteers rather than understanding how and why change is, or is not, happening. For example, placement descriptions are not typically created or validated with the wider community, so they are not informed by the experiences of local youth groups, farmers and residents. This makes it difficult to know with any certainty that volunteer action is relevant and effective in changing people's lives. In response, the research described here sought to introduce ways of plugging knowledge gaps about the impact of volunteer efforts on social and environmental outcomes.

Systemic action research and its interpretive basis

Systemic action research (SAR) (Burns 2007) provides the methodological basis to support volunteers to monitor and assess impact. As an approach to social development, action research can be used to change things for the better (Greenwood and Levin 1998), through the production of practical knowledge (Reason and Bradbury 2001) that is useful to people. It can be carried out by individuals who adopt an enquiring approach to their assumptions and actions. It can also happen when people join together to explore issues of a mutual interest or it can be used more systemically as a tool to prompt a whole community, organisation or network to engage in experimental cycles of action and reflection.

SAR can be thought of as providing a learning architecture for embedding action in change processes (e.g. at the project level) within an analysis of how wider systems (e.g. political processes, institutional practices, and the social and cultural systems of a community) are organised. A systemic perspective views life and efforts to change it as inherently complex. Practitioners working in a systemic way seek to understand the connectedness, relationships, contexts and feedbacks that help to explain why some patterns of behaviour are resilient, some re-establish themselves and some change altogether. This often involves extending enquiry beyond a single group or a single case to bring in different perspectives and to build as complete a picture as possible to describe what is going on and how to best influence it: 'Good systemic work is dependent on a strong network of group-based inquiries that are in turn dependent on strong reflective practice at the individual level' (Burns 2007: 16). By bridging action research and systemic thinking, efforts are made to bring to light the assumptions and relationships that structure the way things get done while supporting actors within the system to continually make sense of their efforts and the (intended and unintended) effects they have.

SAR (Burns 2007) shares a number of principles with other interpretive approaches to research and evaluation. For instance, it rejects prevailing tendencies in social scientific research and programme evaluation to use data to demonstrate that x leads to y, rather than to understand what is happening and why (Bell and Aggleton 2012). It is interested in systems of meaning, trying to go beyond Geertz's (1973) idea of 'thin description' (what you can observe) to generating 'thick description' (focusing on the meaning behind actions). It searches for patterns in thought and behaviour (e.g. by identifying social norms) that may explain energy for or resistance against change, extending inquiry beyond an individual or group so it is situated in a context and proactively seeking multiple perspectives (Genat 2009). Finally, SAR incorporates the knowledge it generates from considering multiple realities and systems interactions into cycles of learning and action, whereby observation and reflection informs planning and action, and action informs the next round of reflection. The overall aim therefore is to create a social learning process in which participants are involved in the data collection and sense-making processes (see Figure 10.1).

SAR has been described as a participatory research approach (Burns 2012) because it encourages actors in the research process to interrogate their own assumptions between intent, action and effect, so that 'people "see" and "feel" the connection between things; they "know" that it is related to their experience; they are "energised" and "motivated"' (Burns 2007: 53). The on-going and cyclical nature of this learning process means people are encouraged to make adjustments to their interpretations of the wider systems of which they are part and that influence and get influenced by their social actions.

Training volunteers in systemic action research

The cycle of volunteers that took part in the study between March and May 2013 were asked to take stock of previous volunteer efforts by carrying out a capacity

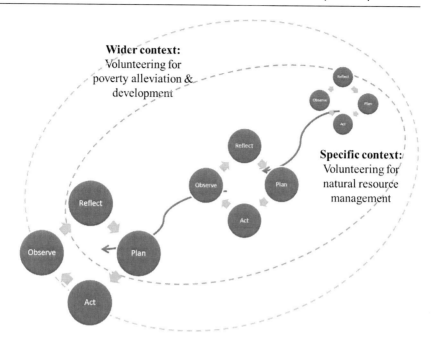

Figure 10.1 Systemic action research as an approach to understanding and enhancing volunteer action

and needs assessment of existing and recently established youth organisations located within the boundaries of the watershed. This created an opportunity to infuse programmatic thinking with locally grounded explanations about programme impact, issues and priorities going forward.

The immersive nature of the volunteering programme means the volunteers are well positioned to make use of interpretive methods. They are set up to engage with local people and embed themselves in community life, naturally blurring distinctions between the observer and the observed so typical of positivist paradigms (Ellen 1984). But effective volunteers – such as interpretive researchers – are not purely a function of their immersion or connectivity to local actors; ways of being and interacting are important for realising and sustaining discernible social and environmental change (Aked 2014).

Over three days, ten UK volunteers, nine Filipino volunteers and three Filipino volunteers from the previous cycle learned and experienced different approaches and techniques from interpretive research, participatory approaches and systemic thinking (see Table 10.1).

In addition, the volunteers learned skills in interviewing, translation, validation, documentation and ethics. The training blended theory with practice. By the end of the three-day period volunteers had used all the tools they had learned about, reflecting on what worked and what had not as a basis for planning their

Table 10.1 Tools and techniques included in the volunteer training

Tool/technique	Principles-based learning	Action-based learning
Storytelling Adapted from www.globalgiving.org/storytelling	Using open-ended questions Giving people the tools to analyse their own stories Using informal spaces and interactions to learn	Reviewed a storytelling form designed as a community and complexity-based feedback tool Used informal approach to collect stories from the community
Storyboard Adapted from www.proveandimprove.org/tools/proveit.php	What is participation and whose knowledge counts? Talking to local people before a project/activity is designed Involving local people in the evaluation of an initiative or activity	Used the storyboard as a group of volunteers to map out how they think their efforts will make a difference Facilitated a session with a local youth group to help them think through their own story about how their actions will make a difference
Social network mapping Adapted from www.netmap.wordpress.com	Weak and strong ties Resource flows between actors Understanding and disrupting power relations	Used individually to visually map who helps them as volunteers to achieve their goals Group work to look for patterns across the social network maps
Systems mapping of local issues Adapted from Burns (2007)	A systemic view of development Assets as well as needs Distributive versus command-and-control leadership Validating abstractions with different stakeholders	Used in small groups to categorise and visually map links between issues, stakeholders, observations, unanswered questions and opportunities for action

work. Follow-up support was provided remotely over the phone and directly at a mid-phase review in which the group was facilitated to analyse collectively the insights generated and to consider possibilities for communicating and acting on these. Towards the end of the three-month placement, work was undertaken to understand what, if any, difference the SAR training had made to the day-to-day work of volunteers. Insights were gathered from several sources, including a group session to map experiences against the global theory of change for the ICS programme, a series of six semi-structured interviews with volunteers, informal ad hoc discussions with one of the ICS Programme Supervisors, and an anonymous evaluation of the training completed by the volunteers.

Reviewing, learning and adapting

A SAR approach introduced new research and sense-making techniques for reviewing the use of volunteering for social and environmental change within the ICS programme. It enabled volunteers and other programme actors to monitor the suitability of project activities and make use of their insights to adapt project work to local realities while *in situ*.

Assessing appropriateness of project activities in the first action-learning cycle

At the training stage, few of the volunteers had engaged with community members (other than their host homes) about the local realities of conserving and managing the watershed. During the action-based learning components of training, volunteers went to the local market, bus stop and local stores to start informal conversations, use open-ended questions and collect stories from resident adults. They used a storyboard exercise (see Table 10.1) with a local youth group to gain knowledge about issues, interests and challenges from young people's own perspectives. With permission, they began to use this information to situate environmental issues within a wider social context. For example, one of their 'systems maps' – a visual map linking issues, stakeholders and observations (see Table 10.1) – plotted how the opinions and actions of young people are often disregarded by adults because young people are not perceived as being capable or serious (see Figure 10.2).

On mapping their own social networks (see Table 10.1), volunteers realised the centrality of the VSO programme supervisors and host homes in providing support and initial connections in the wider community. The process of reviewing their social networks revealed how some volunteers had received more help from supervisors in their work placements than others, and prompted discussion about how to be effective in three months when supervisors have heavy workloads. Together, these sorts of insights made up the first major action-learning cycle. Volunteers had adopted an inquiring approach to their experiences and had gathered knowledge from residents to reflect on some of the social dynamics affecting environmental outcomes.

At the end of training, volunteers revisited the storyboard they had made together to consider how their activities contributed to bringing about change. At this stage, volunteers had new information about the change context and ideas about the sorts of actions they could take. It became clear from the immediate (within 2 months), medium-term (within 2–6 months) and long-term (over a year) changes the volunteers expected to see, that sustainability and some form of legacy were seen as major barometers of success. This was particularly the case given what had been learned about previous efforts by volunteers to work with youth organisations. Conversations with youth leaders revealed that some of the 19 local youth groups on their list had not met since the last cycle of ICS volunteers had left.

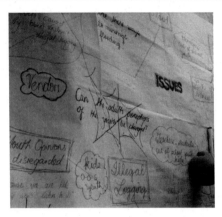

Figure 10.2 A small group of volunteers create a systems map with community-generated insights

A federation to represent all the youth organisations working on issues related to environmental management of the watershed had been initiated three months earlier by the previous volunteers, but no follow-up action had taken place to elect members nor set a vision and remit. The use of the storyboard exercise with the local youth group to explore how their plans would result in change suggested local youth groups faced real barriers to working together. These barriers included lack of meeting space, poor communication, lack of financial resources to cover transport, and non-acceptance by adults, including parents.

The thought processes initiated by the methods used in training also prompted volunteers to reflect on the limitation of their own role and position. In the final session, volunteers spontaneously discussed what was achievable within three months, and what their focus should be. Should they work with a large number of local youth groups or only a few? How should they balance the demands of the placement descriptions they had been given with the work that needed to be undertaken to ensure that youth groups were active and sustainable? Other questions asked were more practical, such as how could volunteers access youth groups attached to schools during the semester break?

The discussion was unexpected, disconcerting, and at times uncomfortable. As participants made sense of the data collected, they realised they had some fundamental concerns about the appropriateness of the activities they had been tasked to do. It was fortunate that this session had been joined by the two ICS programme supervisors who were happy to permit the conversation to unfold. Rather than gloss over the disruption or offer instant solutions, they asked as many questions back as they received from the volunteers. The practice of using interpretive data to reflect and refocus informed what volunteers worked on for the remainder of their placement. Some volunteers re-wrote the placement descriptions they had been given, so they could plan their time according to where they felt they could make the biggest difference. For instance, the volunteers decided to prioritise re-establishing contact with existing youth groups rather than starting afresh with new people. In so doing, the volunteers veered away from protocol within the global ICS programme that proposed that they should only count (and thereby prioritise) work undertaken with new participants of events, trainings, seminars and workshops in reporting frameworks. The local perspectives sought through the SAR process influenced how the volunteers made sense of their role as a form of capacity building that would take concentrated effort with a smaller but consistent group of local actors.

Adapting implementation in subsequent action-learning cycles

The volunteers continued to make use of the principles and methods learned in SAR training over the remaining three months, both in their work supporting local youth groups and in other placement activities such as Community Action Days on particular environmental topics. Overall, it was possible to identify a number of different ways in which the integration of interpretive methods, participatory approaches and systemic thinking in day-to-day project work had affected how volunteers worked and what they did.

Volunteers continued to use informal conversation, meetings and story collection to actively seek community input into project ideas, and this information helped tailor activities to local realities. For example, one group of volunteers responsible for the organisation of a Community Action Day in their municipality found out about existing policy work in local government before making a decision about what to focus on. Rather than campaign about something completely unrelated, the volunteers organised a community procession about waste to support government actions to reduce the use of plastic bags in the market and in local stores. The volunteers went one step further and used the procession as an opportunity to informally interview residents at the market to gather local opinions about an ordinance that would ban plastic bags altogether. As actors who now had the ear of the local government, the volunteers prompted reflection at the community level about proposed changes, and then reported views back to government officers to inform decisions about the policy.

Another group of volunteers made a decision to drop plans to mobilise the community for World Water Day and reorient their efforts elsewhere. Following a request from VSO to organise something to mark the international event, they sought advice from local government officers who suggested a river clean up. The volunteers visited the site and found the river clean. Next, they were advised to plant trees. They talked to local people and realised previous efforts on the part of volunteers to plant trees at the site had not succeeded because of persistent flooding. As the ICS programme supervisor later reflected:

> With the water thing we went about the research in the wrong way. We identified water as the issue and then tried to fit things round it. Rather than figure out what the issue is ... They [the volunteers] interviewed people, they took pictures and we have concluded we are not doing a Community Action Day [CAD] on water. The water was pristine ... The next lot can target the CADs a lot better. They can use these tools to try and find out about things, as opposed to just choosing them.
>
> (ICS programme supervisor)

Volunteers did not only have to challenge the appropriateness of the expectations placed on them, they also demonstrated a willingness to adapt their own ideas about what might be useful based on what they learned. In an account of change linked to the coordination and creation of a new youth group, one volunteer reflected:

> We wanted to do a tree-building activity but we did a needs assessment and the ground was too hard. We were going to do a coastal clean-up but the river was pristine. So we created a calendar of events which is practical: tree planting in the rainy season and coastal-clean up in the summer season when it gets dirty.
>
> (ICS volunteer)

The iterative way in which volunteers went about their work allowed space for assumptions to be challenged and new possibilities to open up. This modelled the action-learning cycles emphasised during training, making efforts more appropriate to local conditions.

The principle of triangulating different stakeholder's perspectives and experiences to create and validate a systemic picture of local issues helped volunteers to uncover new information. For example, frequent visits to the proposed site of the river clean-up for World Water Day revealed the underlying cause of the waste management issue to be the collection of garbage, and not the cleanliness of the water. Residents had paid for collection but because of a dispute between the village leader and the mayor of the municipality the garbage was not being collected. A river clean-up was not going to address the root cause of the environmental problem, which was primarily political.

Efforts by volunteers to find the issues that held most significance or resonance with different stakeholders also helped reassess where to direct energies. In one reflective account, a volunteer talked about how he had built from the initial direction given by their work placement supervisor to make a decision about how to focus his work:

> When I asked specifically for the main problems she [the Volunteer Placement Supervisor] went through the seven environmental problems and listed six of the seven out ... We did the storyboard activity with the first

youth group we met in San Roje high school. We asked what they thought was the main problem in Mabini and they said waste management. After that we went into the community and asked them and they said waste management. So most people agreed it was waste management ... so this is how we came to be working on waste management.

(ICS volunteer)

Incorporating a range of different voices into the assessment and planning process required building relationships in both formal (e.g. government offices) and informal (e.g. at the market) spaces. In a facilitated session to map volunteers' own experience of change to the ICS global theory of change at the programmatic level, the importance of establishing and building relationships was emphasised. Volunteers wanted to include 'connecting organisations through networks' as an outcome of their work, to capture the work they did to mobilise different individuals and groups around a common cause. Some were surprised that relational outcomes were not listed in the global theory of change. A group activity to map these connections identified that volunteers collectively had made over 60 new connections to organisations working locally on environmental issues and had strengthened a further 30 connections. As well as with youth groups, they had engaged with radio stations, Barangay [village] officials, Department for Environment and Natural Resources staff, residents, politicians and Disaster Risk Reduction Management officers.

The insights volunteers generated on the appropriateness and effectiveness of volunteer activities also influenced thinking outside the placement site. For example, the emphasis on the relational aspects of volunteer work triggered further inquiry to identify the qualities of volunteer relationships that make a difference in change processes. One year later an email arrived from a senior staff member of VSO in the Philippines saying that the findings of this work were informing discussion of their theory of change in a monitoring and evaluation workshop. The principal researcher discussed the training in SAR with a counterpart in Kenya, who adopted a similar approach to incorporate training in participatory approaches and systemic thinking into the in-country induction process for the ICS programme. The production of a training pack, in combination with testing different SAR approaches in Ghana, Mozambique and Nepal, has prompted staff at VSO International to consider ways in which they can more firmly embed SAR – and its associated methods – into volunteer training.

Challenges and enablers to learning on the job

Volunteers were positive in their evaluation of SAR training at the end of their placements. Over 85 per cent of the volunteers thought it had helped to make them more effective as volunteers and over 90 per cent said they would recommend something similar to other volunteers.

> It gave the whole team a clearer direction and a better understanding of our role as volunteers in Bohol, Philippines.
> (ICS volunteer, evaluation feedback form)

> For the work we were doing, it gave guidance and knowledge on how to establish the real issue.
> (ICS volunteer, evaluation feedback form)

> It allowed us a means of gathering research that was pertinent in discovering the needs of the community, thus giving us areas of work to focus on.
> (ICS volunteer, evaluation feedback form)

In their end of placement reports, volunteers provided numerous examples of how they had used the tools and techniques. In one or two cases, individuals had gone a step further in the participatory process and trained local youth groups in methods such as story collection and storyboards. This was one example of taking a systemic approach. Volunteers had extended the action research beyond their own reflections as individuals or a group by providing interpretive methods and reflection spaces to community members. This enabled a new set of actors in the change process to interpret and make decisions about how to make better use of volunteering for development.

Overall, using interpretive methods in structured cycles of action and learning was engaging and rewarding. It was energising for the volunteers to understand the relationship between the local context, what they wanted to do, and what they want to achieve. This is quite different to operating in a vacuum of project 'deliverables' where the connections between things are not seen or felt by those who are experiencing and shaping interventions.

The importance assigned in the SAR approach to encouraging volunteers and community actors to be 'active' in their learning about change pathways is supported by research in behavioural psychology. People are more likely to find a course of action purposeful and rewarding if they experience choice with respect to it, efficacy engaging in it, and a connection to those involved in the process (Ryan 2009). The combined qualities of this experience – a sense of autonomy, competency and relatedness – support the psychosocial foundations of people's well-being, which studies show can influence how effective they are at reviewing possibilities and shaping their environments (Fredrickson and Branigan 2005, Thompson and Marks 2008).

This is not to say that working in an iterative way with interpretive data is always easy, or that change is straightforward at the programmatic level. The challenge in facilitating SAR is that it has the power to disrupt, sometimes shaking the foundations of people's belief systems about the wider world and expectations about their role within it. The process of examining root causes, actions and effects against experiences that have occurred in real people's lives demands deep thinking and levels of critical reflection that people are not always used to. The process can dramatically reduce energy levels in a room, especially when people begin to challenge their own and others' assumptions. They can suddenly feel lost or at sea, unsure of themselves, their role and their actions. Within a training environment, it is possible to channel doubt or ambiguity by ending discursive sessions with activities that focus on positives, or chart next steps, so people have concrete things to do with their learning.

It is more difficult to support people to incorporate learning into more effective decision making when confidence dwindles in the field. Despite experiencing a full action-learning cycle during training, it was still unnerving for volunteers when community experiences and locally grounded insights went against what the wider ICS programme advocated or what local officials recommended. Volunteers agonised over the decision (described earlier) to pull the plug on an event to mobilise community action to celebrate World Water Day. The original action had been requested by VSO so they felt a responsibility to deliver. They were also surprised to have received such poor advice from local officials when efforts to triangulate with community members indicated that the river clean-up and tree planting would have little or no environmental impact. The decision to disregard the guidance of people in positions of authority to follow what volunteers themselves had learned from the community took a degree of conviction. It took time for volunteers to feel comfortable in themselves about missing a project 'deliverable', even though doing so made sense from a wider social change perspective.

ICS volunteers were able to remain responsive because they had the support of the locally placed programme supervisors and the facilitator of the SAR. This encouraged reflection and self-critical awareness among volunteers, and created a safe environment in which to change direction or try new things out, even if this meant the occasional false start. Rather than provide solutions about what to do, volunteers were encouraged to trust in themselves, their processes and the conclusions arrived at. This reassurance may have upheld the sense of autonomy, competency and relatedness among volunteers sufficiently to enable both the resilience and behavioural flexibility needed to remain committed and responsive to local realities.

Together, these findings point to the sort of leadership required at the institutional level to engender confidence among front-line workers in social development to act on ideas they develop through new relationships, understandings and perspectives. The act of facilitating systemic action research can lead to a catalysing, bottom-up form of learning and coordination that has been described in the leadership literature as an approach to fostering the conditions for followers to innovate in complex change situations (Marion and Uhl-Bien 2001). In these contexts, where change introduces unpredictability and flux, it has been argued that effective results are not responsive to approaches that impose a single course of action through the use of experts or replication of best practice (Snowden and Boone 2007). Instead, learning architectures and processes are needed to create the conditions for volunteers and other front-line workers to 'probe, sense and respond' (Snowden and Boone 2007: 4). Using a SAR approach, we were able to increase levels of interaction and communication about impact between volunteers and, at senior management level, create insights that resonated more accurately with the local scenario than the global monitoring and evaluation logframe, encourage dissent and diversity in how volunteers approached their work and monitor it for surprising outcomes. Viewed in this way, SAR offered a form of leadership, supporting participants towards new understandings of local realities and their role within them.

The wider implication of this insight is the need for a more sophisticated relationship with theories of change and monitoring and evaluation frameworks in development organisations. A more realistic positioning of theories of change and monitoring and evaluation frameworks as a collection of hypotheses rather than blue prints may permit a more adaptive and appropriate response to implementation. As this study illustrates, interpretive approaches can locate our planning and assessment tools in community and practitioner realities in ways that should strengthen a return on investment. As a group of organisations working to enable development through human exchange, the volunteering sector is uniquely placed to demonstrate the value of rebalancing investment in social development towards people and processes. This study is one small step towards highlighting the benefits of moving away from the indiscriminate provision of technical assistance and rigid output-based results frameworks towards new architectures for learning that can support actors to generate responsive solutions.

Conclusion

In this chapter, I have described a different approach to monitoring progress that trained 22 Filipino and British volunteers in the Philippines to integrate interpretive data into cycles of participatory action and learning. The results of this process were encouraging, with volunteers demonstrating greater knowledge of local development issues, which informed the decisions later taken to deviate from project plans to make their contribution to social and environmental outcomes as relevant and effective as possible. Importantly, these insights were not gained by reducing the complexity of change processes to simplistic explanations about the cause of problems and the volunteers' role in positively influencing these. Rather, volunteers increased their capacity and confidence to integrate insights generated from new relationships, understandings and perspectives into their planning and implementation.

Community-level inputs that called into question programmatic expectations about project deliverables or advice received from local authority figures presented the biggest challenge to volunteers. Findings point to the importance of leadership qualities inherent in an action research approach and the need for a more sophisticated relationship with theories of change and monitoring and evaluation frameworks. This is especially the case in social development organisations striving to chart pathways to impact that go beyond the provision of technical assistance to include the processes that support development actors to learn on the job with local people.

References

Aked, J. (2014) 'How youth volunteer networks translate into relationships for change: participatory systemic action research to explore interpersonal wellbeing processes in the governance of a watershed in the Philippines', *International Society for Third Sector Research Working Paper Series*, IX: 1–45.

Bell, S.A. and Aggleton, P. (2012) 'Integrating ethnographic principles in NGO monitoring and impact evaluation', *Journal of International Development*, 24: 795–807.

Burns, D. (2007) *Systemic Action Research: A strategy for whole system change*, Bristol: The Policy Press.

Burns, D. (2012) 'Participatory systemic inquiry', *IDS Bulletin*, 43(3): 88–100.

Burns, D., Harvey, B. and Aragon, A.O. (2012) 'Introduction: action research for development and social change', *IDS Bulletin*, 43(3): 1–7.

Clarke, P. and Oswald, K. (2010) 'Introduction: Why reflect collectively on capacities for change?', *IDS Bulletin*, 41(3): 1–12.

Ellen, R. (1984) *Ethnographic Research: A guide to general conduct*, London: Academic Press.

Fredrickson, B.L. and Branigan, C. (2005) 'Positive emotions broaden the scope of attention and thought-action repertoires', *Cognition and Emotion*, 19(3): 313–332.

Geertz, C. (1973) *The Interpretation of Cultures: Selected essays*, New York: Basic Books.

Genat, B. (2009) 'Building emergent situated knowledges in participatory action research', *Action Research*, 7(1): 101–115.

Greenwood, D.J. and Levin, M. (1998) 'Action research, science, and the co-optation of social research', *Studies in Cultures, Organizations and Societies*, 4(2): 237–261.

Halpern, D. (2009) *The Hidden Wealth of Nations*, Cambridge: Polity Press.

ITAD, (2011) *Final Mid Term Review Evaluation of DFID's International Citizen Service (ICS) Pilot Stage*. Available at: www.gov.uk/government/uploads/system/uploads/attachment_data/file/67460/eval-int-citz-serv-ics-pilot-stg.pdf (accessed 4 March 2015).

Lough, B.J. and Matthew, L. (2013) *Measuring and Conveying the Added Value of International Volunteering. Forum Discussion Paper*. Available at: http://forum-ids.org/2013/12/forum-discussion-paper-2013-measuring-and-conveying-added-value (accessed 4 March 2015).

Marion, R. and Uhl-Bien, M. (2001) 'Leadership in complex organizations', *The Leadership Quarterly*, 12(4): 389–418.

Marks, N. (2011) 'Think before you think', in R. Biswas-Diener (ed.) *Positive Psychology as Social Change*, Dordrecht: Springer Netherlands, pp. 17–32.

Maxwell, S., Henderson, D., McCloy, R. and Harper, G. (2011) *Social Impacts and Wellbeing: Multi-criteria analysis techniques for integrating non-monetary evidence in valuation and appraisal*, London: Department for Environment, Food and Rural Affairs.

NEF Consulting, (2013) 'The value of money: challenging the preconceptions', *Perspectives*, 2: 1–24.

Ramalingam, B. and Jones, H. (2008) *Exploring the Science of Complexity: Ideas and implications for development and humanitarian efforts*, London: Overseas Development Institute.

Reason, P. and Bradbury, H. (2001) *The SAGE Handbook of Action Research. Participatory Inquiry and Practice*, London: SAGE.

Ryan, R. (2009) *Self-determination Theory and Wellbeing*, Bath: Wellbeing in Developing Countries, University of Bath.

Snowden, D.J. and Boone, M.E. (2007) 'A leader's framework for decision making', *Harvard Business Review*, 1–9. Available at: www.charity-works.co.uk/wp-content/uploads/2013/04/A_Leaders_Framework_for_Decision_Making.pdf (accessed 4 March 2015).

The World Bank Institute, (2013) *Leadership: The World Bank Institute's Leadership for Development Program*. Available at: http://wbi.worldbank.org/wbi/content/leadership-world-bank-institute%E2%80%99s-leadership-development-program (accessed 4 March 2015).

Thompson, S. and Marks, N. (2008) *Measuring Well-being in Policy: Issues and applications*, London: New Economics Foundation.

United Nations Volunteering (2011) *State of the World's Volunteerism Report*, Denmark: United Nations publication.

11

Ethnographic process evaluation

A case study of an HIV prevention programme with injecting drug users in the USA

Yan Alicia Hong, Shannon Gwin Mitchell, James A. Peterson, Carl Latkin and Karin Tobin

Introduction

There is recognition that complex programmes that move beyond a focus on individual-level behaviour change have been central to recent advances in treatment and prevention as part of the global response to HIV (Sumartojo 2000, Rotheram-Borus et al. 2009). Multilevel structural interventions that take into consideration the complex interactions of individuals within social, cultural, economic and political environments have led to more effective and sustained change and effects (Latkin and Knowlton 2005, Ogden et al. 2011). Examples of structural interventions to reduce HIV risks include housing assistance for homeless people, needle exchange programmes for injecting drug users and micro-finance schemes for low-income women (Gupta et al. 2008, Rotheram-Borus et al. 2009). However, with these changes comes the challenge of how best to monitor and evaluate the impact of these structural interventions, as well as understand how successful complex interventions can be adapted and implemented in other settings.

Process evaluation is important when trying to understand the extent to which programmes are delivered as planned, as well as how and why interventions work. Ethnographic approaches to process evaluation are particularly useful when trying to monitor and evaluate complex, structural interventions due to its unique strength in gathering local interpretations to help understand the context and mechanisms of change. In this chapter we focus on an ethnographic process evaluation of an HIV prevention programme among injecting drug users in Baltimore, USA (Hong et al. 2005) to illustrate the benefits of using this approach to improve HIV intervention efforts.

Ethnographic process evaluation

Evaluation research is used to determine whether a programme or intervention has been worthwhile in terms of delivering intended and expected outcomes

(WHO 2000). Most evaluation falls into one of four categories: formative evaluation, process evaluation, outcome evaluation and impact evaluation (Stekler and Linnan 2002). Process evaluation is the least researched and documented of these, particularly in relation to public health programmes (Campbell et al. 2000).

Process evaluation determines whether programme activities have been implemented as intended (i.e. 'fidelity'); it is also used to assess the quality of implementation, clarify causal mechanisms and identify contextual factors associated with different outcomes (Craig et al. 2008). It helps us understand how a successful intervention might be replicated in new contexts, and identify how poor intervention design or improper implementation impacts on programme effectiveness (Stekler and Linnan 2002, Moore et al. 2013). Guidance for process evaluation during complex interventions was recently published in the BMJ (Moore et al. 2015). Typically, process evaluations pose questions about interventions in relation to coverage and process (WHO 2000), and rely on simple quantitative measures to assess implementation (e.g. the number of sessions delivered, the number of participants involved in programme activities). However, such simple measures cannot capture the complexity of structural public health interventions, particularly in terms of changes in intervention context, the quality of implementation, and effectiveness of proposed interventions and mechanisms of change (Moore et al. 2015). Ethnographic process evaluation research offers a holistic approach to doing so (Agar 1996).

The application of ethnographic methods for evaluation of HIV prevention programmes can be traced back to the 1980s at least (e.g. Clatts 1989, Schensul and Weeks 1989, Feldman 1990, Bolton and Singer 1992, Agar 2002). While the application of ethnographic methods in process evaluation is not as common as in formative or impact evaluation, some examples of where this work has been applied include alongside structural HIV prevention programmes in community and clinic settings with drug users in the USA (Hong et al. 2005, Weeks et al. 2015) and Canada (McNeil et al. 2015), female sex workers in China (Weeks et al. 2013, Huang et al. 2015), India (Reza-Paul et al. 2012, George et al. 2015) and Benin (Dugas et al. 2015), and patients attending general clinics in the UK (McMullen et al. 2015).

Ethnographic process evaluation may be defined as the systematic application of ethnographic methods during the piloting and implementation of programmes to assess programme fidelity and quality, and monitor individual and contextual change, with the aim of improving programme delivery and effectiveness. Going beyond the usual simple quantitative documentation of programme dosage and reach, ethnographic process evaluation adopts methods such as ethnographic mapping, participant observation, in-depth interviews and group discussions (LeCompte and Schensul 2010), as well as a detailed analysis of existing programme literature and documentation. In doing so, it aims to obtain a holistic and thorough understanding of the programme and the context in which it is being delivered, the activities of the staff delivering the programme, and perspectives of people receiving the programme.

Like all evaluation activities, successful ethnographic process evaluation requires careful planning and thoughtful design. First, evaluators must have a thorough understanding of the programme theory and assumed mechanisms of change in order to design appropriate evaluation strategies that capture what is happening (Windsor et al. 1984, De Silva et al. 2014). Second, it is important to develop an in-depth understanding of the context in which a programme is being implemented, as this may help understand why an intervention may work in one setting but not another, and understand how to maximise intervention effect (Latkin and Knowlton 2005, Sumartojo 2009). Contextual factors can inhibit or facilitate project implementation, and include issues such as societal relations and structures, cultural traditions, gender norms, practices of stigma, as well as legal and economic policies (Britan 1981, Sumartojo 2009). Third, systematic documentation of the delivery of programme activities – e.g. participant recruitment strategies; programme activity and health communication strategies; dose, duration and reach of programme activities – is required to assess discrepancies between the programme protocol and actual implementation (Hawe et al. 2004, Carroll et al. 2007). This also ensures valid assessment of implementation quality, and enables exploration of mechanisms of change and future adaptation to new circumstances (Glasgow et al. 1999). Finally, ethnographic methods appropriate to the intervention, target population and evaluation objectives require careful selection. Multiple methods are usually employed to monitor programme delivery and capture different perspectives on change (LeCompte and Schensul 2010).

The 'STEP Into Action' HIV prevention programme

During the 'STEP Into Action' HIV prevention programme in Baltimore, USA, ethnographic methods were used to identify and evaluate the factors that facilitated or inhibited HIV prevention message diffusion among injecting drug users. Findings indicated that communication patterns and strategies advocated in training sessions did not translate immediately into the outreach encounter in the drug using communities. The intervention programme was refined and developed based on findings from an ethnographic process evaluation.

The STEP Into Action programme was based on social influence theory and a previously successful HIV prevention intervention (Latkin et al. 2003), and adopted a harm reduction and social influence approach (Tobin et al. 2011). It took the form of a network-oriented intervention that trained injecting drug users to promote HIV prevention and harm reduction within their drug and sexual networks. 'STEP' was the acronym participants were encouraged to use when talking to their networks about harm reduction – 'Stand up and be positive', 'Talk with respect', 'Evaluate the situation', and 'Put a plan into action'.

The study design was a controlled Phase II efficacy trial. Participants were randomly assigned to either an experimental condition (where they received the STEP intervention) or an equal-attention control condition group (where they received the same number of sessions but with a focus on general HIV prevention knowledge). The STEP intervention programme consisted of six sessions – four group sessions that focused on peer mentoring and communication skills, one individual session, and one dyad session (in which a participant brought his or her primary drug or sex partner, referred to as 'partner' in this chapter, or other people in their risk networks, known as 'network member'). Booster sessions were provided after the conclusion of the main intervention phase. During each intervention session, the participants received training from a health educator. After the session, participants practiced what they had learned with their partner. When participants returned to the next session, they underwent a 'homework debriefing' in which they shared their experiences with the rest of the group and the health educator. STEP was tested and revised through five cohorts of pilot studies between July 2003 and January 2004. Although each pilot cohort consisted of the same six sessions described above, significant changes were made to the intervention manual as a result of the ongoing process evaluation and the feedback occurring at the time. All the piloting procedures were approved by the Institutional Review Board of The Johns Hopkins University School of Public Health.

This programme took place in Baltimore, Maryland, which has some of the highest rates of injecting drug use, HIV and sexually transmitted infections in the USA (CDC 2015). Inclusion criteria for programme participants were that they were at least 18 years old, were able to recruit a partner, and self-reported injecting drug use within three months prior to the research. Participants were recruited using word-of-mouth, community outreach, advertising in community newspapers, and flyers on the streets. The number of participants in the pilot sessions varied from five to 11 in different cohorts. Most of the participants were African American (83 per cent), and 69 per cent were men.

Ethnographic data collection and analysis

Data were collected through participant observation and in-depth interviews. One of the evaluation goals was to observe the intervention process. This included the development of session materials, training (i.e. facilitators' presentation of the materials, and participants' reactions to, and interactions with, the materials), participants' ability to communicate the programme's HIV prevention information to their partner or other people in their risk networks, and participants' ability to demonstrate risk reduction behaviours.

After obtaining informed consent from the participants, at least one ethnographer observed the group sessions. During each session break, the ethnographers talked to participants to elicit feedback about the session and build rapport. After several sessions, the ethnographers would ask participants if they were willing to demonstrate skills during outreach activities in the community. Ethnographers then accompanied the participants into the community to observe how they practised the skills they learned. Some of these activities and conversations were audiotaped. Detailed field notes were also taken. For the individual and dyad programme sessions, where the presence of observers was deemed to be too intrusive, sessions were taped and analysed at a later date. During their observations and fieldwork, ethnographers identified opinion leaders and key informants (i.e. those who had extensive community networks). Individual informal interviews were set up with these informants. These interviews usually took place in the street settings, and ethnographers took field notes on their return from the street.

The dataset consisted of tapes and notes of training sessions, fieldwork and interviews in the communities, and in-depth interviews with key informants. These notes, along with other field notes, were uploaded to a database in Microsoft Access. Ethnographers initially analysed the field notes using the themes that paralleled the domains and/or content areas addressed in the session activities and objectives, with an allowance for new themes emerging through the analytical process (Silverman 1993, LeCompte and Schensul 2010).

Once each session of six per wave was complete (i.e. when the training session and the street outreach were completed), the ethnographic team organised all available data and met with the implementation team to discuss how to translate the evaluation findings into possible actions. Through discussions with the project team, decisions were made to refine the training protocol or to reframe the implementation. For each problem we identified in the ethnographic process evaluation, there was a correspondent action to 'fix' the problem.

Ethnographic process evaluation findings

The focus of this chapter is on process evaluation, and particularly on how ethnographic methods can be used to inform the redesign of an intervention programme during pilot implementation. Therefore, we present illustrative findings of those aspects of the intervention that did not work very well in training sessions or the community settings, and how they were altered in light of evaluation findings.

'Getting clean' versus 'harm reduction'

The programme was based on the philosophy of harm reduction, rather than the prevention of drug use (Elliott *et al.* 2005), which acknowledged participants' current risky behaviours and encouraged them to reduce the risks on a step-by-step basis. From the first pilot, ethnographers observed a tension between the beliefs about 'getting clean' and 'harm reduction'. Drug users in the group often expressed that getting clean was their ultimate solution (i.e. once they were clean of drugs, then all other problems in their lives would diminish), whereas facilitators often brushed past the notion of getting clean and talked instead about reducing risks in ways other than abstinence. As one ethnographer observed in his session notes, 'some of the participants were internalising their participation in the group session as treatment or intervention for cessation of their drug use'. Several ethnographers made similar observations while listening to the session tapes. Another noted: 'I have noticed that participants talked about a sense of remorse when they knowingly practice high risk behaviours. This feeling is compounded by a sense of powerlessness to *do anything about it'* (emphasis in original).

To achieve the goal of getting clean, individuals often have to go through many steps of harm reduction. At this point, getting clean and harm reduction are convergent rather than conflicting. Based on this understanding, the intervention language was modified so that the facilitators first acknowledged that getting clean was a positive objective, and then emphasised that harm reduction was one process for achieving their ultimate goal of abstinence while reducing their HIV risk. Throughout the programme, we communicated to participants that getting clean and harm reduction were on a continuum rather than dichotomous categories, and we emphasised that the skills to achieve both beliefs were similar. We changed the training script to show how harm reduction could help them get clean, and that getting clean was often an over-generalisation for all their problems. Instead the training reflected that the skills they learned in the programme, such as social and communication skills, would allow them to address important interpersonal issues and establish a foundation for controlling and ceasing drug use. We also pointed out that there were major life goals that could be enhanced while they were trying to get clean, foremost among them improving relationships with family members and partners. Participants, therefore, were encouraged to discuss their experiences of getting clean and how they integrated the harm reduction philosophy into achieving this goal. They acknowledged that every small positive change they made while trying to get clean is safer for themselves and others.

'Partner' and 'network member'

The objective in the first session of the peer mentor training was to help participants feel that they could become community health educators in their own social networks, and disseminate harm reduction messages to their partners. It was important that they also felt that they could practice what they preached, becoming more cautious with their drug use and sexual practices. The participants were expected to bring their sexual or drug-using partners to the programme and disseminate HIV prevention information to these people. However, the intervention-specific meaning of partner was not clear to participants during the initial sessions. In the first cohort of the pilot phase, participants were told to identify 'a person who they wanted to help'. However, as an ethnographer noted in his observation notes of group sessions, 'for several participants the priority for their efforts "to help" did not reveal skills directly involving the health educator skills ... a link between them "helping others" and the "health educator" identity needs to be explored or established'.

Participants were asked to practise the harm reduction skills with their partner, but observations of the training sessions and street outreach suggested that some participants were not clear about the notion of partner. For example, in the first cohort session, one participant stated that he wanted to assist his three year old daughter, because the child's mother had recently died and he was taking on the responsibility of raising his daughter. In contrast, a female participant practised outreach by initiating a tense conversation of condom usage with a stranger passing her house, whereas her conversation with her partner regarding harm reduction was minimal. In some informal interviews, several participants indicated that when talking about a partner, they thought of only a sexual partner, not a drug use partner, and that they did not tend to use the word partner in their daily conversations.

These observations indicated that what the educator role participants were supposed to assume was either interpreted so broadly as to include everyone they knew, or understood so narrowly as to include only their sex partners. Therefore, the training protocol was revised so that it would be less confusing and more flexible for participants to disseminate the harm reduction messages to people in their risk networks. First, we stopped using the word partner in the group sessions and encouraged participants to identify network members that they listed in a network interview. We also invited several 'harm reduction educators', who had graduated from previous intervention programmes, to share their experiences of learning and disseminating harm reduction skills to their sexual partners, drug use partners, and other people in their risk networks. In addition, during the homework debriefing participants were encouraged to share their experiences of disseminating harm reduction messages among their network members, so that the facilitators could help them stay on track and the session participants could learn from each other.

'Stay positive' versus 'Sometimes you gotta go hard'

Originally, the 'S' in STEP stood for 'start positive and stay positive', which encouraged the health educators to look at the positive side of behaviours for themselves, their partners, and other community members, and avoid any negative comments. In a group session when participants discussed their previous homework assignment, one participant commented that 'sometimes you gotta go hard' (i.e. be more assertive about the harm reduction messages), because many times the situations in the streets or communities did not allow him merely to stay positive. He provided an example of trying to disseminate the safe drug-splitting procedure (i.e. splitting the drug dry on a piece of paper, rather than using the same injecting equipment to share the drug) to his drug use partner, who ignored his advice and continued preparing drugs in a shared cooker. Finally he 'went hard' and insisted on this safe procedure, and his partner gave in and began to listen to his suggestion. Other participants, however, shared their positive experiences of staying positive. One suggested that he told his friends that 'the life you save is your own'. Another expressed a sense of accomplishment from working as a health educator in the community, stating 'helping somebody creates a domino effect, when I help someone else, who helps someone else.'

These observations of negative and positive experiences of working as a health educator in the community suggested that some participants had interpreted being positive narrowly as being nice to everyone all the time. Feedback also suggested that staying positive alone was not an adequate tool for participants who encountered many hard situations in the street. Through informal interviews with key informants and observations in the streets, ethnographers noted that in the community of drug users, whose ideologies differed from mainstream values, identifying or promoting oneself as a positive model without acknowledging the realities in the communities might stimulate negative "sniff" (e.g. disregard, contempt). Therefore it is critical to be respectful while being positive.

Based on these observations, we changed the letter S in STEP to 'stand up and be positive', with an emphasis on having a positive attitude toward life. Staying positive involved being respectful, rather than telling others how to run their lives, and believing in oneself and others. We encouraged participants to initiate conversations about safe drug use or sexual practices with their network members by first acknowledging positive steps that their network members were taking already. Rather than saying, 'it's stupid to share needles/cookers', the conversation should start with how the network felt and understanding their own concerns. Group problem solving activities were designed to allow participants to focus on the skill of standing up and being positive. Participants were read a scenario and asked to identify the positive aspects of the individual's behaviour. Eventually, participants began to describe conversations within their own networks in terms of first acknowledging the positive aspects of their networks' behaviours.

Communication skills in training sessions versus communication in the streets

Through some individual interviews with participants, we learned that communication was the most cited barrier for health educators. For example, several participants mentioned that they had difficulty bringing up the subject of condoms and safe sex with their partners, because they thought their partner would get suspicious of their sudden interest in using protection. Some mentioned that their partners did not want to discuss the programme, because they felt that if the participants got clean they would end up leaving their drug-using partners, so they avoided discussing any issue regarding harm reduction. Others exchanged the ideas of 'what made it easy to go out and practice (what they learned in the intervention sessions)'. One said being 'straight up' helped (i.e. just be straightforward to start the conversation); it was often perceived as being difficult to initiate conversations, but when they were in the conversation, they felt more comfortable.

During the early pilot sessions, the communication skills taught focused on active listening. Many participants responded that these skills were not very effective when they had conversations with their peers. Some participants mentioned being nervous, because they did not want to 'get into other people's business', or they didn't want to take the risk of 'getting cursed out'. During community outreach, two participants told an ethnographer that in real life they rarely picked up the topic of HIV, especially in interactions involving injection. They also suggested that 'if there is something "in it" for someone they will tend to listen'.

Based on the ethnographers' observations and participants' suggestions, we changed the communication skills from focusing on active listening to focusing on talking with respect and evaluating the situation through asking open-ended questions and incorporating the notion of stand up and be positive. Conversations could start with respect and concern of the network's current situation, and then gradually move to a discussion on how to reduce risks in their injection or sexual behaviours so as to have a safer lifestyle.

We also created conversation starters to help initiate non-confrontational conversations. Some were different facts about HIV or HIV prevention, including, for example, 'did you know cold water works better than hot water in cleaning needles?' Another conversation starter focused on the use of novel condoms, such as polyurethane male condoms and a condom marketed specifically to an urban clientele named 'the Jimmy Hatz'. These conversation starters seemed natural to the setting and during street outreach we found that participants could initiate conversations more easily by using these conversation starters.

Good metaphor versus useful tools

In the session on injection-related HIV risk reduction, we used an 'injection risk ladder' to help participants understand the different levels of risk involved in drug use. For example, splitting drugs dry or using new needles each time you inject were considered safe drug use practices and were placed at the bottom of the injection risk ladder. In contrast, using someone else's needle without rinsing it is an unsafe practice and, therefore, placed on top of the ladder. During the session, participants found this risk ladder very interesting and actively identified the levels of risk using the ladder. The injection risk ladder served as an effective teaching aid for the facilitators as well as a useful metaphor for the participants to describe methods of reducing risks of HIV acquisition and transmission.

However, in the informal conversations with participants after the session, some participants expressed the concern as to whether risk was always the factor in decision making. They asked how they could constantly remind themselves about the level of risks in situations where consequences were not the first thing in their mind, especially when they were holding the drugs in their hands. Our observations in shooting galleries suggested that how to split drugs equally was a big concern for many participants who shared drugs and shot up together. Drug users understood that sharing needles was risky, but many still shared cookers or used dirty needles to prepare and split drugs. The two most popular methods of drug sharing are wet and dry methods. Dry-splitting methods were rarely used because of the difficulty of measuring dry drugs and the loss of drugs due to paper absorption. Wet splitting (i.e. splitting the drug in solution) was commonly used because of the perceived ability to split drugs equally.

Based on these observations, we changed the injection risk ladder from numerous items on the ladder to only a few items, and incorporated getting clean at the bottom of the ladder. We also added more emphasis on practices of safer splitting. We made a video of different safe splitting methods and asked participants to practise some of the methods in the sessions. We also provided tools and supplies that they would need for each method. For dry splitting, we gave participants laminated cards with square grids so that drugs could be divided easily without any loss due to paper absorption. Due to the success of this method in helping to split drugs equally, participants named this paper the 'Even Steven'.

The second method was called the 'norm-ject'. One clean syringe without a needle (i.e. a norm-ject) with ounce markers was used only to draw up the water and to measure the drugs. Drugs were cooked in one fixed clean cooker, and then the norm-ject was used to draw up the drugs and squirt the drug equally to other cookers. Participants were initially not very enthusiastic about this splitting method, because 'it is too complicated and takes up too much time'. Ethnographers introduced this method to some opinion leaders in the shooting galleries and found it could be potentially successful. Video demonstrations and practices in the training sessions further reduced the anxiety of applying this method. We distributed norm-jects to participants and their network members with a card explaining their use. Participants reported increased acceptance of this method, and even gave it a new name, the 'New Jack'.

Conclusions

This study illustrates an ethnographically informed process evaluation that was carried out to pilot a network-oriented peer outreach HIV prevention programme. We have presented how to use a systematic ethnographic data collection strategy – consisting of participant observation, in-depth interviews and group discussions to help refine and improve a programme through small, regular changes.

In this study, programme success and sustainability depended on the dissemination of the harm reduction messages through social networks. Therefore, it was crucial to develop a culturally and linguistically appropriate programme that could motivate the participants to begin and continue harm reduction conversations with their partners and other people in their risk networks. The best way to ensure that the intervention materials were relevant and effective, and could be disseminated was to observe participants' social interactions within the training sessions, as well as with other people in their drug use settings. By using ethnographic methods in process evaluation we were able to ensure that the programme was being implemented with local, in-depth insight from programme participants.

Ethnographic evaluation methods have unique advantages in terms of gathering information that could not be captured easily by surveys. In complex multilevel structural interventions, there is often a gap between the research protocol and actual programme delivery. A gap also exists between what occurs in the intervention session and what occurs in reality on the street. Insight into these gaps is not usually captured through simple quantitative process measures, especially when the intended programme activities are so deeply ingrained in social and cultural practices that are unique to a particular group of people. Yet, process data collected through ethnographic methods can help bridge these gaps by gaining vital local insight, observing the differences, and adjusting the intervention to people's practices that are specific to a particular local context. As such, ethnographic process evaluation enables developing culturally appropriate and effective interventions, and lessons learned in one context can facilitate the difficult process of implementing effective programmes in other socially and culturally different contexts.

References

Agar, M. (1996) 'Recasting the "ethno" in "epidemiology"', *Medical Anthropology*, 16(4): 391–403.

Agar, M. (2002) 'How the drug field turned my beard gray', *International Journal of Drug Policy*, 13(4): 249–259.

Bolton, R. and Singer, M. (1992) *Rethinking AIDS Prevention: Cultural approaches*, Philadelphia, PA: Gordon & Breach Science.

Britan, G. (1981) 'Contextual evaluation: an ethnographic approach to program assessment', in R. Conner (ed.) *Methodological Advances in Evaluation Research*, Beverly Hills, CA: SAGE, pp. 47–60.

Campbell, M., Fitzpatrick. R., Haines, A., Kinmonth, A.L., Sandercock, P., Spiegelhalter, D. and Tyrer, P. (2000) 'Framework for design and evaluation of complex interventions to improve health', *British Medical Journal*, 321: 694–696.

Carroll, C., Patterson, M., Wood, S., Booth, A., Rick, J. and Balain, S. (2007) 'A conceptual framework for implementation fidelity', *Implementation Science*, 2: 40.

CDC (2015) *HIV among African Americans*. Available at: www.cdc.gov/nchhstp/newsroom/docs/cdc-hiv-aa-508.pdf (accessed 23 July 2015).

Clatts, M. (1989) 'Ethnography and AIDS intervention in New York City: life history as an ethnographic strategy', in National Institute of Drug Abuse (ed.) *Community-Based AIDS Prevention: Studies of intravenous drug users and their sexual partners*, Rockville, CT: National Institute of Drug Abuse, pp. 225–233.

Craig, P., Dieppe, P., Macintyre, S., Michie, S., Nazareth, I. and Petticrew, M. (2008) *Developing and Evaluating Complex Interventions: New guidance*. Available at: www.mrc.ac.uk/documents/pdf/complex-interventions-guidance (accessed 22 July 2015).

De Silva, M., Breuer, E. and Lee, L. (2014) 'Theory of change: a theory-driven approach to enhance the Medical Research Council's framework for complex interventions', *Trials*, 15: 267.

Dugas, M., Bédard, E., Batona, G., Kpatchavi, A.C., Guédou, F.A., Dubé, E., Alary, M. (2015) 'Outreach strategies for the promotion of HIV testing and care: closing the gap between health services and female sex workers in Benin', *Journal of Acquired Immune Deficiency Syndromes*, 68(Suppl. 2): S198–S205.

Elliott, R., Csete, J., Wood, E. and Kerr, T. (2005) 'Harm reduction, HIV/AIDS, and the human rights challenge to global drug control policy', *Health and Human Rights Journal*, 8(2): 104–138.

Feldman, D. (Ed.) (1990) *Culture and AIDS*, New York: Praeger.
George, A., Blankenship, K.M., Biradavolu, M.R., Dhungana, N. and Tankasala, N. (2015) 'Sex workers in HIV prevention: from social change agents to peer educators', *Global Public Health*, 10(1): 28–40.
Glasgow, R.E., Vogt, T.M. and Boles, S.M. (1999) 'Evaluating the public health impact of health promotion interventions: the RE-AIM framework', *American Journal of Public Health*, 89(9): 1322–1327.
Gupta, G., Parkhurst, J.O., Ogden, J.A., Aggleton, P. and Mahal, A. (2008) 'Structural approaches to HIV prevention', *Lancet*, 372(9640): 764–775.
Hawe, P., Shiell, A. and Riley, T. (2004) 'Complex interventions: how "out of control" can a randomised controlled trial be?', *British Medical Journal*, 328: 1561–1563.
Hong, Y., Mitchell, S.G., Peterson, J.A., Latkin, C.A., Tobin, K. and Gann, D. (2005) 'Ethnographic process evaluation: piloting an HIV prevention intervention program among injection drug users', *International Journal of Qualitative Methods*, 4(1). Available at: http://ejournals.library.ualberta.ca/index.php/IJQM/article/view/4450 (accessed 19 June 2015).
Huang, Y., Muessig, K.E., Zhang, N. and Maman, S. (2015) 'Unpacking the "structural" in a structural approach for HIV prevention among female sex workers: a case study from China', *Global Public Health*, 10(7): 852–866.
Latkin, C.A. and Knowlton, A.R. (2005) 'Micro-social structural approaches to HIV prevention: a social ecological perspective', *AIDS Care*, 17(Suppl. 1): S102–S113.
Latkin, C.A., Sherman, S. and Knowlton, A. (2003) 'HIV prevention among drug users: outcome of a network-oriented peer outreach intervention', *Health Psychology*, 22(4): 332–339.
LeCompte, M.D. and Schensul, J. (2010) *Analyzing and Interpreting Ethnographic Data*, Walnut Creek, CA: Altamira Press.
McMullen, H., Griffiths, C., Leber, W. and Greenhalgh, T. (2015) 'Explaining high and low performers in complex intervention trials: a new model based on diffusion of innovations theory', *Trials*, 31(16): 242.
McNeil, R., Kerr, T., Lampkin, H. and Small, W. (2015) '"We need somewhere to smoke crack": an ethnographic study of an unsanctioned safer smoking room in Vancouver, Canada', *International Journal of Drug Policy*, 26(7): 645–652.
Moore, G.F., Raisanen, L., Moore, L., Din, N.U. and Murphy, S. (2013) 'Mixed-method process evaluation of the Welsh National Exercise Referral Scheme', *Health Education*, 113(6): 476–501.
Moore, G.F., Audrey, S., Barker, M., Bond, L., Bonell, C., Hardeman, W., Moore, L., O'Caithain, A., Tinati, T., Wight, D. and Baird, J. (2015) 'Process evaluation of complex interventions: Medical Research Council guidance', *British Medical Journal*, 350: h1258.
Ogden, J., Gupta, G. R., Fisher, W.F. and Warnerd, A. (2011) 'Looking back, moving forward: towards a game-changing response to AIDS', *Global Public Health*, 6(Suppl. 3): S285–S292.
Reza-Paul, S., Lorway, R., O'Brien, N., Lazarus, L., Jain, J., Bhagya, M., Fathima, M.P., Venukumar, K.T., Raviprakash, K.N., Baer, J. and Steen, R. (2012) 'Sex worker-led structural interventions in India: a case study on addressing violence in HIV prevention through the Ashodaya Samithi collective in Mysore', *Indian Journal of Medical Research*, 135: 98–106.

Rotheram-Borus, M.J., Swendeman, D. and Chovnick, G. (2009) 'The past, present, and future of HIV prevention: integrating behavioral, biomedical, and structural intervention strategies for the next generation of HIV prevention', *Annual Review of Clinical Psychology*, 5: 143–167.

Schensul, J.J. and Weeks, M. (1989) 'Ethnographic evaluation of AIDS-prevention programs', in National Institute of Drug Abuse (ed.) *Community-Based AIDS Prevention: Studies of intravenous drug users and their sexual partners*, Rockville, CT: National Institute of Drug Abuse, pp. 110–120.

Silverman, D. (1993) *Interpreting Qualitative Data: Methods for analyzing talk, text and interaction*, Thousand Oaks, CA: SAGE.

Steckler, A, and Linnan, L. (eds) (2002) *Process Evaluation for Public Health Interventions and Research*. San Francisco, CA: Jossey-Bass.

Sumartojo, E. (2000) 'Structural factors in HIV prevention: concepts, examples, and implications for research', *AIDS*, 14(Suppl. 1): S3–S10.

Tobin, K.E., Kuramoto, S.J., Davey-Rothwell, M.A. and Latkin, C.A. (2011) 'The STEP into Action study: a peer-based, personal risk network-focused HIV prevention intervention with injection drug users in Baltimore, Maryland', *Addiction*, 106(2): 366–375.

Weeks, M.R., Li, J., Liao, S., Zhang, Q., Dunn, J., Wang, Y. and Jiang, J. (2013) 'Multilevel dynamic systems affecting introduction of HIV/STI prevention innovations among Chinese women in sex work establishments', *Health Education & Behavior*, 40(Suppl. 1): S111–S122.

Weeks, M.R., Kostick, K., Li, J., Dunn, J., McLaughlin, P., Richmond, P., Choudhury, S., Obidoa, C., Mosher, H. and Martinez, M. (2015) 'Translation of the risk avoidance partnership (RAP) for implementation in outpatient drug treatment clinics', *Journal of Psychoactive Drugs*, 22: 1–9.

WHO (2000) *Process Evaluations*. Available at: http://whqlibdoc.who.int/hq/2000/WHO_MSD_MSB_00.2e.pdf (accessed 22 July 2015).

Windsor, R.A., Baranowski, T., Clark, N. and Cutter, G. (1984) *Evaluation of Health Promotion and Education Programs*, Mountain View, CA: Mayfield.

12
Using the Reality Check Approach to shape quantitative findings
Experience from mixed method evaluations in Ghana and Nepal

Dee Jupp

It was in 2011 that the field team of young Nepali researchers came back to town to start their debrief with me. They were tired after staying four nights in the homes of villagers and their long, wet trek from Num in the Koshi Hills, but this did not dampen their eagerness to challenge me: 'We thought we were supposed to go to the poorest community, wasn't that the plan?' 'Yes', I replied limply, 'the secondary data we used indicated it was.' 'But', they almost screamed at me, 'everywhere we saw young boys gambling on *carrom*[1] and Ludo even at six in the morning, and there's lots of drinking of imported beer' (I noted their strong emphasis on the word 'imported'). 'The school kids walk around with thousand rupee notes in their pockets, they all have the latest mobile phones, new houses are being constructed everywhere.' Now they were all talking at once. 'They buy food rather than grow it, employ people from outside to work for them and …' This last was their final blow. 'They say their priority need is a bank in the community.' We calmed down and spent the next two days reviewing systematically and reflexively the information the study team had painstakingly gathered during their Reality Check Study in Num. But, the well triangulated conversations, observations and interactions they had made during their time in the community made it very clear that this community was indeed not poor, despite what the statistics told us. And this was an epiphany for us all.

The Reality Check Approach

An initiative of the Swedish Embassy, Bangladesh, the Reality Check Approach was first developed in 2007 by Dee Jupp, Helena Thorfinn and Esse Nilsson for use as a qualitative longitudinal study approach to track the Sector Wide Approaches in primary education and primary health in Bangladesh (Lewis 2012). It extends the tradition of listening studies (Anderson *et al.* 2012) and beneficiary assessments (Salmen 1998, Ruedin and Shutt 2013) by combining together elements of these approaches with periods of time spent living with people, usually those who are directly experiencing poverty. At the core of the Reality Check Approach is the immersion of the researcher in families and households to engage with, listen to, observe and document their voices, opinions and experiences. Reality Check Approach studies intend to channel these voices into policy dialogue so that future policy and practice is better geared to real needs and the local context. Like other qualitative styles of work, the approach focuses on the 'how' and 'why' rather than 'what', 'when' and 'how many'.

The process of immersion (living with households and joining in their lives) is core to the approach and is regarded as an essential element. Immersion changes the dynamic of the relationship of the outsider with host families and communities (Hammersley and Atkinson 2007). It creates opportunities to experience first hand what people mean about, for example, the difficulties collecting water, the behaviour of service providers, the poor light with which to study, the impact of continuous rain on their livelihoods and the hardships associated with tilling drought-affected land. It also provides an opportunity for detailed observation of, for example, household dynamics, child–parent behaviour and relationships, and daily routines (DeWalt and DeWalt 2002). Most importantly, it enables a relaxed and trusted context for conversations and enhanced understanding of how people live their lives (Feldman et al. 2003). By spending a considerable amount of time with the household and their neighbours, less extractive forms of communication can be used. By staying with a family, the power distance between the outsider and the family diminishes (Ebbs 1996). By purposely staying with the most disadvantaged, older people, children and poorer, marginalised community members, often 'unheard' in conventional evaluations and studies, are brought to the fore.

The Reality Check Approach is best understood as an 'approach' rather than a formal methodology or a strict set of tools, methods or techniques. It can be seen as a set of guiding ideas and principles that can be built into an implementation plan based on the particular context and purpose. Four key principles underpin this way of working: depth, respect for voice, flexibility and simplicity (Lewis 2012). Crucially, a Reality Check Approach study aims to document, in depth, the experiences and perceptions of local people. A variety of techniques may be used to do this – including observation, participating in family activities, conversation, stories, drawings, photographs, accompanying people on visits to service providers – to provide detailed information not usually available through conventional monitoring and evaluation systems or formal research. The basic premise of the approach is the importance of listening. This respects what people have to say about their situation, and attempts to document people's views in ways that allow their voices to be properly heard by those higher up in the policy system, in government, by development partners or by civil society organisations. Team members do not stick to a set question format, sample or schedule, which makes it possible to follow up and cross-check what people say, and to respond flexibly to new and unexpected insights. Rigour is achieved by 'triangulating' people's stories and other information gathered during the research. A study is intended as a simple, direct and immediate type of 'pulse taking'. It aims to utilise a less complex, 'light touch' approach than those often used in the large-scale surveys common in quantitative research or evaluation. It takes less time when compared to the long duration required by most forms of qualitative anthropological ethnographic fieldwork. A Reality Check Approach study simply tries to use some basic but effective data collection methods to document poor peoples' views and perspectives as clearly as possible (Lewis 2012).

These principles make the approach slightly different from many conventional styles of research, information collection, and monitoring and evaluation, even while the approach combines elements from each. For example, engaged listening and observation helps overcome the limitations of survey data based on short interviews that offer breadth but may lack depth and contain inaccuracies or oversimplifications. The idea of 'learning' is preferred to that of 'finding out', while 'conversation' is preferred to an 'interview'.

The careful construction and preparation of a Reality Check Approach team is key to its success. The members of the team must be 'people persons', who are friendly, warm, open and able to put others at ease. They must be able to put aside their own assumptions and suspend judgement (Bernard 1994). Advance preparation involves reflecting on behaviours and attitudes that may hinder or enable people to talk and express themselves openly and safely. Informality and ease of conversation in everyday situations are central to this approach. This is far removed from public space events in which people are invited or self-select, where overt power dynamics play out, in which people feel differentially confident and secure and where conformity often dominates.

The photo in Figure 12.1, taken during a Reality Check Approach study in Indonesia in 2014, illustrates something of the comparative advantage of the Reality Check Approach. Researchers just 'hang out' with people (Bernard 1994, DeMunck and Sobo 1998, Beazley 2003). On the left are the ubiquitous 'cool young men' who eschew formal public events. Then there is a young mother with a small child who said, 'I can't go to meetings even if I want to, I'd be told off because the kids were disturbing', and a teenage girl who told us, 'we are not allowed to attend meetings. The elders think we have nothing to contribute because we are only young'. There is also an older woman who feels that attending a meeting is boring and far away from home; she explained that she cannot sit for too long. The man in the middle is the neighbourhood joker and laughed that he would not be welcome at a meeting. But here they all are, chatting with us outside in the shared courtyard.

Notes are never taken in front of people and conversations are never recorded as these processes would immediately distort the special spaces of interaction created. An insistence on ordinariness is achieved through efforts to reduce the peculiarity of our homestays as well as the power relations between ourselves and the families with whom we live. We think we have achieved this when our host families explain to their neighbours why we are there. In Rwanda in 2011, one family member explained, 'they are not guests, they have to live the same way as we do, see look at the blisters on her hands – she worked hard in the field this morning'; in

Using the Reality Check Approach 175

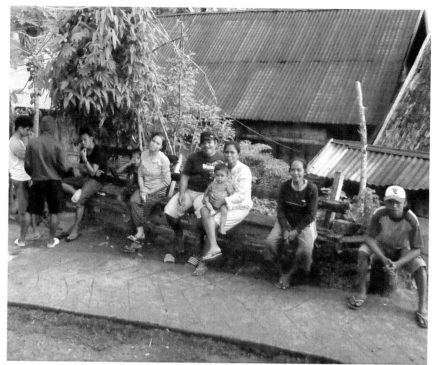

Figure 12.1 Chatting and hanging out with a range of villagers, Sulawesi, East Indonesia, 2014

Source: Photograph taken with participants' permission to reproduce.

Bangladesh in 2012, someone said, 'he ate simply and only what we normally eat'; and in Nepal in 2014, a girl said, 'at first I was shy but after he stayed the night on the floor and walked with me to the fields, I could talk to him just like my brother'.

Experiences using the Reality Check Approach

The following case studies – from Nepal and Ghana – illustrate the benefits of using the Reality Check Approach at different stages of monitoring and evaluation around interventions. The first describes how it was used in a mixed methods longitudinal evaluation in Nepal as a means to provide a theory of change based on people's perspectives and insights to better inform the design of survey instruments. The second demonstrates how the approach is being used alongside annual conventional quantitative surveys to complement and enrich the findings in evaluations in Nepal and in Ghana. The third example illustrates a more unusual use of this style of work, as the only primary data element of a mixed method retrospective study in Nepal to assess the impact of development aid.

Improving the design of evaluation frameworks and instruments

The Reality Check Approach has been used before an evaluation study begins in order to develop a theory of change constructed from people's perspectives rather than those of the project staff, and to improve the design of survey instruments. A Reality Check Approach had been commissioned as an element of a mixed methods monitoring, evaluation and learning component for the DfID-supported Rural Access Programme in Mid and Far West Nepal. The quantitative elements of this research centred on a household study based on the Nepal Living Standards Survey instrument. This was extended by further questions considered to be relevant for a programme designed to enhance access to markets, health, education and local government services. The sampling frame for the survey included direct and indirect beneficiaries living on or within new or maintained roads as well as those living more than five hours walk away. The sample size was 3,200 households, representing the largest and most detailed household survey ever to be conducted in this part of Nepal.

A scoping Reality Check Approach study was conducted at the end of 2013 to gather insights to enhance the design of the household survey questionnaire based on local perspectives. There were three main areas of enquiry, including understanding people's perception of poverty, their aspirational change and issues related to responding to household surveys. Researchers stayed with 12 households living in poverty in two districts. The findings led to the creation of a 'people's theory of change'. Significant differences were noted between this and the project theory of change, with the study data providing a means to make changes to the latter. One of the most important points of departure was the perception of people that increased rural access would lead to greater opportunities for migration, while the project had suggested that out-migration would decrease. The people's theory of change also noted a number of concerns about increased rural access, including: the potential for more antisocial behaviour (drinking, gambling); an increase in crime as 'strangers' had greater access to the location, and illegal activities such as logging and drug smuggling; displacement of traditional culture, skills and livelihoods, such as increased consumption of snack food, displaced portering work, disintegration of traditional reciprocal labour arrangements as people became increasingly concerned with cash income earning, and displaced local artisan work with increased cheap imports; and abandonment of the elderly and fragmentation of families. The people's theory of change had given special emphasis to access to networks and information as an outcome of enhanced rural access. As a result of insights from the study, two new modules were added to the survey. These captured the potential negative impacts that road construction and maintenance might bring to the region, as well as access to information and grievance/complaints procedures.

The scoping study was also able to provide advice on the structure of the questionnaire (e.g. leaving education and caste-related questions to the end of the survey to avoid people feeling uncomfortable), the behaviour of enumerators (e.g. which questions people would have difficulty answering, when was the best time to conduct the survey, and that few difficulties should be anticipated related to the gender of the enumerator and the respondent). It pointed out that certain questions needed rewording and needed additional coded response alternatives. For example, options for health seeking did not include private providers and informal providers such as the *dai* (traditional midwife) and *dharmy* (spiritual healer).

Enriching findings from evaluation surveys

In Northern Ghana, the Reality Check Approach is being used as part of a third party mixed methods monitoring, evaluation and learning programme alongside the implementation of the Millennium Village Project, 2011–2017. The overarching goal of this project is to make progress against the Millennium Development Goals through an integrated package of interventions dubbed the 'big push', addressing the immediate capital deficits in a locality with a view to providing the enabling conditions for local economies to become resilient and self-sustaining. The evaluation adopts a 'difference in difference' design whereby Millennium villages are matched with both 'nearby' and 'far away' control villages using community-level characteristics summarised by a propensity score. A number of quantitative survey instruments and observations are used, including a household questionnaire, adult female and male questionnaires, blood tests, cognitive tests for children, easy and advanced education tests, and anthropometry. These are complemented by three qualitative strands: participatory rural appraisal sessions with men and women; an institutional assessment using key informant interviews; and the Reality Check Approach study 'to ground truth and qualify the findings of the quantitative survey' (Masset *et al.* 2013: 15), which offers an 'interpretive lens' to provide understanding of people's attitudes and behaviours to explain the numbers.

The implementation of the baseline quantitative instruments preceded the Reality Check Approach study but the findings were not available before the study commenced. Arguably, this was apposite. We were able to stay in the homes of villagers in treatment and control villages without knowing what the survey had revealed, and without knowing whether they were in a treatment or control village. We stayed in six villages, with 20 of the poorest households for four days and nights, interacting with them, their neighbours, local power holders and local service providers they came into contact with. Conversations were held with more than 800 people. The findings were analysed by the team, and a report was written based on this. Only then did the quantitative and qualitative streams come together for a workshop in June 2013. This sort of joint reflection is rare. More often qualitative and quantitative elements of an evaluation remain parallel initiatives, often producing separate reports that appeal to separate audiences. Thanks to enlightened leadership that brought researchers out of their comfort zones, this was to be a truly mixed methods process. The team leaders of all the evaluation elements spent two days studying the data. It was at this point that the qualitative elements came into their own as interpretive lenses. There were many 'ah ha' moments shared during that workshop as we tried to make sense of the data. The interpretive insights provided around consumption patterns, school going, health seeking behaviour and migration were some of the most significant.

Engel curves (Lewbel 2008) are powerful economic analysis tools that describe the relationship between household expenditure on particular items (e.g. food) in relation to total expenditure. Commonly it is found that expenditure on food does not increase proportionally as a share of expenditure but rather becomes less. The Engel curves derived from the baseline survey seemed to defy Engel's Law as food expenditure was found to relate linearly, rather than proportionally, with total expenditure. This was dismissed by the survey team as 'almost certainly measurement error'. But the leads of both the qualitative streams refuted this: 'but we found people here delay funerals … sometimes for years because of the huge burden of feeding mourners … they also avoid going to other social obligations which require food contributions when they cannot afford them.' We drew on other qualitative findings that showed a massive decline in livestock holding by the poor compared to previous generations, and reminded our colleagues that 'contributions to social gatherings are often meat which poorer households now have to buy in'. We concluded our argument that 'this apparent defiance of Engel's Law is a result of delayed consumption'. We had, after all, spent time with families who explained that they did not go to family funerals because they had nothing to contribute and delayed those for their immediate family because they said they could not 'do it properly and respectfully'. Support also came from other studies, such as another qualitative study that reported that the funeral rites of the Kasena people who live in northern Ghana can be postponed for years:

> [Funeral rites] take place sometime after burial of the deceased, the time lapse depending on the family circumstances – consensus among the immediate kin and elders about when to hold the rites and, more importantly, the availability of quantities of foodstuff necessary for the rites.
> (Awedoba and Hahn 2014: 52)

While the interpretation of the consumption data differed and was not resolved, there were several other areas where the Reality Check Approach study provided important explanatory insights into survey trends. The baseline report fully integrated qualitative and quantitative findings (Masset et al. 2013). We were well aware of reports that claim to combine quantitative and qualitative data, but tend to relegate the qualitative data stories to text boxes, perpetuating the perception that qualitative research provides anecdotes. We insisted that this report would be written collectively 'without boxes' so that statements from the quantitative data would be explained by findings from the qualitative research within the main narrative of the report.

The quantitative data showed that a statistically significant larger proportion of girls attend school than boys at all education levels, and higher literacy rates among girls. Findings from the Reality Check Approach study concurred, noting that boys were more likely to drop out of school to work on the farm and herd animals. However, the reasons for dropping out of school that had coded answers in the survey omitted a number of reasons identified in our study. These included bullying, feeling too old to go to school (as a result of late enrolment or high number of repeat years of schooling), finding school too difficult, being 'not the school type' (i.e. not studious), school being boring, fear of corporal punishment (with boys, in particular, being more likely to experience punishment at school for bad behaviour, poor attendance and poor academic achievements and concomitant demotivation), and the lessons being too difficult to follow. All of these important explanations were subsumed as 'other' in the questionnaire. The questionnaire suggested that reasons might include the 'need' to work or help on the farm, implying that the decision to drop out is primarily an economic one. We felt this was a loaded question as boys told us that they simply preferred not to go to school, wanted to be seen as an adult and wanted personal pocket money.

According to the survey findings, 80–90 per cent of households own mosquito nets but malaria incidence remains rather high. The Reality Check Approach study enabled insight into the reasons for these disparities. It found that most households had nets – sometimes more nets than the number of household members, and sometimes still in polythene wrappers. Less than a quarter of people used them because they had to sleep outside due to the high night temperatures (often in the high 30s in February and March) and felt that the nets, which impede even the slightest breath of air, prevented sleeping. The research team members did not use mosquito nets either as they also found it impossible to sleep. Families told us that they might use them in the rainy season when mosquitos disturb their sleep but had not made a connection between nets and malaria prevention.

This experience illustrates that the Reality Check Approach study not only provided important behavioural insights into the quantitative data (e.g. the use of mosquito nets) but that findings challenged assumed explanations (e.g. the Engel curve) and suggested extended, more appropriate potential answers to be included as coded answers in the survey (e.g. the reasons for school drop-out). It also pointed to problems with administering the survey. For example, our study revealed that both men and women hide cash expenditures from each other, so reliance on one member of a household for this information during survey completion would lead to unreliable results. Like many surveys, it assumed that people have one main livelihood, but our study revealed otherwise. The increasing need for cash (for health insurance, school supplies, dry cell batteries and lighting fuel, and farming inputs) in what had until recently been essentially a cashless society, has compelled families to search for multiple cash income sources, a concomitant reduction in traditional reciprocal labour arrangements and sale of higher proportions of produce than before. The survey also asked people to 'show me where members of the household most often wash their hands', but the Reality Check

Approach study found that people do not wash their hands in isolation – they tend to take baths, but rarely just wash their hands. There was also a range of questions that were not included in the survey at all, in particular, around crime.

Following the scoping study in West Nepal for the Rural Access programme discussed above, the Reality Check Approach was also used in parallel with a household survey in West Nepal 'to help explain the findings from the household survey' (Itad 2014: iv). The study was particularly helpful in explaining survey findings that appeared to be contrary to conventional wisdom. For example, the survey found that people in remote villages earned more money than expected and more than in less remote areas. The baseline report noted, 'this is not consistent with the generally held belief that the outer and therefore more remote zones have less economic opportunity and therefore lower household income potential' (Itad 2014: 15), and might have fallen victim to the 'measurement error' explanation used in Ghana. But one of the Reality Check Approach teams had trekked for four days to reach their study locations where there are still no roads. The field notes describe the findings and confirm that the survey data was likely to be valid:

> We found a high level of public poverty with poor access to services and markets and poor connectivity to the outside world. People felt neglected by the Government, remote and cut off. But the people here were 'cash rich'. Families had good cash incomes, mostly from cross border trade with China, although people were reluctant to talk too much about this. Chinese traders come to buy a range of at least six different medicinal herbs. By paying a small 'fee' to the Community Forest Committee, families said they could gather herbs over a period of 1–2 months and expect to earn about GBP2,700. We observed extensive opium cultivation too and, although conversations around this were difficult, the cultivation was not hidden. Significantly, the villagers always used US dollars to discuss money, never Nepalese rupees. They said they no longer need to migrate to India for work. Portering too is lucrative, especially using pack animals, as the village now has a new trail connection with a major district town. A single mule can carry a load at a rate of GBP16 from the district town for local hirers, and more for outsiders, providing a typical monthly income per mule of GBP75–100. People here invest in gold as savings, with much evidence of this wealth in the jewellery worn by the women. The only shops in the village were two gold dealers. Families said they had enough food stock to last them the year. Bottled alcohol consumption was high with families saying they spent an average of GDP100 per month.
>
> (Field notes, W. Nepal, 2014)

The second surprise from the survey was that Dalit households were not more income poor than other groups. The study provided some clarity on this:

Traditionally landless, Dalits have always needed employment and have been working in India for generations. Many shared with us that they have accumulated savings and have purchased land and houses, especially from others in the village who have left for the Terai. This study indicates that often they had assets such as TVs and mobile phones when their Chettri or Brahmin neighbours did not. In one study site, Dalits were in a position to be the main money lenders in the village, especially where large loans were required (for example, to service broker and transport costs for overseas migration to Japan or Korea). Most of the Dalits with whom the study team stayed or interacted did not see themselves as poorer than others in the village (except in Humla, where the difference was acute). Some had been able to set up shops and were making good livings but the majority were continuing the tradition of migration for work.
(Reality Check Approach Team 2014: 14)

Further survey findings were examined from the perspective of our study. The survey indicated that the majority of respondents said that they used health posts 'rarely', or that use was 'not needed'. However, study findings suggest that, rather than leading to the assumption people have rather good health or high levels of stoicism, the 'not needed' category may mask a preference for private medicine shops. These medicine shops, which in Nepal are often run by qualified pharmacists, are preferred because people can pick up medicines easily and quickly, and the shops are open long and regular hours and are well stocked. This is often in direct contrast to the experiences at government health centres.

Understanding change and impact from local people's perspectives

Returning to the epiphany in Nepal mentioned at the beginning of this chapter, it was not so much that the statistics were so misleading; that happens, even though these seemed to shock the Nepali Development Studies graduates who made up the bulk of the research team. The surprise resulted more from the apparent pace of change, from the 2010/11 Nepal Living Standards Survey data (GRM International 2013) that we were using. Furthermore, the significant observed changes had almost nothing to do with development aid. By going into communities as independent researchers, without either the theories of change or the normative frames of reference of development projects that had been implemented in the region, we stumbled on a significant driver of this change: the local production of the spice, cardamom, which had been missed by nearly all the evaluations and studies done before. The Reality Check Approach study had been commissioned within a multiple methods study looking at 40 years of development interventions to evaluate the long-term impact of development assistance in East Nepal. The major part of this study was a comprehensive secondary data review of a large volume of project and programme implementation, monitoring and impact assessment documents, population datasets (focusing on agriculture, education, health, finance, transport and communication), and numerous independent quantitative and qualitative studies. Not one of these studies documented the early introduction and rise of cardamom production, which according to the local people was the undisputed driver of social and economic change (GRM international 2013: 166).

This hugely significant finding only became apparent by spending time immersed in local communities. Its significance is well illustrated by the comment, 'cardamom is our identity, no cardamom no life' (young man, Num, Koshi Hills). The study discovered that the change began when a local farmer in Num brought cardamom from Ilam to Num in 1983. The following extracts from field notes demonstrate that far from being a deprived area, as the survey data suggested, Num is now flourishing:

> The entrepreneur farmer grew the cardamom as an experiment on his own land and over the next ten years the entire neighbourhood adopted the practices so that it is now the main income source. By the time of the Reality Check Approach study, 30 years later, every household is said to grow a minimum of 200kg and many grow ten times this amount. The minimum of 200kg will guarantee an income of GBP2,700 per year. The houses all have zinc roofs and many have small retail outlets. People have reduced their livestock and paddy land as they can now afford to buy these commodities. A primary school teacher who cultivates a little over two acres of cardamom makes more than GBP67,000 profit each year. They send their four children away to college and have been able to purchase a tractor and retail shop, which further contribute to their income. Another family produces 400kg of cardamom per year from their half acre plot with a profit of about GBP5,350. Like others he has reduced his livestock to just two goats. So prosperous are these farmers that they employ seasonal workers through outside contractors to harvest for 15–30 days in September through to November. Since many brokers regularly come to Num to purchase cardamom, this has opened opportunities to sell other high value crops including the *yarshagumba* (said to be an aphrodisiac), *chiraito* (medicinal herb) which, while wild in the past, is now being cultivated. While other study villages mostly indicated a net out-migration, Num is experiencing the opposite. 10–13 houses are being built each year. The latest building under construction is a new police station paid for by community contribution because, as a young cardamom farmer noted, 'we need a bank here in Num rather than have to travel to Khandbari' and the bank cannot be established until there is a police station. Although in the 1990s many families had sons working abroad (said to be 70%), now only an estimated 10% of households do. Nobody said they are dependent on remittances any more.

With high incomes, it was hard for the study team to find someone willing to porter, and finally negotiated a rate of five times the Nepal minimum wage. Previous interest in servicing the tourist trade has waned and trekking companies arranging visits to the Makalu Barun national park bring in their own porters and guides and arrange camping rather than using the lodges and guesthouses which Num people used to provide.

(Field notes, Nepal, 2013)

Conclusions

Qualitative research without quantitative can be insightful but vague; ... quantitative without qualitative can be precise but may be wrong headed, misdirected and contrived.

(Kalinowski *et al.* 2010: 33)

The above quotation illustrates the value of methodological pluralism in good quality evaluation research. Qualitative and quantitative approaches need to draw inspiration from each other and provide a more considered analysis when thoughtfully combined. The experiences described in the case studies indicate that it is not enough to conduct multiple method research when genuine mixed methods can offer so much more. Ethnographically informed interpretive studies that seek to understand people's local realities and aspirations, and the context and relevance of interventions with the minimum of etic distortion, offer greater local insight than other qualitative methods in a mixed methods evaluation study.

The Reality Check Approach seeks to enrich description of context and phenomena, provides in-depth insight into the relevance and experience of development interventions, uncovers overlooked elements of change, and flags up areas for further research. These studies also remind those carrying out quantitative studies that they should not ignore their own biases and the impact of the behaviour of enumerators by hiding behind statistical method.

In particular, the Reality Check Approach lends itself to use at different stages in the evaluation process. It is relatively quick, and can be readily integrated into evaluation timelines. Before the conduct of household surveys, a scoping study can develop a theory of change from people's perspective and can provide important local insight into design and administration of survey instruments. During evaluations, Reality Check Approach studies can provide important, alternative and local explanations of data emerging from surveys. As a relatively agile and low cost form of evaluation study, the Reality Check Approach can be used effectively long after project interventions to review what local people think was relevant and significant, what change has been sustained, and what contributed to processes of change during social development programmes.

Note

1 *Carrom* is a popular board game across East Asia. It is similar to billiards except discs rather than balls are used and these are flicked using fingers.

References

Anderson, M.B., Brown, D. and Jean, I. (2012) *Time to Listen: Hearing people on the receiving end of international aid*, Cambridge, MA: CDA Collaborative Learning Projects.
Awedoba, A.K. and Hahn, H.P. (2014) 'Wealth, consumption and migration in West African society: new lifestyles and new social obligations among the Kasena, Northern Ghana', *Anthropos*, 109: 45–55.
Beazley, H. (2003) 'Voices from the margins: street children's subcultures in Indonesia', *Children's Geographies*, 1(2): 181–200.
Bernard, B.H. (1994) *Research Methods in Anthropology: Qualitative and quantitative approaches*, Walnut Creek, CA: AltaMira Press.
DeMunck, V.C. and Sobo, E.J. (1998) *Using Methods in the Field: A practical introduction and casebook*, Walnut Creek, CA: AltaMira press.
DeWalt, K.M. and DeWalt, B.R. (2002) *Participant Observation: Guide for field workers*. Walnut Creek, CA: AltaMira Press.
Ebbs, C.A. (1996) 'Qualitative research inquiry: issues of power and ethics', *Education*, 117(2): 217–222.
Feldman, M., Bell, J. and Berger, M. (2003) *Gaining Access: A practical and theoretical guide for qualitative researchers*, Walnut Creek, CA: AltaMira Press.
GRM International (2013) *Research into the Long-Term Impact of Development Interventions in the Koshi Hills of Nepal*, London: GRM.
Hammersley, M. and Atkinson P. (2007) *Ethnography: Principles in practice*, London: Routledge.
Itad (2014) DFID Nepal Rural Access Programme. *Monitoring, Evaluation and Learning Component: Baseline report*, Hove: Itad.
Kalinowski, P., Lai J., Fiddler, F. and Cumming, G. (2010) 'Qualitative research: an essential part of statistical cognition research', *Statistics Education Research Journal*, 9(2): 23–34.
Lewbel, A. (2008) 'Engel curve', in S.N. Durlauf and E. Lawrence (eds) *The New Palgrave Dictionary of Economics*. Blume: Palgrave Macmillan. Available at: www.dictionaryofeconomics.com/article?id=pde2008_E000085 (accessed 25 March 2015).
Lewis, D. (2012) *Reality Check Reflection Report*, Stockholm: Sida.
Masset, E., Jupp, D., Korboe, D., Dogbe, T. and Barrett, C. (2013) *Millennium Villages Impact Evaluation: Baseline summary report*, Hove: Itad.
Reality Check Approach Team (2014) *Nepal Rural Access Programme Baseline Report*, Hove: Itad.
Reudin, L. and Shutt, C. (2013) *SDC How-to-Note Beneficiary Assessment*. Bern: SDC.
Salmen, L.F. (1998) 'Towards a listening bank; a review of best practices and the efficacy of beneficiary assessment', *Social Development Papers*, 23: 1–18.

Part IV

Understanding impact and change

13

Innovation in evaluation
Using SenseMaker to assess the inclusion of smallholder farmers in modern markets

Irene Guijt

Introduction

SenseMaker is a narrative-based research method that aims to elicit personal micro-narratives to help understand what matters to whom. This chapter focuses on its use to understand change from the perspectives of those who are rarely, if ever, heard in mainstream evaluation research. Such voices might include small-scale coffee producers in Colombia sharing stories of risk to foster more inclusive business models, or urban citizens in Vanuatu explaining how parliamentarians' decisions impact their lives. SenseMaker is one of several emerging options – including Outcome Mapping and Outcome Harvesting (Earl *et al.* 2001, Wilson-Grau 2015) and systems thinking (Hummelbrunner 2011) – that are making monitoring and evaluation practice better able to deal with complex situations and interventions.

Much evaluation in the international development sector deals with non-linear, multi-actor, unpredictable and long-term change processes, and an expansion of the associated methods repertoire is critical. Traditional monitoring and evaluation frameworks and related methods are increasingly recognised as inadequate when coping with this kind of complexity (Stern *et al.* 2012, Befani *et al.* 2014). Many such frameworks – and related methods – have multiple failings (Guijt 2008, Ramalingam *et al.* 2014). They may assume that causal pathways and information needs are knowable prior to project or programme implementation, and are stable over place and time. Monitoring and evaluation protocols and formats are frequently framed in terms of simplified hierarchical action plans that distort and reduce the messy realities and partnerships in which interventions are nested. The creation of too simplistic a set of cause–effect logics can prohibit agile adaptation during implementation, despite the inevitability of changes in contexts and social relationships. The critical processes needed to transform information into actionable insights – such as analysis, critical reflection, interpretation and communication – are often assumed to occur automatically, without requiring explicit methodological attention. A balanced picture of what is often a complex reality is assumed to emerge from chosen indicators, with little influence from power relations between those involved in monitoring and evaluation (and the context of these relationships) on the quality of evaluation design or implementation process, or its outcomes.

Complexity-aware options are needed to capture unanticipated emergent results and to acknowledge that interventions change over time, to be of use in situations where a credible counterfactual based on a predetermined set of variables is neither useful nor feasible. One stream of methodological innovation in evaluation focuses on listening to how local people experience impact, and ensuring these insights are regularly incorporated. Such interpretive methods assume an interdependence between people, how they make meanings, and their interactions with the world around them. As Rowlands (2005: 84) explains, 'interpretive researchers thus attempt to understand phenomena through accessing the meanings participants assign to them'.

SenseMaker is one method (aided by the use of software of the same name) that recognises that narratives may allow better access to contextualised knowledge about behaviours and actions than questions and answers (Snowden 2010). This method gathers many micro-narratives about life experiences and enables respondents to make sense of these themselves (cf. Snowden 2010, Casella et al. 2014). This chapter illustrates how SenseMaker can be useful for (impact) evaluation, by focusing on one case study that assessed the inclusion of smallholder farmers in markets that currently operate in ways that exclude these farmers as valued and sustained sellers (Deprez et al. 2012).[1]

Connecting smallholders to inclusive markets

This study was undertaken by a Belgium-based non-governmental organisation called Vredeseilanden (VECO) that strives for more viable livelihoods for organised small-scale farmers through improved income from sustainable agriculture. The organisation focuses particularly on sustainable agricultural 'value chain' development that connects largely low-income farmers to modern markets in ways that benefit them. The study involved the application of SenseMaker to help VECO understand how to assess its impact in terms of fostering a more inclusive way of doing business between different actors in the modern market chain. Value chain development is a complex process in which different actors – smallholder farmers, processors, traders, retailers and consumers – work together to achieve shared goals, while subject to government policies, environmental aspects and market dynamics. Learning to navigate this complexity in a sustainable and equitable manner requires an organisational and individual capacity development process, policy shifts, and changes to the relationship between farmers and other chain actors.

Value chain development requires a planning, monitoring and management approach to understand the complex processes in which individuals and organisations are engaged in markets. To complement an existing participatory learning and accountability system, VECO decided to pilot SenseMaker within its Inclusive Modern Markets programme (Deprez et al. 2012). During initial pilot studies, VECO sought to understand the impact on smallholder farmer inclusion by looking at issues relating to 'ownership', 'voice', 'risk' and 'reward', and the extent to which these are experienced by different chain actors. Since the initial pilot studies, VECO has reframed its use of SenseMaker around five impact areas that measure inclusive business: chain wide collaboration, effective market linkages, fair and transparent governance, equitable access to services, and inclusive innovation (Lundy et al. 2014).

Two very different cases were chosen for the pilot work, although both involved smallholder farmers organised into cooperatives, selling produce to a private company. These differed in context, product, geographical scope, complexity, type of farmer organisation, type of buyer and market. In Southern Ecuador, plantain bananas are collected by members of a farmers' cooperative and transported to West Ecuador to be processed into banana chips. These Fair Trade certified banana chips are then sold to a French buyer, who sells them on to French and Belgian supermarkets. The second case study involves tea production in northern Vietnam by a group of farmers who were just starting up a cooperative. The tea is collected and bought by a local tea processing company, and sold nationally.

VECO's interest lay in understanding the inclusiveness of the value chain itself, rather than the attribution of causal links between the VECO programme and changes in the two value chains. As such, SenseMaker was used to reveal the inclusiveness of business relationships through the eyes of smallholder farmers, and provide insight into how VECO might measure the impact of its work in the future (Deprez et al. 2012).

How SenseMaker works

SenseMaker is the name used to describe both a method and accompanying software that facilitates local people to generate and analyse data. Stories are collected from hundreds or thousands of individuals, either through face-to-face interviews or online data collection. Each conversation collects an account or story about a particular issue, as well as the respondent's interpretation and analysis of their story. SenseMaker has evolved largely from use for diagnostic and planning purposes, but is described here in terms of its utility for understanding people's perspectives on the changes brought about by specific interventions.

Designing the question framework

Any evaluative process is guided by questions. In SenseMaker, stories are elicited using a prompting question to help people share a meaningful story. The choice of question depends on the knowledge needed. For impact evaluation, open-ended questions that elicit 'outcome' stories rather than evaluative statements are useful. This can happen before and after interventions in order to understand perspectives on change over time. During this particular VECO study, interest lay in assessing how farmers, staff of private companies and others involved in supporting the value chain experienced their involvement in value chains. The following prompt was formulated to invite a story of change from the farmers:

> Think about the agricultural value chain in which you are actively involved. Think of a specific moment or event (that happened in the last six months) when you felt particularly encouraged or concerned about producing tea and selling to the company/buyer. Please describe what happened briefly. Who was involved? Why did it happen?

Prompts were tested with intended respondents in the context in which the evaluation took place to ensure that questions asked generate micro-narratives from respondents that illustrate impact or change. If left too broad, very general stories may make subsequent analysis less insightful. If too specific, prompts can inhibit the type of open-ended inquiry that is desired.

Next, those using SenseMaker identified a predefined series of questions that were asked to enable the respondent to interpret, analyse and give significance to different aspects of the narrative they had just provided. These questions establish what is known as a 'signification framework'. Multiple-choice questions are included to gather information about the respondent (e.g. gender, age, degree of engagement with the programme being evaluated) and about the story (e.g. how the story made the person feel, its core themes and where it took place). Three specific types of questions – 'triads', 'sliders' and 'stones' – were also used to examine the more nuanced nature of people's experiences.

As illustrated in Figure 13.1, 'triads' are triangles with three variables constituting the points of the triangle. The apices are constructed as evenly balanced labels (worded in positive, negative or neutral terms), with the centre of the

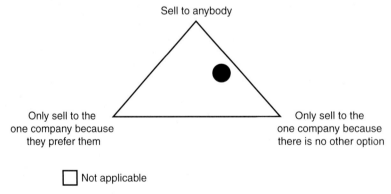

Figure 13.1 A triad question about autonomy in the value chain
Source: Adapted from Deprez 2015.

triangle representing a balance where all responses are equally present. The respondent is asked to mark a spot in the triangle to indicate how the story shared relates to each of the three labels. In this example, farmers sharing experiences of marketing their Fair Trade produce were asked to place a dot in the triangle to indicate their sense of power to decide which retailer to sell to. This question illustrates the extent of power of farmer voice.

'Sliders', also known as 'dyads' or 'polarities', are used by SenseMaker to construct patterns in relation to a certain quality, such as shared decision making, trust, or a result area (e.g. profitability). As illustrated in Figure 13.2, visually, these questions provide a sliding scale between two extremes, with a 'zero point' in the middle. This type of visualisation encourages respondents to be more thoughtful than with a four or five point rating scale. The visual might look like Figure 13.2 or may simply take the form of a line along which the respondent marks their response. In this example, farmers and other actors in the tea and banana chip chains were asked to indicate the extent to which their story was one of shared or unilateral decision making – an aspect of chain-wide collaboration.

Question: In your story, the chain in characterised by ...

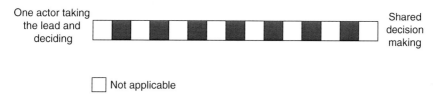

Figure 13.2 A slider about the degree of shared decision making
Source: Adapted from Deprez et al. 2012.

Question: In your story, in the case of [type of risk M / P / T] ...
Drag your symbol and position where it belongs according to you

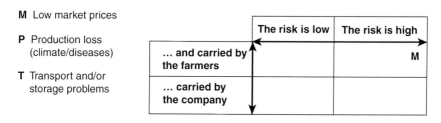

Figure 13.3 A 'stones' question about risk sharing
Source: Adapted from VECO 2015.

Figure 13.3 illustrates the use of a question type called 'stones' that enables respondents to undertake a comparative assessment of several elements of a narrative. Farmers were asked about how different types of risks (from low to high) are shared by farmers or by companies. The respondent places each risk – or 'stone' – onto a grid or matrix where he or she feels it best fits in relation to their story. If a farmer placed the stone (labelled low market prices, or 'M') as per Figure 13.3, it would indicate that his/her story concerned a situation where the risk of low market prices was high, and that the risk was carried by the farmer rather than being shared with the company buying his/her product.

When SenseMaker is used for evaluation purposes, I have found it useful to adopt a question framework that incorporates questions that are descriptive (i.e. what has changed), causal (i.e. what might explain the changes) and evaluative (i.e. whether the changes are valued or not). Multiple-choice descriptive questions might focus on the theme of the shared narrative (e.g. agricultural inputs, production, processing, trading), as well as the feelings of the person sharing the narrative (e.g. proud, encouraged, indifferent, ashamed, confident, angry and/ or sad). Combining the answers can reveal patterns about which themes are experienced with more positive or more negative feelings (evaluative question). When carried out over time, patterns of change can be assessed. Causal questions could include triads about voice, shared decision making, and so forth, as these are all variables that could explain the extent to which inclusion of smallholder farmers in markets has become more possible, and is being experienced as such by farmers.

Signification frameworks are more robust when they are developed with input from many stakeholders, informed by existing theory or knowledge about the topic of interest, and then tested *in situ*. Such testing makes it more likely that questions are clear and meaningful for the topic and respondent, and that the length of question set (around 20–30 questions) is manageable for respondents. Fewer questions help maintain the interest of the story sharer, but a more limited set of questions can also reduce the analytical options and depth of insights.

Collecting stories and signifiers

Story collection by interviewers and self-coding by respondents can occur in a variety of ways. People can share stories in individual interview settings, with collection being either paper-based or on smartphones or tablets. Stories can also be collected and self-coded in groups. In the pilot studies in Ecuador and Vietnam, stories were collected through facilitated group sessions (Deprez *et al.* 2012). In Ecuador, data was collected from 75 farmers via two rounds of story collection, each lasting two days. In Vietnam, 144 respondents were reached through one round of story collection over a five day period. In both countries, VECO staff guided farmers through the questions, as they wrote their experiences and related responses on printed survey forms. The data was subsequently entered into an online database – known as 'Collector' – that offers a replica of the paper survey forms. In more recent studies, VECO has been collecting stories and answers directly, individually or in group settings, into the online database via tablets.

Two additional issues are important to ensure high quality data collection: sampling and training. The use of a well-defined sampling frame will make it very clear whose perspectives are and are not informing the analysis. This was decided by VECO prior to commencing each of the studies, and primarily involved smallholder farmers, with other input from other chain actors (e.g. farmer organisation leaders/staff, buyers, traders, processors or service providers).

Due to the use of personal stories and the unusual way in which triads and sliders work, training of researchers, enumerators or fieldworkers who will collect the stories is also critical. Training ensures that prompting questions are asked in a way that does not lead respondents, and that triads, sliders and stones questions are used effectively to gather respondents' interpretations and analyses of their original stories.

Analysis and use

Once the stories and answers to the analytical probing questions have been entered into the online database, further analysis can begin. This usually involves two steps. Step one consists of SenseMaker software-aided visual pattern detection, to uncover the extent and nature of impacts, and explanations for these patterns. This task is best undertaken by people who have been trained to use the SenseMaker software. It generates patterns to support sensemaking – or the analytical process that is required to interpret the data set. Each triad, slider and stones visual output is examined in light of the full data set. A single triad may be parsed for different variables to compare patterns. For example, the pattern created by combining all the data produced by the question in Figure 13.1 could be viewed twice – one with positive stories and another with negative stories – to see whether the distribution of stories changes, or to examine how autonomy over who to sell to has a positive or negative influence on farmers' experiences. In the case of VECO, five staff members were introduced to the software and its various applications during a one-day workshop, and undertook the subsequent analysis (Deprez *et al.* 2012).

The second analytical step involves making sense of the data through an iterative process of scrutinising visual patterns and stories relevant to these. Sitting down with visual patterns that have potential value, and clusters of stories associated with these patterns, is an important part of this process. Who does this is important – those involved need to understand the context within which different perspectives have been uncovered, so that analytical 'aha' moments can occur when examining story clusters. In this case study, different stakeholders – including 20–30 farmers, VECO staff, and representatives from the private company and government – were invited to a two-day workshop to discuss the initial patterns.

There are different ways to structure the interpretation process. One option is to ask people to cluster visual insights into those that confirm existing programme strategies or theories of change, those that challenged them, and those they simply did not understand. These discussions can help programme staff to identify what to keep on doing, what to do differently, what to stop doing, and what new ideas might be worth trying to ensure impact is achieved. Flipping between stories and statistics bridges the qualitative and quantitative information divide, leading to statistical data backed up by an explanatory narrative.

SenseMaker's interpretive and evaluative basis

In 2008, when I first encountered SenseMaker, several features seemed to help overcome some of the limitations of monitoring and evaluation practice. At that time, predefined indicators seemed the only route to shaping evaluation systems, based on the incorrect assumption that it is possible to know fully in advance what it is one needs to find out. Where was the space for emerging insights and for new impacts or changes? Why were unintended consequences rarely given sufficient attention? Why were performance-oriented processes so prevalent? Why was there so little space for approaches that focused on learning and improvement? Methodologically it seemed an either/or choice was needed between quantitative or qualitative representation of data, situated in a deeply problematic debate that gave preference to so-called 'gold standard' methods that privileged quantitative data above those in which individual, human voices were heard. SenseMaker offered an alternative to this.

Taking complexity seriously

Much monitoring and evaluation practice is based on the assumption that what needs to be measured is knowable ahead of time through simple and predictable cause–effect relationships. This has spawned multiple variations of logic model and results-oriented evaluation protocols. However, real-life project settings are often subject to quite different cause and effect relationships, thus requiring the identification of different approaches to generating evidence, undertaking analysis and planning action that are valid for different conditions (Snowden 2010). For example, it makes little sense using only predefined indicator-based approaches when evaluating the impact of interventions in complex environments for which the overarching goal may be clear, but the predicted pathways to reach the goal will inevitably evolve over time (Snowden and Boone 2007). SenseMaker was developed to fill the gap created by the paucity of options to understand complex environments. Data are processed as they emerge, to assess the dispositions for change and stagnation that exist in a particular situation, and to identify possible programmatic responses. In complex and chaotic situations, rather than measuring and categorising, short cycles of experimentation (probe–sense–response) are useful in advancing towards the intended impact of an intervention or programme. This principle aligns well with the growing interest in international development in tight feedback loops – cycles of action, data collection, learning and adaptation – to enable continual and quick experiential learning (cf. Andrews *et al.* 2012).

Voices at scale

SenseMaker recognises that people most often share and give meaning to their lives through discussion and narratives in the form of stories about personal experiences (Snowden 2010, Casella *et al.* 2014). Two issues of scale need consideration here: the first relates to whose voices count, and the second relates to how many of these voices matter. It is important to help bring voices that are never or seldom heard into the decision-making process. With VECO, local farmers had never been asked systematically and at this scale about their experiences of risk sharing and pride in, or ownership of, their product. During the work undertaken, local farmers were included in the evaluation, which was designed to facilitate their involvement in decisions about, for example, pricing stability or quality standards.

SenseMaker works with micro-narratives. Multiple micro-narratives hold the potential to paint a nuanced picture or mosaic of experiences that may not be achieved through other more in-depth qualitative studies involving fewer respondents. The aim is to gather multiple perspectives about a multitude of experiences that influence people's actions in the system or community being transformed and evaluated. Moreover, those living or working in a particular context may have access to some but not all of the relevant information; hence there is merit in pooling a large range of experiences, perspectives, motivations and values around the topic of inquiry (Hutchins 1995).

Surprise and ambiguity

While those involved in programmes and projects, as implementers or funders, need to be willing to challenge what they believe to be true, they also need to be open to surprises and consciously seek them (Guijt 2008). Evaluation frameworks and methods are very good at finding out what people know, or think they need to know. Information about predefined indicators, targets and milestones can sometimes provide 'evidence that disconfirms cherished expectations' (Weick and Sutcliffe 2001: 155). Such a 'mismatch-based surprise' (Lorini and Castelfranchi 2007: 134) may trigger further investigation to clarify the source of the discrepancy. But reconsideration of beliefs can also come from 'astonishment in recognition' (ibid.: 134), which constitutes the random, unexpected, unplanned encounters and events that occur as activities unfold and people interact. SenseMaker can generate both kinds of surprise. Users can look at visual patterns and stories to check whether a predefined expectation is met or not, verifying whether there is a match or mismatch. Users can also explore the data, parsing and linking and comparing different subsets while remaining open to experiencing moments of deep cognitive dissonance.

Reducing the intermediating bias of evaluation professionals

Geertz (1973: 9) wrote that 'what we call our data are really our own constructions of other people's constructions of what they and their compatriots are up to'. Because of this, the more the 'we' can be taken out of the process, the more people's own versions of their worlds can be seen and heard. However, when it comes to analysing narrative data, traditionally evaluators undertake the process of analytical coding themselves, often using predefined or emergent categories. In contrast, SenseMaker works on the basis that those who share their stories are best qualified to interpret what their own narratives mean. This 'self-signification' provides people with the opportunity to put their stories into context. The 'self-tagging' of respondents' stories aims to avoid evaluator biases during the initial stages of data interpretation. It helps those wanting to understand impact get more 'inside the world of those generating it' (Geertz 1973: 9). The person sharing the story decides what it means. When responding to the questions within a signification framework, respondents add meaning to their story, and in doing so they open the door to their worlds.

Analysing smallholder farmers' stories

Findings from the pilot studies in Vietnam and Ecuador illustrate how SenseMaker generated smallholder farmers' perspectives about their inclusion in modern markets (Deprez *et al.* 2012). Following the two step analysis process explained above, visual analysis was undertaken to examine the extent to which

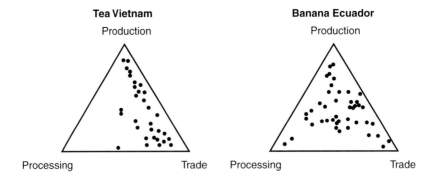

Figure 13.4 Smallholder story trends for production, trade and processing
Source: Adapted from Deprez *et al.* 2012.

smallholder farmers' narratives focused on three different aspects of their business: production, processing and trading (see Figure 13.4). These patterns were then parsed for positive and negative feelings, to understand where farmers were experiencing successes or problems in relation to more inclusive business.

In Vietnam, results showed that production and trading were critical stages – around two thirds of stories related to trading. Stories indexed against positive emotions by the respondents were evenly distributed between production and trading. However, stories associated with negative emotions – notably frustration, anger, worry, sadness – were linked more closely to trading. Feedback on these results – the visual patterns and related stories – generated significant reflection and debate among farmers, farmer leaders and the company on issues specifically related to payment schedules and price setting. Through use of a triad question that asked who sets the prices paid to farmers, analysis of narratives indicated that farmers are the least powerful actor in setting prices for tea; private companies were largely responsible for setting payment schedules, together with other middlemen, leaving farmers vulnerable to price fluctuations (Deprez et al. 2012).

> I remember one day in June, I picked tea to sell to The Company at its gate. The lady buyer of the company said 'your tea is not really good, I can pay you only 3600 dong [GBP0.11] for a kg'... One day later, I also picked tea and brought it to The Company and sold it at a higher price, 3800 dong [GBP0.12] a kg. After that, I carried tea to sell here again, the buyer said that she could pay me only 3500 [GBP0.11] per kg. What happened made me sad and I wish that The Company could have a system to stabilise the tea price for farmers.
>
> (Smallholder tea farmer, Vietnam)

> In the morning of June 25, 2011, Mr Lam, the collector [middleman], notified us the price of 2200 dong [GBP0.07] a kg. I picked tea and carried it to his house for selling. In the morning, I sold it to him at 2200 dong [GBP0.07] a kg as informed, but the price in the afternoon was down to 1800 dong [GBP0.05] per kg. I asked him why did there exist two different price levels on the same day? We argued with each other and he replied because my buyer price level is going down, I have no way of reducing the level as well. I got frustrated and decided to transport it to The Company and sold it at 2500 dong [GBP0.08] for a kg.
>
> (Smallholder tea farmer, Vietnam)

In contrast, 15 stories from Vietnamese tea farmers indicated that there was an opportunity to contribute to shaping payment schedules. Nine of these came from one village that sells tea directly to the collector with whom they agree on payment, indicating the importance of increasing effective market linkages, and fair and transparent governance.

Workshop discussions – including farmers and company directors – about these results led to some immediate changes around pricing in particular. For example, one company director, upon hearing about the effects of multiple daily fluctuations in prices, proposed putting up a sign at the factory of the price of tea for each day and not changing it. This is a strategy that he has since implemented.

In the banana chips chain in Ecuador, farmer organisations were seen as having more power in price setting than in the Vietnam case, with visual patterns pointing to an equal number of stories about farmers and private companies setting the price, with a clear cluster of stories balanced between the two (Deprez et al. 2012). However, discussion of the results identified problems about the division of roles and expectations between grassroots farmer organisations and the cooperative: who is in charge of commercialisation? Who determines the quotas and when these should be met? Who delivers to the company? How are payments organised and scheduled?

Findings from the pilot studies in Vietnam and Ecuador pointed to the ability of SenseMaker to generate smallholder farmers' perspectives about change relating to their inclusion in modern markets. In doing so, this method provided interesting information to assist VECO to unpick the less tangible elements of its influence in value chain development, as well as develop new ideas for future impact measurement (Deprez et al. 2012). Consequently, VECO has initiated other applications of SenseMaker, including a focus on smallholder farmers' production and sale of rice in Senegal, cacao in Indonesia and coffee in Congo. These studies are helping VECO build a differentiated understanding about the impact of its chain-focused work on smallholder farmers' experiences of inclusion in markets (Deprez 2015).

Since the pilot studies, VECO has also shifted its analysis process from systematically working through each triad, slider and multiple choice question, to clustering patterns around the principles it is seeking to impact (Deprez, pers. comm., 20 April 2015). Such analysis allows VECO to build a more nuanced understanding about where in the chain, and why, it is having an impact in terms of smallholder farmers' involvement in more inclusive business.

The challenges of evaluation innovation

Beyond the VECO project, SenseMaker has been used by others to undertake diagnostic studies for project design, to create baselines for impact studies, to conduct retrospective studies on outcomes that help rethink underlying theories of change, to deepen understanding about intended impacts, and to undertake focused evaluations of short-term initiatives. These experiences point to a number of conditions that help to ensure that SenseMaker works well when trying to understand change and impact.

In terms of evaluation design, it is important to establish a clear sampling frame, and use a purposive mix of descriptive, causal and evaluative questions to elicit evaluative conclusions about the programme being assessed. As pointed to in other literature about interpretive and ethnographic analysis processes (e.g.

Bell and Aggleton 2012), it is also important to gather other sources of information to allow for triangulation of findings.

Work is also required to make the data collection process both feasible and ethically sound. For example, for large projects, investment in a data collection modality (paper vs technology; individual vs group) that can be implemented with local capacity is needed to ensure wide and diverse utilisation of SenseMaker in different contexts. When gathering paper-based data, transcription must be both accurate and affordable. Where longer term data collection is envisaged, such as in the application of SenseMaker to pre- and post-intervention analyses of change, ethically sound, secure and confidential data storage systems need to be established and used routinely. Greater consideration of the ethical requirements for data storage and access is required, with thought about how long stories can be stored safely, who is allowed to access them for analysis, and ensuring that respondents are always asked to consent to their involvement in projects with a clear understanding about these issues.

Using SenseMaker well requires strong commitment and skill to ensure that previously unheard voices remain central in evaluation work. This is, of course, not unique to this evaluation approach. Enumerators and researchers require sufficient training and experience in communicating with local people, research facilitation and data analysis, in order to gather the stories, enable local people to interpret these stories, and analyse and convey what the story patterns have to offer organisations using this approach. In this way, SenseMaker challenges the role of the evaluation professional, who is initially hired for his or her methodological and subject matter expertise, but is then asked to uncover local interpretations and analyses. Evaluators leading the SenseMaker approach must also be confident and experienced in facilitating discussions with those commissioning the evaluation to come to actionable priorities and strategies to support the continuation of existing programme activities, and identify those that need to be stopped and those that are new.

SenseMaker does not suit all organisations or all monitoring and evaluation applications. The approach has been met with scepticism and blank expressions from those who favour more mainstream monitoring and evaluation methodological traditions that tend not to be geared towards embracing complexity. The method challenges such evaluation approaches in many ways, including how to understand impact in a way that is different to usual predetermined logic models. The approach can take some people and organisations outside their comfort zone by introducing ambiguity into the local-led sensemaking process. For example, in the design phase, stakeholders involved in shaping the question framework are asked to let go of the idea of standardised indicators, letting concepts and principles guide the process rather than targets and milestones. This continues into the sensemaking phase itself, where researchers or enumerators elicit micro-narratives and let respondents interpret these stories of change based on their own understandings of local contexts and experiences. Organisations concerned with upward accountability may be less keen to invest in a way of working that actively seeks to prioritise many, diverse, local perspectives of change, from the vantage point of those whose lives are intended to improve from development efforts.

Conclusions

In this chapter, I have illustrated how SenseMaker offers a valuable and unique contribution to evaluation practice. It complements more mainstream monitoring and evaluation approaches that are better suited to what is knowable and what we know we need to know. For VECO, the method has provided interesting information and insights in relation to impact measurement, particularly in relation to the less tangible aspects of smallholder farmer inclusion in markets. Using SenseMaker in a one-off event generates potentially interesting insights, but its real power for learning about change lies in continuous story capture. If stories are collected on a regular basis using the same signification framework, one could observe shifting patterns of impact and change over time.

The method has captured the attention of many organisations due to its potential to combine the in-depth interpretive, qualitative insight found in micro-narratives and anecdotes, and quantitative analysis at large scales. As an approach, it can bring voices seldom heard into decision making, explicitly seeking the unexpected, reducing evaluator biases, providing timely and continuous feedback, and aggregating patterns of impact across diverse contexts. The growing attentiveness in international development with different forms of feedback – including listening to experiences and preferences of citizens or clients and acting on these (Guijt 2014) – suggests that interest in SenseMaker is only likely to grow.

Recognising that most social development programmes take place in complex environments means questioning the core foundation of accepted monitoring and evaluation practices and framings, typically based around predictable logic models of change. Complex problems cannot be tamed by ignoring them, or trying to understand them through theories relying on known inputs, outputs and outcomes. The field of evaluation needs novel ways to hear what local women, men and children have to say about development efforts that seek social change for their benefit, and to do this at scale. Where development efforts have become more about procedures and protocols rather than relationships, adopting an interpretive approach to evaluation can re-humanise efforts by hearing about how people's lives have been impacted. As illustrated in this case study, SenseMaker offers a new interpretive option to understand local people's perspectives on change and programme impact.

Note

1 Other examples of the use of SenseMaker can be found here: http://cognitive-edge.com/sensemaker.

References

Andrews, M., Pritchett, L. and Woolcock, M. (2012) 'Escaping capability traps through problem-driven iterative adaptation (PDIA)', *Working Paper 299*. Available at: www.cgdev.org/sites/default/files/1426292_file_Andrews_Pritchett_Woolcock_traps_FINAL_0.pdf (accessed 21 May 2015).

Befani, B., Barnett, C. and Stern, E. (2014) 'Introduction: rethinking impact evaluation for development', *IDS Bulletin*, 45(6): 1–5.

Bell, S.A. and Aggleton, P. (2012) 'Integrating ethnographic principles in NGO monitoring and impact evaluation', *Journal of International Development*, 24: 795–807.

Carr, N.G. (2015) 'Anti-anecdotalism', in J. Brockman (ed.) *This Idea Must Die: Scientific ideas that are blocking progress*. New York: HarperCollins, p. 128.

Casella, D., Magara, P., Kumasi, T.C., Guijt, I. and van Soest, A. (2014) 'The Triple-S Project Sensemaker® experience: a method tested and rejected', *Triple-S Working Paper 9*. The Hague: IRC.

Deprez, S. (2015) *Voices that Count. Using micro-narratives to organise systematic and real-time feedback on the inclusion of smallholders in modern markets*, Leuven: VECO.

Deprez, S., Huyghe, C. and van Gool Maldonado, C. (2012) *Using Sensemaker to Measure, Learn and Communicate about Smallholder Farmer Inclusion*, Leuven: VECO.

Earl, S., Carden, F. and Smutylo, T. (2001) *Outcome Mapping: Building learning and reflection into development programs*, Ottawa: International Development Research Centre.

Geertz, C. (1973) *The Interpretation of Cultures*, New York: Basic Books.

Guijt, I. (2008) *Seeking Surprise: Rethinking monitoring for collective learning in rural resource management*. Published PhD dissertation. Wageningen University, Wageningen, The Netherlands.

Guijt, I. (2014) Week 50: Feedback loops – new buzzword, old practice? Available at: www.betterevaluation.org/blog/feedback_loops_new_buzzword_old_practice (accessed 8 May 2015).

Hummelbrunner, R. (2011) 'Systems thinking and evaluation', *Evaluation*, 17(4): 395–403.

Hutchins, E. (1995). *Cognition in the Wild*, Cambridge, MA: MIT Press.

Lorini, E. and Castelfranchi, C. (2007) 'The cognitive structure of surprise: looking for basic principles', *Topoi*, 26(1): 133–149.

Lundy, M., Amrein, A., Hurtado, J.J., Becx, G., Zamierowski, N., Rodriquez, F. and Mosquera, E.E. (2014) *LINK Methodology: A participatory guide to business models that link smallholders to markets*. Available at: http://ciat-library.ciat.cgiar.org/articulos_ciat/LINK_Methodology.pdf (accessed 20 May 2015).

Ramalingam, B., Laric, M. and Primrose, J. (2014) *From Best Practice to Best Fit: Understanding and navigating wicked problems in international development*, London: Overseas Development Institute. Available at: www.odi.org/sites/odi.org.uk/files/odi-assets/publications-opinion-files/9159.pdf (accessed 8 May 2015).

Rowlands, B. (2005) 'Grounded in practice: using interpretive research to build theory', *The Electronic Journal of Business Research Methodology*, 3(1): 81–92.

Snowden, D. (2010) 'Naturalizing Sensemaking', in K.L. Mosier and U.M. Fischer (eds) *Informed by Knowledge: Expert performance in complex situations*, New York: Psychology Press, pp. 223–234.

Snowden, D.J. and Boone, M.E. (2007) 'A leader's framework for decision making', *Harvard Business Review*, November: 1–10.

Stern, E., Stame, N., Mayne, J., Forss, K., Davies, R. and Befani, B. (2012) *Broadening the Range of Designs and Methods for Impact Evaluations*. Working Paper 38. Available at: http://r4d.dfid.gov.uk/Output/189575 (accessed 8 May 2015).

VECO (2015) SenseMaker Signification Framework 'Inclusive Business', Leuven: VECO.

Weick, K. and Sutcliffe, K. (2001). *Managing the Unexpected: Assuring high performance in an age of complexity*, San Francisco, CA: Jossey-Bass.

Wilson-Grau, R. (2015) *Outcome Harvesting*. Available at: www.betterevaluation.org/plan/approach/outcome_harvesting (accessed 5 March 2015).

14

The use of the Rapid PEER approach for the evaluation of sexual and reproductive health programmes

Eleanor Brown, Rachel Grellier and Kirstan Hawkins

In sexual and reproductive health research, the role of naturalistic qualitative enquiry – the study of people's behaviours and life experiences in their natural settings, and the multiple, socially constructed meanings that people bring to them (Lincoln and Guba 1985) – has been the subject of intense debate, particularly within a push for a greater results-based focus (White 2009). Typically, it has been argued that too rigid a focus on measuring outcomes has resulted in limiting the types of methods and evidence that programmes can use, which means that we cannot see the process of change, understand causality, or identify and measure unexpected outcomes (Bell and Aggleton 2012). Conversely, critiques of the previous use of participatory research techniques have argued that there was little solid evidence on whether development spending was 'doing any good or not' (White 2009: 8). By implication, methods were not producing the kind of evidence that could be counted as a rigorous measurement of 'impact'.

In this chapter, we share lessons learned from evaluating sexual and reproductive health programmes using the Rapid Participatory Ethnographic Evaluation and Research (Rapid PEER) method. The benefits and challenges of this qualitative approach are discussed using two case studies in Papua New Guinea and the UK. These illustrate the value and importance, both for programme staff and the wider sexual and reproductive health community, of the ethnographic data obtained through Rapid PEER and how this information can be used to strengthen and explain, rather than replace, quantitative outcomes.

Understanding sociocultural logic

In 2002 Price and Hawkins (2002) published details of a new methodology that they termed the Participatory Ethnographic Evaluation Research (PEER) approach, using ethnographic principles to answer questions crucial to sexual and reproductive health research more rapidly. The PEER method aims to work with 'insiders' within a social network to collect data, privileging 'emic' perspectives on the measurement of change and impact. Price and Hawkins (2002) argued that economic–rationalist models of human behaviour in reproductive health, in which fertility behaviour is understood as driven by an attempt to maximise scarce resources, resulted in abstracting individuals' behaviour from the sociocultural and political context in which decisions about reproductive health are made. These models frequently result in conceptions of declines in fertility as dependent on the diffusion of Western ideas, primarily through the spread of information or education. This ignores the fact that global advances (and reversals) in people's rights to enjoy sexual health and well-being have been made on the back of wider arguments about people's rights and needs to access sexual and reproductive health services. Fundamentally, reproduction is a 'political' process, grounded within gender-based power relations and maintained within local knowledge and health systems. Programmes and research to measure their impact need therefore to understand the internal sociocultural logic employed within the daily lives of the people that they intend to serve.

PEER was designed to understand and measure the processes of change that programmes aimed to achieve. Since its development, the approach has been used throughout the programme cycle, including formative research, programme monitoring, and evaluation of change and impact (Price and Hawkins 2002, Hawkins et al. 2004). The method has been found to be especially useful for 'researching the un-researchable', including highly sensitive issues or communities where the strength of traditional norms or patterns of stigma mean that individuals find it hard to talk openly about the internal 'truths' that form their inner worlds.

If aid programmes and interventions aim to catalyse positive change, evidence of 'impact' must include cataloguing positive and negative change, and highlight lessons to guide further interventions (Batliwala and Pitman 2010). Research methods need to capture change as it emerges, and develop powerful lines of enquiry about the process of change. As Batliwala and Pitman (2010) argue, this is particularly pertinent for programmes and interventions that aim to strengthen women's rights, where the particularities of power shifts and implications for women's reproductive choices need to be better understood at many different points throughout the programme cycle. With respect to sexual and reproductive health issues, control over women's reproductive choices is mediated by structural and contextual factors in complex and powerful ways that need to be better understood.

To date, over 50 formative research and impact evaluation studies have been conducted using this method, focusing especially on sexual and reproductive health issues. The usefulness of the methodology lies primarily in generating data on the internal sociocultural logic of communities under study, which programme staff can then use in specific ways: in advocacy, for understanding how specific health areas are framed and understood; in programme learning, for assessing how programmes are perceived and in what ways they can improve programmes and interventions; and lastly, for impact evaluation, for exploring how change is defined and what public good it is perceived as creating (Batliwala and Pitman 2010).

What is Rapid PEER?

Rapid PEER was developed as an adaption of the original 'full' method for the purpose of programme evaluation. As with the original approach, the rapid version works by using pre-existing networks of trust (Price and Hawkins 2002). Ordinary members of the target population or community (anyone who has not undertaken a paid or voluntary role within the project) are recruited to be PEER researchers. These researchers are trained in basic conversational interviewing skills and research ethics. A small number of broad questions are agreed during the training workshop and translated into the language of 'everyday' conversation between friends. Following this, data collection and initial data analysis are completed within five days. During this time, these researchers interview two to three friends over a period of 48 hours, using the questions developed during training to structure the conversation, on an individual basis. If possible, the interviewee should be someone outside the interviewer's immediate family.

A key feature of Rapid PEER is that data is collected in the 'third person' and that no notes are taken during the interview. Questions deliberately do not ask about the interviewee's own knowledge or behaviour, and instead ask what other 'people like them' do, say or believe, although researchers and their friends may incorporate their own experiences into their narratives. Direct personal experience is not attributable. This lack of attribution enables participants to provide insights into behaviour and experiences that deviate from accepted norms and values more openly. Thus the focus is less on building consensus around specific issues than on understanding a full range of behaviours and the factors underpinning them.

Detailed individual debriefings with researchers take place no more than 48 hours after they have finished the interviews. A qualitative research specialist and the researchers meet to recall, review and discuss the data that has been collected on a one-to-one basis. It is at this point that detailed notes are taken by the research specialist. During a final workshop the research findings are fed back to the PEER researchers, allowing the research specialists to validate their analysis, and enabling further exploration of the data and joint analysis of the implications of findings with community members for programmatic practice.

Rapid PEER relies heavily on story-telling to generate 'thick description' (Geertz 1973: 3) of complex social realities. This harnesses the power of qualitative narrative and story-telling – in other words, gossip – which is often dismissed as 'anecdotal' evidence but which, in reality, often informs and influences people's opinions and decisions in their daily lives. An added benefit is that these stories can often be used to develop training and communication materials for future use within the programme.

Trust between researchers and project participants is essential to producing reliable research findings, and trust is maintained in several ways. This includes the use of third person narratives so that direct personal experience can never be attributed (although PEER researchers and their friends may actually be talking about themselves), as well as through shared ownership of the research process at critical stages, including verbal explanation and interrogation of the narrative data. In practice, this joint-ownership, non-threatening approach means that researchers become increasingly willing to discuss issues that are never normally raised in public. They also have the opportunity to explore these issues within a safe and controlled environment. PEER researchers, who seldom have 'voice' outside, or sometimes within, their communities often say that contributing to and helping with the evaluation makes them feel valued.

The benefits of the method are that the ethnographic data provide in-depth insights into the daily lives and practices of research participants living in marginalised and hard-to-reach communities. This approach has been shown to produce rich data on issues such as risk behaviour, stigma and discrimination, sexual networking, abortion, and how people perceive access to and quality of services. The use of broad questions enables interviewees and researchers to locate a programme or intervention within the wider context of their social worlds, thus identifying underlying drivers of and challenges to behavioural change associated with programme activities. The impacts and unintended consequences of actions made are more likely to be revealed than through use of structured interview schedules. Crucially, however, the method does not provide generalisable population-based data. The sample size is, of necessity, small and the information obtained is highly detailed and context specific. However, it does produce actionable programmatic findings within a very short timescale, with a study sometimes being completed in less than two weeks.

The following two case studies provide clearer insight into both the strengths and limitations of the Rapid PEER approach. The first concerns an evaluation of a 'marital training programme' for the reduction of HIV and concurrent sexual relationships in Papua New Guinea. The second highlights experiences from base and endline studies on the practice of female genital mutilation in the UK, conducted within groups where this practice is known to be highly prevalent in countries of origin.

The Tokaut na Tokstret marital training programme in Papua New Guinea

The *Tokaut na Tokstret* (translated as 'talk out and talk straight') programme, administered by Population Services International in Papua New Guinea, was a four day relationship training workshop for married couples. The aim was to reduce new infections of HIV by building more respectful relationships between couples, by increasing correct condom use and perception of personal risk related to sexually transmitted infections and HIV, and reducing concurrent sexual relationships. The fostering of respectful relationships was addressed through separate sessions for men and women on empathy, intimacy, communication, cheating, conflict resolution, gender roles and improved understanding of reproductive anatomy. The evaluation was commissioned to understand attitudes to sexual relationships and sexual health related issues, how the project was making a difference (or not), and how the intervention could be improved (Grellier *et al.* 2011).

Up to ten community members (including a mix of male and female individuals) were recruited as researchers at each of three sites – Bunum Wo (Western Highlands), Itubada (Southern Highlands) and Ambugo (Oro) – where the training had been delivered. Researchers interviewed two friends each. Training took place during a one-day workshop, in which conversational prompts were translated from Tok Pisin (the local *lingua franca*) into the everyday language used within the researchers' own social networks. Data was collected during debriefing sessions conducted over three to four days per site, and reviewed during a final workshop. In total, 31 researchers interviewed 49 friends, generating 80 narrative interviews.

The narratives provided information on outcomes against the project indicators, such as addressing high levels of sexual risk through reducing the number of concurrent sexual relationships and increasing condom use in sexual relationships outside of cohabiting couples. They also revealed how and why certain aspects of the intervention had worked, which components had limited effect due to cultural inappropriateness, and what aspects of the programme were simply rejected. In addition, interviewees described the programme as having significant unintended benefits at household level. One of the most valuable outcomes of this evaluation was increased understanding of the process of change brought about by the intervention and how information and skills obtained through the programme were used and adapted by men and women to achieve mutually beneficial outcomes. These processes were considerably more complex and culturally specific than had been realised by programme staff.

Many narratives described how better communication and negotiation skills were bringing about positive change in the quality of married relationships:

> The big difference is to do with the attitude of helping because before we didn't have time to listen to each other. Men and women would stand far away from each other and just scream back and forth. But PSI said that this way of communicating is not good because it will destroy your family. You must communicate well between each other. Talk kindly to each other and this will not make your wife or husband get cross with you and you will understand each other even better and not get cross all the time. This is the big thing that I have learned from the training and I am following this in my family.
>
> (Female researcher, Itubada)

Frustrations within marriage were frequently related to sex. Women were generally angry with husbands for demanding sex when the wife was tired after working in the field all day, while husbands were perceived to have often spent their day relaxing, socialising and drinking. Another cause of resentment was that husbands were perceived to spend the majority of their wages on beer, cigarettes, betel nut and other women. This meant that the household often went without food, clothes and other necessities. This resentment led to a vicious circle of women reluctant to have sex with their husbands, who then sought out and spent money on other sexual partners, which led to further resentment and hostility from wives (see Figure 14.1).

The research narratives described how husbands and wives initially changed their behaviour as a calculated approach to achieving pragmatic personal gain. In time, however, participants described how the knock-on benefits increased and led to a more peaceful and enjoyable domestic environment. Not only was there a substantial decrease in gender-based violence and partner concurrency, but there were also unintended improvements in nutrition, household savings, women's access to resources, and improved outcomes at school for children, as men increasingly handed more substantial amounts of their wages to their wife for spending on household goods. One PEER researcher explained how and why the process of change occurred within households:

> [He said that] "we never understood each other. If I talked, she would not agree with me. But after the training she came to agree with me and we communicated. I also came to agree with her. Something that improved was that we were discussing when to have sex, and how to budget money: if we have 100 Kina [£24.63] we agreed to spend 50 Kina [£12.30] and to save 50 Kina [£12.30]"... Sometimes if the wife is very busy then the husband will complete his tasks first and then he would help his wife. They have five children and the husband usually helps his wife by babysitting the children, he plays with them and talks to them and distracts them so that the wife completes

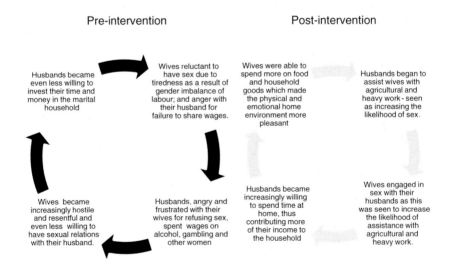

Figure 14.1 Self-reported changes by male and female PEER researchers pre- and post-programme intervention

her jobs like washing clothes or working in the garden ... He said 'communication is important because if my wife asks me to go and fetch water and I refuse, then in return if I ask her for something (sex) she will say "you always disobey me. Why should I help?"'

(Female researcher, Itubada)

Drawings feature strongly in the Rapid PEER approach. At the beginning of the researcher training workshop, participants draw pictures of aspects of their everyday lives. At the final researcher workshop, drawings were also used as a way of enabling researchers to express in a non-verbal way what an intervention has meant to them. Examples of some of the drawings are illustrated in Figure 14.2.

While the drawings in Figure 14.2 do not directly reflect any individual component of the initiative or refer to any particular outcome or indicator, they use locally appropriate symbolism to explain, very powerfully and eloquently, the project's overall impact on life within the household. As one researcher explained:

> We have two pictures: the left is before the training, the right is after the training. When the training did not happen this [first picture] is how the family lives. The dots represent the tears of the family. Husband stands by himself and wife stands by herself. Around them are two girls and one boy child. Husband always goes drinking and when he comes home he fights with the mother so they don't stay together. They go their separate ways. After training [second picture] they have changed their way of living. Now they are working and living together. This drawing of everyone in the canoe represents everyone living peacefully together. In the canoe the husband sits at the back and steers the canoe, and the wife sits in the front. In between the husband and the wife are the children. They have in the canoe: sago to represent food, fish, firewood, an axe for cutting firewood, bush knives and arrows (for hunting protein). They have everything they need.

(Male researcher, Itubada)

Another unexpected finding from the evaluation concerned the components of the training that participants did not like. The training focused on developing sexual intimacy between couples to reduce concurrency – it had been felt that sexual 'boredom' or dissatisfaction was one of the drivers of men (and sometimes women) seeking sexual relationships outside marriage. In order to reduce this, information on different sexual positions was provided together with information on men and women's reproductive systems. Many participants found descriptions of human anatomy deeply upsetting, as established norms on sexual propriety meant that men and women often did not openly talk about the opposite sex's bodies. The information on sexual positions was described as inappropriate and undesirable since it was perceived as being for sex with sex workers:

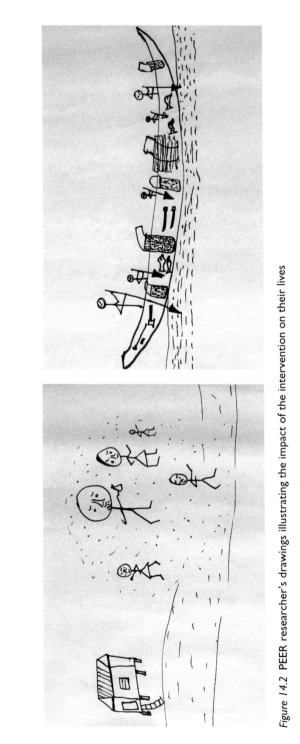

Figure 14.2 PEER researcher's drawings illustrating the impact of the intervention on their lives

In our custom, if I want to describe a woman's or man's private parts I have to describe them in parables, otherwise it's like cutting that person with an axe on the head. We don't discuss about these things openly and it's very hard to talk about it.

(Male researcher, Itubada)

The Rapid PEER approach identified that most of the programme objectives such as improving couple communication and reducing concurrent relationships were being achieved, and that these were having a further unintended impact on household well-being, particularly in terms of increased access to education for children as a result of reduced conflict within the household. The evaluation also highlighted how marital relationship training could be better aligned with contextual perceptions of sexual relations within marriage, and not be seen to undermine traditional norms.

Tackling female genital mutilation in the UK

The Female Genital Mutilation Special Initiative aims to strengthen prevention of this practice in the UK through a community-based approach, and is funded by three funders (Trust for London, Esmée Fairbairn Foundation, and ROSA The Fund for Women and Girls). Up to 16 projects were funded in 2010, and often operated in a complex environment for prevention in the UK. While female genital mutilation (FGM) is illegal in the UK, anecdotal evidence strongly suggested that the practice was on-going. A core aim of the initiative was to build women's confidence to 'speak out' against the practice, and to strengthen the prevention of FGM. The first phase of the project ran from 2010–2013, with an evaluation conducted in August 2013.

The interim report of the initiative in 2011, one year after project inception, confirmed other policy analysis that identified government FGM prevention efforts as being poorly integrated with wider child and adult safeguarding procedures, and badly coordinated and with little to no reporting or detection of cases of female genital mutilation itself (Roy *et al.* 2011). A raft of policy instruments were introduced over the course of 2011–2014 which spelt out in no uncertain terms that the practice was to be considered a form of child abuse, and fully integrated into safeguarding procedures that included the better detection of girls at risk by frontline workers such as GPs, midwives, teachers and social workers (RCM *et al.* 2013). Concomitantly, and in response to a push from activists, the practice gained a higher media profile. However, little was known at this time about how these multiple prevention efforts were being perceived among the communities affected by the practice. A key challenge for the evaluation was to obtain information on attitudes towards female genital mutilation in view of social taboos and the high levels of stigma surrounding this practice.

The evaluation used mixed methods, including in-depth interviews with project leads and key stakeholders, a review of the projects' monitoring data (which collected data on numbers reached, and qualitative observation data on project activities), a PEER project conducted at baseline (2010), and a Rapid PEER assessment at the end (2013) of the first phase of the initiative, before launching into a second phase of funding (Options UK 2013).

Given difficulties in talking about female genital mutilation, it was felt that an interpretive approach was an appropriate method for collecting data on the ways in which FGM was being talked about, and how discourse shifted over the course of the project (as an indicator of the strength of support for continuing or ending the practice). Furthermore, as the method does not involve direct personal attribution, respondents were able to talk about support or rejection of FGM, and women who had themselves been subjected to the practice would not be required to report on their own personal and deeply traumatic experiences. The method could also collect narrative data on how the project itself was being perceived, as well as reporting on wider community views of efforts by others, since it asked about what 'other people' were saying and collected perceptions of community-level views.

Over 260 people participated in the baseline and endline studies, with 70 researchers interviewing two to three friends each. The ages of respondents ranged from 16 to 65 years of age, with an average of 32 years. About half had children. Respondents ranged from a wide range of ethno-linguistic groups reflecting the diversity of female genital mutilation affected communities with which funded projects work, including Sudan, Guinea, Gambia, Somalia, Uganda, Nigeria, Eritrea, Ethiopia and Yemen.

In the baseline study it was found that female genital mutilation was not openly discussed within social networks, even within communities in which it was known to be highly prevalent in countries of origin. However, people often reported that there was still strong pressure to 'circumcise' their daughters. Grandmothers, in particular, applied pressure, and might arrange for a daughter to be circumcised without the parent's consent, often outside the UK. In some instances, women reported that they were afraid to return to their countries of origin, where they could claim little protection. While awareness of the legal status of FGM was relatively high, there was still a widespread perception that some forms of the practice were 'acceptable', specifically 'less severe' forms (Type I or II, according to the WHO classification) that did not involve infibulation but did involve partial or full excision of the clitoris. Respondents reported varying perceptions of who supported FGM within the local community. Data revealed that support for FGM was more closely linked to perceptions of the need to affirm cultural identity.

In the endline study, specialists led a one-day refresher training with the funded project workers that covered consent, basic interviewing skills, planning a study, and a review of the final questions. The questions included were: What do people in our community say about FGM? How has this changed over the last three years? Do people want to end the practice (why or why not)? How has the project impacted on our community and their opinions of female genital mutilation/circumcision? Where can people affected by female genital mutilation/circumcision go for support and information? Project leaders then selected and re-trained two to five researchers in each project site, who each interviewed two friends.

The endline narrative data revealed the extent to which the practice had become talked about with greater confidence. The 'noise' around FGM, including the media attention and the 'safe spaces' created by the projects had enabled women and men from communities to discuss it more openly, despite the taboo status that it held at project inception. The data also showed a plurality of arguments being used to counter support for FGM. There were, however, strong generational differences in people's positioning on the issue, with older women in particular often staunch supporters of the practice as intrinsic to cultural identity, but with younger people more confidently rejecting the practice.

> It is much easier for people to discuss FGM without shying away and avoiding it as it is such a sensitive topic. In the beginning of the project it was an avoided topic and seen as rude to talk about circumcision. However, over the course of the project there has been a massive shift. However, there are still those that will walk out of a room where they hear FGM being discussed.
> (Female researcher, Bolton)

> More and more women speak out against FGM practice – before, everyone used to be silent, maybe afraid.
> (Female researcher, London)

Increased awareness of the UK Law on FGM and the harmful health impacts of the practice were often deployed by projects in the first instance, as they provided powerful counter-arguments to local support for the practice. The project data showed, however, that often women did not associate health symptoms that they were experiencing with the effects of female genital mutilation, and that access to clinical care was important for beginning to recognise the harms associated with the practice. However, disconnecting the practice from religious justifications for its continuation had also facilitated progress in countering views of the practice as a religious duty, to maintain women's sexual purity:

> Mainly, the religious groups have been vocal and clear it is not a religious practice and that has changed people's perception and how people perceive the practice ... Religious people and young people, who grew up in the UK, are often among those who do not want to continue. For young people who grew up in the UK ... they have friends from other Islamic countries and when they discuss this with them, they soon find out it is not an Islamic practice. That has influenced them, and also having greater access to information.
> (Female researcher, London)

Young women's voices were particularly strong in rejecting the practice, seeing it as a violation of their right to make decisions about their bodily integrity. In some instances, this had clearly helped young women to reject the practice even when they were under strong pressure to consent to it being done.

> Young people are absolutely against FGM. My niece went to Somaliland with her aunt and her relatives started to make plans to circumcise the niece but she refused and her mother, who was not with her but in the UK, called the family and asked them to leave her alone if she did not want to be circumcised. She came back unharmed.
> (Female researcher, London)

The above quotation illustrates an apparent generational difference in gender-based hierarchy. With respect to efforts to prevent female genital mutilation, it underlines the importance of a focus on strategies that can further support young women (as young mothers protecting their daughters, or as young women at risk themselves) to reject the practice. In the next narrative, an older woman's support for FGM is not reversed, but her power to make decisions on whether to conduct the practice within the family are questioned and resisted:

> My grandmother used to bully that one sister who did not have FGM and call her names and say things like 'you are stinking because that "thing" is still on you'. Nowadays, my older sister has four children and none of them have been cut. My grandmother cannot bully everyone, and there is so many of them who are not circumcised in the family. We also have been trying to explain to her that being uncircumcised is really not a problem. It seems that she is accepting the situation. Of course, she is not happy about the situation but she is not as aggressive and abusive as she used to be.
> (Female researcher, London)

Younger women within these narratives also talked about the importance of women's sexuality, especially within marriage. This is an important counter-argument, as those who support female genital mutilation viewed it as intrinsic to maintaining a cultural heritage, and in some cases genital cutting was justified as offering protection against the more liberal sexuality of mainstream UK culture. Young women's voices rejected these views. Significantly, their opinions were also echoed by young men in these narratives, who asserted that they would not insist on marrying a woman who had been circumcised. Both young men and young women talked about the importance of both partners enjoying a sexual relationship and that female genital mutilation prevented this:

> Young girls feel future husbands should love them for them, regardless of them not being circumcised.
> (Female researcher, London)

> The majority of men are against the practice and they will tell you openly they would not like to be married to circumcised women, but they would not make a big fuss out of this, or FGM in general, but it would not influence their choice of partner. It is not a breaking point.
>
> (Female researcher, London)

> There are many young people who are not all being influenced negatively like most parents claim. They should see that young people are achieving great things. FGM is not required to raise brilliant daughters.
>
> (Female researcher, London)

Endline data found that attitudes towards the practice had shifted, and that fear of detection and heightened awareness of the harms caused by it had resulted in some people deciding not to perform FGM on their daughters. However, there were also still some very strong supporters of the practice, who sought to maintain a cultural tradition intrinsic in their eyes to their definition of womanhood:

> When it comes to the community, there is a split on FGM with some wanting it and some saying it's a bad practice. Women like myself think FGM provided women with dignity and kept them in check to behave and not divert from their religious beliefs. Many people in the community know FGM is not connected to religious practices and use this as an excuse to disregard who we are. FGM is part of who we are as women and this identity should not be lost.
>
> (Female researcher, Liverpool)

While there had been progress in creating safe spaces in which the harms of the practice could be discussed, both the project reports and the Rapid PEER results showed that it was often still difficult for many women who opposed it. Those who supported FGM often stated that they did not believe that it would be detected, or that the government would take any action. Lack of prosecutions for FGM was widely known about, but lack of intervention on the part of government agencies and child protection staff also allowed support for the practice to continue unchecked.

> Most people are aware of the law on FGM and that a 14 year sentence is attached but many people in the community say, 'how will the government detect this?' and they are right, how will they? I think the UK Government's view on FGM will not influence many but condemnation in the community by important leaders, women and political figures will actually reach the community and change the mind-set of many people.
>
> (Female researcher, Liverpool)

In contrast, many more people in these narratives wanted to see FGM end as a practice. They perceived the lack of government response as a form of neglect, which essentially overlooked rights abuses within minority ethnic communities. Younger women were especially scornful of the lack of a tougher stance on FGM, and were clear about the harms it causes.

> They know that it is illegal, that is why it is done in such a secret way but the government needs to speak out.
> (Female researcher, Manchester)

> I see FGM like domestic abuse, which no one really talked about but everyone knew it was happening.
> (Female researcher, Liverpool)

Overall, this Rapid PEER evaluation provided important insights into how people in communities affected by FGM viewed efforts to improve prevention. The case study demonstrates the usefulness of the method for gaining insights into highly sensitive issues, including gaining the views of those who still supported maintaining an illegal practice. Data elicited were useful programmatically, in demonstrating how and in what ways the projects had shifted attitudes towards FGM, and in delineating which future groups the projects should work with, namely young women and men. The data also underlined the importance of using community champions to advocate for change while also using a culturally affirmative approach.

Finally, the approach provided a range of data that had a much wider remit for advocacy and policy engagement. The data were clear in arguing that many viewed the lack of intervention by government as a form of neglect, and provided much needed evidence on the demand among people in affected communities (and most importantly, among young women at risk of female genital mutilation) for tougher government intervention. The data from younger women in particular showed how important it was for FGM prevention that the identification of cases and prosecution should be seen to 'work', to support those who question the practice and resist pressure to perform it.

Concluding comments

The two case studies described here demonstrate how an interpretive approach utilising ethnographic principles can enable the rapid collection of data on sensitive issues and from highly marginalised or vulnerable groups. The use of simple, broad questions enables an evaluation of a programme's impact on the daily lives of those it aims to reach, along with the sometimes unintended consequences of programme interventions. In both cases described, PEER researchers and respondents provided very significant insights into how the programmes gained, and sometimes lost, cultural legitimacy while challenging and changing traditional gender-based values and behaviour.

To be used most effectively, however, it is crucial to understand the different types of data that these methods can yield, and what they do not. Interview narratives focus on gathering perceptions of 'what is being said about' an issue by specific population groups within a community. Whether or not these community perceptions are factually correct is not important – the fact that something is perceived to be true is what is significant in terms of understanding programme impact and planning for future intervention. Rapid PEER works especially well with people who have little voice within or beyond their community, and for issues where stigma or shame preclude open public acknowledgement and thus easy measurement using quantitative survey-based approaches. Importantly, however, data collected via this approach cannot be used to enumerate respondents or their attitudes, although it can help those who use it to reach conclusions concerning the strength of consensus and variations within the data.

As indicated above, the use of these methods can produce useable data quickly, often within a week. This rapidity also makes it highly adaptable to programme monitoring. The method enables flexibility around the framing of the issues under study and the design of research evaluation questions, and enables respondents to identify what they perceive to be the most significant consequences, both negative and positive, of the programme. These may or may not coincide with the perceptions of programme developers and staff, and the strong use of narratives and stories enhances understanding of how and why such discrepancies arise and can be used to stimulate discussion about future project development. As these case studies illustrate, the method provides valuable evidence on how programmes can shift to harness 'insider' perceptions and align themselves more to the people's own interests and concerns.

References

Batliwala, S. and Pittman, A. (2010) *A Critical Overview of Current Monitoring and Evaluation Frameworks and Approaches*, Toronto: AWID.

Bell, S.A. and Aggleton, P. (2012) 'Integrating ethnographic principles in NGO monitoring and impact evaluation', *Journal of International Development*, 24: 795–807.

Geertz, C. (1973) *The Interpretation of Cultures*, New York: Basic Books.

Grellier, G., Saville, E., Topurua, O. and Kumie, D. (2011) Rapid PEER Qualitative Evaluation of the HIV Prevention and Control in Rural Development Enclaves Project: "TOKAUT NA TOKSTRET!" Marital Relationships Training. Available at: www.psi.org/wp-content/uploads/drupal/sites/default/files/publication_files/PSI%20PNG%20Rapid%20PEER%20MRT%20Evaluation.pdf (accessed 19 October 2015).

Hawkins, K., Pokharal, D., Sthapit, S. and Subedi, H. (2004) *A Step-by-Step Guide to Key Informant Monitoring: A participatory and community-based monitoring, empowerment and advocacy tool*, Kathmandu: Nepal Safe Motherhood Programme and Options Consultancy Services Limited.

Lincoln, Y. and Guba, E. (1985) *Naturalistic Enquiry*, Newbury Park, CA: SAGE.

Options UK (2013) *The FGM Initiative: Summary of PEER Research Endline of Phase One*, London: Options UK, Trust for London, Esmée Fairbairn, ROSA the UK Fund for Women and Girls.

Price, N. and Hawkins, K. (2002) 'Researching sexual and reproductive behaviour: A peer ethnographic approach', *Social Science and Medicine*, 55: 1325–1336.

Roy, S., Ng, P., Larasi, L., Dorkenoo, E. and McFarlane, A. (2011) *The Missing Link: A joined up approach to addressing harmful practices in London*, London: Imkaan.

Royal College of Midwives (RCM), Royal College of Nursing, Royal College of Obstetrics and Gynaecology, Equality Now, UNITE (2013) *Tackling FGM in the UK: Intercollegiate recommendations for identifying, recording, and reporting*, London: Royal College of Midwives.

White, H. (2009) *Some Reflections on Current Debates in Impact Evaluation*, The International Initiative for Impact Evaluation, Working Paper No. 1. Available at: www.3ieimpact.org/media/filer_public/2012/05/07/Working_Paper_1.pdf (accessed 16 March 2015).

Using interpretive research to make quantitative evaluation more effective

Oxfam's experience in Pakistan and Zimbabwe

Martin Walsh

This chapter examines Oxfam's use of interpretive research to deepen the findings of project evaluations based on the use of quantitative survey methods. It describes two pilot studies of this kind. The first sought to understand the success of a community-based disaster risk management project in Pakistan; the second traced the multiple impacts at household level of a smallholder irrigation scheme in Zimbabwe. These studies employed different qualitative and participatory research methods to tease out local understandings and explanations of project impacts. In both cases, the rich information that this interpretive and (in the Zimbabwe case) ethnographic research generated was then used to (re)interpret the quantitative findings of existing evaluations in order to generate programme insights and lessons for development practice (Walsh and Fuentes-Nieva 2014, Walsh and Mombeshora 2015).

By analysing these two pilot studies I hope to highlight the lessons that Oxfam has learned about combining interpretive approaches to research with a quantitative model of evaluation. There is relatively little consensus among practitioners about the best ways in which to do this, or even whether it is feasible in the first place. The 'quantitative turn' in the evaluation of development interventions that privileges the use of experimental research designs based on randomised controlled trials has polarised debate (Shaffer 2011, Eyben *et al.* 2015). It has also fostered a renewed interest in alternative approaches to evaluation based on ethnographic principles and participatory processes (Bell and Aggleton 2012, Cornwall 2014). However, rather than seeing these as incommensurable or competing paradigms, Oxfam's experience suggests that the intersubjective and interpretive modes of enquiry that characterise ethnographic research (and participatory methods that are used in the same spirit) can be integrated with experimental approaches in order to generate more effective learning for programmes.

Evaluation and accountability: Oxfam's effectiveness reviews

Oxfam is an international confederation of 17 affiliates working together with partners and local communities in more than 90 countries around the world. The largest and oldest affiliate is Oxfam GB. Like many UK-based NGOs, it has been drawn into the audit culture (Strathern 2000) in response to both internal and external pressure and inducements to demonstrate greater accountability through the systematic and rigorous evaluation of its humanitarian and development programmes and campaigns and advocacy work.

For many years, all of Oxfam GB's programmes have been subject to standard procedures of monitoring and evaluation. The typical monitoring and evaluation cycle includes the collection of baseline information, definition of indicators, regular progress reviews and the commissioning of independent end-of-project reports. Implementing this system consistently across hundreds of projects worldwide poses a huge challenge, as does translating it into effective programme learning. In 2010, responding to the new accountability agenda of government and other donors (Eyben et al. 2015), senior management supported the introduction of a 'Global Performance Framework' whose purpose was to 'to promote effective, results-focused, and accountable programme management' (Oxfam GB 2010: Preface). An important component of this was the development of a parallel system of evaluation based on the operationalisation of global indicators through 'effectiveness auditing' (for details see Hughes and Hutchings 2011). This represents a direct response to the need to demonstrate accountability using robust measures of impact.

This new system of global auditing that operates independently of the regular monitoring and evaluation processes was begun in 2011–12. Every year a random sample of mature projects worldwide is selected for effectiveness review. Random sampling averts possible accusations of bias, while the choice of mature projects ensures that they have had time to have measureable impacts. Projects that have been implemented at local level and allow for the measurement of impacts on a large number of direct beneficiaries are evaluated using a quasi-experimental research design. This involves the administration of household surveys to intervention ('treatment') and comparison ('control') groups, and the use of statistical analysis (multivariable regression and propensity score matching) to compare them and assess the evidence for project impacts on key outcomes, such as different aspects of women's empowerment (Bishop and Bowman 2014). A small number of such 'large n' quasi-experimental studies have been conducted by Oxfam staff every year since 2011–12, and in the process their methodology has continued to be developed and refined.

The random sampling of projects and the publication of the resulting Project Effectiveness Reviews reflect the importance of this approach for establishing the accountability of the organisation and its programmes. Efforts are also made to ensure that the effectiveness reviews feed back into project and programme learning, and where possible, project teams and partner organisations are involved in the process of evaluation. However, end-of-project evaluations often come to conclusions at odds with those of effectiveness reviews based on research undertaken earlier in the project cycle. There are various reasons for this, in addition to the fact that they are undertaken at different times using different methods. End-of-project evaluations usually address all of a project's objectives and its theory (or theories) of change, whereas effectiveness reviews are more likely to focus on particular project components and activities that can be measured using global indicators that in some cases derive from a different theory of change. The closer involvement of project staff in the monitoring and evaluation cycle and end-of-project evaluations also tends to ensure their greater relevance to country programmes, as well as consonance with their views. Although it is recognised that integrating the two approaches to evaluation would be ideal, this has yet to happen.

When the effectiveness reviews were first being planned, it was suggested that it might be useful to select some for further in-depth investigation using a more interpretive approach that engaged with people's own understandings of project impacts. This 'drilling down' was originally conceived as a way of explaining interesting and/or unexpected quantitative results. Planning for the first study began in late 2012. The rest of this chapter describes both pilot studies and the evolving process of research that has led to planning more. It soon became evident that not only was interpretive research often necessary to explain the results of effectiveness reviews, but it could also throw up interesting results of its own. The two studies have generated important lessons for the practice of evaluation, as well as for programming in Oxfam.

The Pakistan study: information flows faster than water

Oxfam's Community-based Disaster Risk Management and Livelihoods Programme in Pakistan was co-funded by the European Commission and ran for four years from June 2008 until mid 2012. Its aim was to reduce the vulnerability of participating communities by reducing the loss of life and assets, and promoting livelihood resilience in times of extreme flooding. In 2011, the programme was selected for inclusion in the first batch of effectiveness reviews. The review examined the work of two implementing organisations in two districts in Punjab Province. Field research was undertaken in December 2011 and focused on two key areas of interest: the extent to which households possessed characteristics ensuring their resilience to the impacts of climate change and in particular flooding, and their actual response to the extreme floods that hit Pakistan in July–September 2010. A household survey was administered to representative samples of 341 households in 57 villages targeted by the programme (the intervention group) and 400 other households in 63 similar villages in adjacent areas that were not (the comparison group). Propensity score matching and multivariable regression were used in the statistical analysis of the survey results to reduce bias in the comparisons made between the two groups. Following analysis the report of the effectiveness review was published in June 2012 (Hughes 2012).

The effectiveness review identified a number of large and positive differences between the intervention and comparison households. Households participating in the programme scored more positively on most of the resilience characteristics that the survey measured (these characteristics included variables relating to livelihood viability, the potential for livelihood innovation, access to contingency resources and support, and social and institutional capability). There was also strong evidence that they experienced less asset loss during the catastrophic floods of 2010, which were the worst in Pakistan's recorded history. In particular, they increased their ownership of farm equipment and various household items, as well as improving toilets and roofing. They also managed to cultivate more land over time. The same respondents were also found to be more aware of their villages' disaster management plans, and had participated more than others in disaster preparedness meetings. But there was no indication that the programme had positively affected livelihood diversification and motivation among the supported households to pursue alternative livelihood strategies.

The effectiveness review alone was unable to explain why the programme had these contrasting impacts, and recommended further research to find out why. The Community-based Disaster Risk Management and Livelihoods programme therefore became the subject of the first in-depth follow-up study, which, as well as explaining the findings of the effectiveness review, was designed to draw further programme lessons from it. An independent consultancy team, experienced in resilience-related issues, was commissioned to undertake participatory and investigative research to this end. They were asked to explain the different effects that the effectiveness review had attributed to Oxfam's programme, including the lack of livelihood impacts (for details see Walsh and Fuentes-Nieva 2014).

Research was undertaken in the UK and Pakistan in February–March 2013, using a number of qualitative methods. In addition to a literature review of relevant documentation, nine semi-structured interviews were held with Oxfam advisers, and a 'learning history' workshop conducted in Islamabad with five staff in the country office. Learning history is an action research practice designed to bring the history of a development initiative to life by charting the experiences of those involved in it (Roth and Bradbury 2008). As a learning tool it is used to deepen participants' understanding of how change has happened within programmes, institutions and communities; to adapt strategies, programmes and theories of change; and to foster a more critical and reflective way of thinking and acting. In the Islamabad workshop, a participatory map and timeline of key events and activities during and after the programme was developed. This was refined following probing about the reasons for events and the roles of those involved. Further reflection led to the identification of significant phases and important lessons that had been learned at different times in the history of the programme. Finally, additional insights and lessons were drawn from a review of the whole workshop process.

On the basis of their reading of project documentation (including the effectiveness review), key informant interviews and the learning history workshop with Oxfam staff, the consultants developed a number of hypotheses to test in the field. A series of propositions derived from these were written into a questionnaire that was pretested with Oxfam staff in Islamabad and the two partner organisations before being used to guide nine focus group discussions in Rajanpur and Muzaffargarh Districts. Separate discussions were held with staff of the partner organisations that had implemented the programme, government officials (including directors of relevant district departments), community-based organisation forums (umbrella organisations) in the programme areas, and community-based organisations and their members who had participated in the effectiveness review. Some of the groups comprised no more than two, three or four participants, fewer than the number usually recommended for focus group discussions (Krueger and Casey 2000, Laws et al. 2013). In all cases, however, careful note was made of participants' responses to the propositions that were put to them, and these were recorded, translated, annotated, sorted and systematically analysed with reference to the hypotheses that the consultants had developed.

The consultancy team deliberately chose to interview programme participants at the different levels of governance involved in developing community-based flood management and resilience in programme villages. This research design recalls the contemporary practice of multi-sited ethnography, which is especially common in the anthropology of organisations and development institutions (Marcus 1995, Falzon 2009). In other respects field research was rather less ethnographic in style. Resource and time constraints meant that during the follow-up study it was not possible to conduct interviews at household level in either the intervention or comparison villages. However, the community-based organisation members who were interviewed in groups did include householders who had participated in the programme, and their responses form part of the resource of narrative data that was gathered at different levels of its governance. While focus groups are rarely included in guides to anthropological research, their use is spreading, and group interviews have long been considered part of the ethnographic toolbox (Kratz 2010). Needless to say, the interview protocol developed by the consultants was rather more structured than that typically used in either group interviews or focus group discussions (Laws et al. 2013).

The consultants' report to Oxfam was finalised in May 2013. The next step was for Oxfam's researchers to condense this into a much shorter and more accessible learning document that also incorporated the results of the effectiveness review. This required further research in the form of a quick literature review of recent Oxfam work on resilience and related issues as well as integration with insights from an end-of-project evaluation and those garnered by Oxfam's Head of Research during a visit to Islamabad in March 2013 to discuss the programme with Oxfam country staff and the partner organisations that had implemented it.

As a result, the consultants' findings were reordered and in effect reanalysed to highlight what were felt to be the most important lessons that could be drawn from them. This proved quite challenging: whereas the consultants had examined and discussed a wide range of issues pertaining to programme practice and resilience in Pakistan, Oxfam researchers focused on the most striking example of programme success, the effective response of participating communities to the 2010 floods. Because the consultants had not been able to conduct semi-structured interviews at household level, there was less information available on people's experiences of these events than might otherwise have been desirable. However, triangulation between the different available sources of evidence, including quantitative survey results and the records of focus group discussions, did provide sufficient data and a clear explanatory narrative.

This narrative formed the basis of the resulting Oxfam research report, 'Information flows faster than water: how livelihoods were saved in Pakistan's 2010 floods' (Walsh and Fuentes-Nieva 2014). The main argument of this report, as summarised in accompanying blog posts (Walsh 2014a, 2014b), ran as follows. When the 2010 floods struck, households participating in the programme received an average of two days' advance warning of the floods, which was twice as long as comparable households outside the programme. They therefore had more time to get ready and evacuate, and, as the effectiveness review showed, they lost far less grain and far fewer livestock and other farming assets as a result.

The programme had only been operating for 18 months, so how did households achieve this level of preparedness so quickly? Oxfam's local partners, the Doaba Foundation and the Help Foundation, had bridged the gap between villagers and authorities when it came to early warning of flooding. As one focus group participant said:

> We did not know how to access different line departments and were not aware of laws and policies. The partner organisation helped in developing linkages with these departments; now we have [government officials'] mobile phone numbers and also invite them to our [community-based organisation forum] events.
>
> (Chenab Forum discussion)

Local people felt empowered to demand information from government authorities about river flows and levels, and in language they could understand. Once received, this information was swiftly disseminated through the participating communities and people trusted the information enough to act on it. According to another focus group participant:

> Once, we started to evacuate our families and assets to the shelter, and other villagers in the [non-project village] said 'Are you mad? The river is almost dry!' But we got correct information in advance of them and advised them to do the same.
>
> (Chenab Forum discussion)

Early warning information 'flowed faster than water', and communities were able to evacuate in good time. This success was achieved because of the participatory and rights-based approach that both partner organisations had used in implementing the Community-based Disaster Risk Management and Livelihoods programme in local communities. Among other things, they had recognised the importance of communication and the development of a shared discourse and knowledge of entitlements among programme participants, empowering them to act and make use of appropriate technologies in a timely fashion (for details see Walsh and Fuentes-Nieva 2014). Many NGOs in Pakistan have the same capability, and in the wider region the value of participatory disaster risk reduction has been well established for many years, if not always put into practice. As such, this is an approach that can be readily reproduced elsewhere.

However, while the programme did an impressive job in saving local livelihoods, efforts to diversify them were less successful. This was largely because the programme was not designed to tackle the very considerable structural (social, economic, institutional and gendered) constraints to livelihoods diversification in these communities. Even if it had, it would not have been able to impact significantly on local power relations in the four-year time frame available. Different aspects of this were reflected in comments made during the focus group discussions (for more detail and quotes see Walsh and Fuentes-Nieva 2014).

The research report drew a number of lessons from this analysis for resilience-building and related programming. It also made a number of methodological recommendations for future effectiveness reviews and mixed methods studies of this kind (Walsh and Fuentes-Nieva 2014: 15). Although no specific mention was made of the relative lack of qualitative data about individuals and their households, the absence of such detail was keenly felt during report writing and affected the style of subsequent communications about the research that are thin on human interest stories and quotes. As a result, research for the second pilot study was designed somewhat differently.

The Zimbabwe study: turning water into well-being

The second in-depth study followed on from an effectiveness review of the Ruti Irrigation Project in Zimbabwe. This project was funded directly by Oxfam from May 2009 to March 2012. Its aim was to contribute to sustainable livelihoods and resilience to climate change among poor and vulnerable households in the drylands of Gutu District in Zimbabwe's Masvingo Province. The project focused on the development of a 60 hectare surface irrigation scheme in which 270 farmers, many of them women, were given individual plots of land to cultivate and were supported with a variety of agricultural inputs and training. It was hoped that the resulting year-round harvesting of crops would also indirectly benefit up to 50,000 people in the surrounding area by providing them with a more diverse and secure source of food.

In 2011, the project was randomly selected for an effectiveness review, and field research for this was undertaken in October that year while the project was still running. A household survey was administered to 70 households that were full participants in the irrigation scheme (the intervention group) and 162 other households that had been selected to join the scheme but were yet to harvest any crops on it (the comparison group). The same statistical techniques were used as in the Pakistan study and, following analysis, the report of the effectiveness review was published in June 2012 (Bishop 2012).

As might be expected, survey results showed that production of maize, a local staple, had more than doubled among households participating in the irrigation scheme. There was also some evidence to suggest that these households were more food secure and had a higher standard of living than non-participants, though there was less difference than might have been expected. In contrast, there was much stronger evidence to show that households participating in the scheme had acquired significantly more assets. The effectiveness review recommended that further research be undertaken to explain these mixed findings, as well as to assess the food security impact of the project on the wider community, a question that it had not addressed.

The Ruti Irrigation Project was therefore selected as the subject of the second pilot follow-up study. This time it was recognised that there was a need for further quantitative as well as qualitative research. Quantitative data were required so that the number of indirect project beneficiaries and extent of food security impacts could be estimated. In-depth household-level research of the kind that had been lacking in the Pakistan study was needed to understand exactly how people had benefited from increased agricultural production and how its impacts were perceived. This study was also different from the previous one in that Oxfam staff from both the country and regional offices took part in fieldwork. They were also more involved in the analysis of the results.

Following a scoping visit to Ruti by Oxfam researchers, a Zimbabwean anthropologist and development consultant was employed to find out what impacts the scheme had on the households of both scheme members and others in the wider community. He was also asked to find out how widely these impacts had spread and why, and what people's own explanations were for any variation in impacts, gendered and otherwise, within and between their households. Fieldwork was undertaken in Gutu and Buhera Districts by the consultant and an assistant researcher in March–April 2014. Their research, which Oxfam staff facilitated, was based on a number of methods, beginning with a literature review of project documents and other sources, including crop production data from the scheme.

Fieldwork began with nine key informant interviews with district and government department officials and others involved in the development and administration of the scheme. These were followed by four focus group discussions, three with farmers from different phases of the irrigation scheme (a total of 32 men and women, some of them also irrigation committee members), and a fourth with eight farmers who were not members of the scheme. Discussions focused on farmers' own perceptions of life before and after the scheme. They were also used to generate lists of male and female irrigators and non-irrigators who lived at different distances from the scheme. These lists were then used to draw up a purposive sample of farmers for individual interview, making sure that this included both scheme members and non-members living in different kinds of households.

In total 22 irrigators (17 male heads of household and five women) and 11 non-irrigators (eight male heads and three women) were interviewed at length using the standard procedures of semi-structured interviewing, following a checklist of topics but also allowing the conversation to develop in line with participants' own observations (Nichols 1991, Pratt and Loizos 1992, Laws et al. 2013). At the beginning of each interview the interviewees were asked to outline their life histories, before describing the variety of impacts the scheme had upon them and their households, whether they were scheme members or not. As well as eliciting qualitative information about life before and after the beginning of the irrigation scheme, quantitative data on household demographic and socio-economic characteristics were also recorded, including age and gender composition, education levels and asset ownership. As in the key interviews and focus group discussions, the researchers also asked about decision making and the changing nature of gender relations in the household, the role of children, and the impact of external events including weather extremes on livelihoods and farming on and off the scheme. Notes were also made on anything of interest that was observed or happened during the interviews.

The consultant's report was finalised in May 2014. It included translated transcripts of all the individual interviews, which provided particularly detailed material for analysis and have given the final research report its title: 'Turning water into well-being: how an irrigation scheme changed lives in a Zimbabwean dryland' (Walsh and Mombeshora 2015). Here, for example, is a 49 year old widow's statement about the impacts of the scheme on gender relations in general:

> Life after the scheme was established has now changed for the better despite the fact that we still face acute shortage of water in the scheme. We are now producing food not only for domestic consumption but for sale as well. We are now growing high value crops such as tomatoes, beans and wheat which not only bring income but also improve our health. The scheme has also empowered us widows but has also removed the stigma attached to single mothers and widows regarding ownership of land. Women are now proud owners of land in the rural areas and land that they can call theirs[,] a thing unheard of in the past. Unlike in the dry land areas where women own land through their husbands, women in the scheme own their land and this land can be put [into a] will and can be inherited by their loved ones upon death. In the scheme we can also produce crops all year round and have cash in terms of income. We also use the scheme as collateral security to borrow from others. The scheme

also helps us physically since we work throughout the year. In the past we never visited or socialised with our folks in [another ward] but with the introduction of the scheme, we now make several visits to the ward to see our friends and share ideas.

(Female irrigator, Ruti Irrigation Scheme)

The collected interview transcripts from this study provide numerous insights such as this into local perceptions of the impacts of the irrigation scheme, allowing us access to people's voices and a wealth of information about their changing lives that could only be guessed at from the results of the effectiveness review and glimpsed in the records of the key informant interviews and focus group discussions.

As well as asking interviewees directly how their lives had been affected by the scheme, the researchers also inquired what had happened to their harvests of irrigated crops. They recorded the decisions taken about different harvests, including the amounts consumed, given away, bartered and sold. They did the same for crop sales, recording how the resulting income had been used in each case and what the further consequences of these decisions had been. This produced a lot of detailed information about the forward linkages of crop production on the scheme, including its impacts on household decision making and gender relations, and the spread of benefits to neighbours, friends and relatives in the wider community who were not irrigated plot owners themselves. Some individual illustrations of this are given in the final report of the study (Walsh and Mombeshora 2015).

These data showed how and why the scheme's impacts had spread both locally and more widely. It proved more difficult, however, to put a figure on the total number of people and households affected. The mapping of individual households' harvests and their forward linkages was incomplete: it would have taken far too long to collect comprehensive information from all of the interviewees, even if they had been able to recall it and had the patience to do so. In the absence of household data that could be extrapolated, only very rough estimates of the wider extent of project impacts were available. An end-of-project evaluation undertaken by Oxfam staff in Zimbabwe estimated that the scheme had the potential to provide sufficient food every year for approximately 3,000 people in the two neighbouring wards, a figure that falls far short of the 50,000 targeted by project planners. Additional calculations made for the follow-up study produced a comparable number. This suggested that while the project had significant impacts, in numerical terms these were limited by both the relatively small size of the scheme and the lack of an efficient marketing system for some of the main cash crops grown on it, a constraint that many interviewees complained about.

While recognising that it had some limitations, the ethnographic and interpretive research undertaken for this study provided a much richer account of impacts at household and community level than the effectiveness review survey was able to. To begin with, it explained why the survey had underestimated the impact of the project on participants' livelihoods: this was because its comparison group included many people who were also benefiting from farm inputs provided by the project and employment opportunities on the scheme. In other words, they did not constitute an independent comparison group. More importantly, the in-depth study demonstrated that the irrigation scheme had done a lot more than contribute materially to sustainable livelihoods and resilience among both participants and non-participants. In addition to enhancing food security and increasing farm incomes and employment, it had fostered social cohesion and well-being by impacting positively on gender relations as well as relations between kin, neighbours and friends. More than one interviewee declared that the project had 'increased the love' in their household, or words to that effect. It is difficult to imagine this kind of analysis and detail emerging had the Zimbabwe study not used the methods that it did.

Conclusions: lessons and next steps

The editors of this volume began an earlier paper (Bell and Aggleton 2012) by pointing to some of the limitations of quantitative 'results-based' methods of impact evaluation ('attribution analyses') as compared with more conventional approaches to monitoring and evaluation that are embedded in programme practice. The subsequent focus of their argument and the accompanying case study is on the ways in which the latter can be improved by adopting an ethnographic approach: 'We propose that using [ethnographic] principles to underpin qualitative evaluation holds the potential to enable practitioners to learn about programme impact and, through, feedback, improve programme design and delivery' (2012: 799). The two pilot studies described in this chapter likewise provide support for the use of interpretive and/or ethnographic methods in evaluation. They show, moreover, that this use need not be restricted to qualitative evaluation, but that interpretive and ethnographic approaches can also be productively combined with quantitative evaluation. The follow-up studies in Pakistan and Zimbabwe were not only successful in explaining quantitative results that the effectiveness reviews could not explain, but they also highlighted important issues that earlier evaluations had missed. They did so by drawing directly on people's own perceptions of project impacts, their explanations for these, and their views on how practice might be improved. In the process, what had become mixed methods evaluation was also turned into programme learning.

In the course of undertaking the two pilot studies, lessons were also learned about how their methodology could be improved. The contrast between the Pakistan and Zimbabwe studies shows clearly that focus groups discussions, like many other methodological shortcuts, are no substitute for in-depth interviewing and observation in the field. The semi-structured interviews conducted in Zimbabwe, although relatively few in number, provided a wealth of information about the experiences of individual farmers and the impacts of the irrigation scheme on their lives and livelihoods. This level of detail was lacking in the Pakistan study, although the learning history workshop and focus group discussions conducted there did provide valuable insights into the interaction between different levels of programme governance that was essential to its success. In both cases the triangulation of data collected using different methods was very important, as was the extra effort expended on analysis, synthesis and interpretation. At the same time it is evident that much more could have been achieved if the qualitative and quantitative components of research had been more fully integrated. Ideally, basic ethnographic research (including literature review) should precede and inform the design of surveys. This would, for example, have prevented the mistake made when the wrong group of farmers was selected for comparison in the Zimbabwe effectiveness review.

Integrated mixed methods research poses a number of challenges in terms of logistics and cost, and is not feasible in every circumstance. Oxfam is, however, continuing to explore its use in evaluation, particularly when its cost can be covered by programmes and justified by the importance of the learning that results. At the time of writing (June 2015) three more in-depth studies are in the pipeline, linked to effectiveness review surveys in Uganda, Ethiopia and Bolivia. The first two of these are funded as part of Oxfam GB's WE-Care ('Women's Empowerment and Care') initiative, and will focus on gender equality and the issues surrounding women's unpaid care work. Fieldwork for the Uganda study is already underway, and being conducted by an experienced researcher following an explicit ethnographic protocol that includes participant observation in a purposive sample of local households. Looking further ahead, plans are also being made for piloting programme evaluations that integrate the methods of the effectiveness reviews and in-depth studies with the standard framework of monitoring and evaluation and end-of-project evaluations. While the specific results of this are difficult to predict, it is expected that this ongoing research will continue to generate important lessons for Oxfam's programmes and evaluation practice, and will consolidate the role of ethnographic and interpretive research in these.

References

Bell, S.A. and Aggleton, P. (2012) 'Integrating ethnographic principles in NGO monitoring and impact evaluation', *Journal of International Development*, 24: 795–807.

Bishop, D. (2012) *Ruti Irrigation Project Effectiveness Review: Full report*. Oxford: Oxfam GB. Available at: http://policy-practice.oxfam.org.uk/publications/effectiveness-review-ruti-irrigation-project-zimbabwe-247851 (accessed 22 June 2015).

Bishop, D. and Bowman, K. (2014) 'Still learning: a critical reflection on three years of measuring women's empowerment in Oxfam', *Gender and Development*, 22(2): 253–269.

Cornwall, A. (2014) 'Using participatory process evaluation to understand the dynamics of change in a nutrition education programme', *IDS Working Paper No. 437*. Available at: www.ids.ac.uk/publication/using-participatory-process-evaluation-to-understand-the-dynamics-of-change-in-a-nutrition-education-programme (accessed 22 June 2015).

Eyben, R., Guijt, I., Roche, C. and Shutt, C. (2015) *The Politics of Evidence and Results in International Development: Playing the game to change the rules?* Rugby: Practical Action.

Falzon, M.A. (2009) *Multi-sited Ethnography: Theory, praxis and locality in contemporary research*, Farnham: Ashgate.

Hughes, K. (2012) *Pakistan's Community-based Disaster Risk Management and Livelihoods Programme – effectiveness review: Full technical report*. Oxford: Oxfam GB. Available at: http://policy-practice.oxfam.org.uk/publications/effectiveness-review-community-based-disaster-risk-management-and-livelihoods-p-247231 (accessed 22 June 2015).

Hughes, K. and Hutchings, C. (2011) *Can We Obtain the Required Rigour without Randomisation? Oxfam GB's non-experimental Global Performance Framework*. New Delhi: International Initiative for Impact Evaluation. Available at: www.3ieimpact.org/en/evaluation/working-papers/working-paper-13 (accessed 22 June 2015).

Kratz, C.E. (2010) 'In and out of focus', *American Ethnologist*, 37(4): 805–826.

Krueger, R.A. and Casey, M.A. (2000) *Focus Groups: A practical guide for applied research*, Thousand Oaks, CA: SAGE.

Laws, S., Harper, C., Jones, N. and Marcus, R. (2013) *Research for Development: A practical guide*, London: SAGE.

Marcus, G.E. (1995) 'Ethnography in/of the world system: the emergence of multi-sited ethnography', *Annual Review of Anthropology*, 24: 95–117.

Nichols, P. (1991) *Social Survey Methods: A fieldguide for development workers*, Oxford: Oxfam.

Oxfam GB (2010) *Oxfam GB's Programme Framework*, Oxford: Oxfam GB.

Pratt, B. and Loizos, P. (1992) *Choosing Research Methods: Data collection for development workers*, Oxford: Oxfam.

Roth, G. and Bradbury, H. (2008) 'Learning history: an action research practice in support of actionable learning', in P. Reason and H. Bradbury (eds) *Handbook of Action Research*, London: SAGE, pp. 350–65.

Shaffer, P. (2011) 'Against excessive rhetoric in impact assessment: overstating the case for randomised controlled experiments', *Journal of Development Studies*, 47(11): 1619–1635.

Strathern, M. (2000) *Audit Cultures: Anthropological studies in accountability, ethics and the academy*, Abingdon: Routledge.

Walsh, M. (2014a) 'How livelihoods were saved in Pakistan's 2010 floods', Oxfam Policy & Practice blog. Available at: http://policy-practice.oxfam.org.uk/blog/2014/05/how-livelihoods-were-saved-in-pakistans-2010-floods (accessed 22 June 2015).

Walsh, M. (2014b) 'Lessons from Pakistan's 2010 floods', Dossier on 'Ensuring access to water', Fairplanet blog. Available at: www.fairplanet.org/dossier/ensuring-access-to-water/#chapter-7 (accessed 22 June 2015).

Walsh, M. and Fuentes-Nieva, R. (2014) *Information Flows Faster than Water: How livelihoods were saved in Pakistan's 2010 floods*. Oxford: Oxfam GB. Available at: http://policy-practice.oxfam.org.uk/publications/information-flows-faster-than-water-how-livelihoods-were-saved-in-pakistans-201–317457 (accessed 22 June 2015).

Walsh, M. and Mombeshora, S. (2015) *Turning Water into Wellbeing: How an irrigation scheme changed lives in a Zimbabwean dryland*, Oxford: Oxfam GB.

16

Can qualitative research rigorously evaluate programme impact?

Evidence from a randomised controlled trial of an adolescent sexual health programme in Tanzania

Mary Louisa Plummer

Introduction

The merits of well-conducted qualitative research are widely recognised. Qualitative interviews involve more rapport building between interviewer and respondent than is possible in brief, survey interviews, which can contribute to increased trust and more honest reporting of sensitive issues (Fenton et al. 2001). The semi-structured nature of qualitative research creates the possibility of new and unanticipated findings that are provided in the subjects' own voices and conceptions, rather than researchers' preconceived wording. Qualitative studies can result in relatively in-depth, nuanced and valid understandings of difficult-to-research topics (e.g. Agadjanian 2005). These attributes are valuable when studying highly secretive issues, such as adolescent sexual behaviour. They are also useful when evaluating a programme's impact, especially as programme participants may falsely report attitudes and behaviours which they know have been promoted by programme implementers (Devine and Sevgi 2004). Participant observation – when a researcher lives and works among members of a target population for an extended period of time – can be particularly effective in collecting valid data on sensitive behaviours, because it relies on researchers' observations of everyday life and their informal conversations with people, rather than self-reported information in formal interviews (Pool 1997).

To date, qualitative research has been used mainly for programme development, process evaluation and interpretation of quantitative impact results, and only rarely has been considered suitable for direct assessment of programme impact (Prowse 2007). One reason for this is that qualitative data are time-consuming to collect and analyse, so the research usually only takes place on a fairly small scale, involving perhaps a few dozen interviews or subjects. It is difficult to know whether a small group may differ in significant ways from the broader population, so qualitative findings are not assumed to be representative on a large scale, unlike structured quantitative data collected from hundreds or thousands of subjects. In addition, qualitative data are collected in a narrative form that can be unwieldy and complex to organise, analyse and interpret, unlike the more systematic and straightforward nature of quantitative data analysis.

This chapter questions some of the assumptions above. For example, can qualitative research be conducted on a large enough scale, with carefully selected sites and subjects, to produce both valid and representative impact data? How truly representative is quantitative research of sensitive data likely to be, if widespread bias leads to consistent under- or over-reporting across a population? This chapter examines such questions by assessing the accuracy and representativeness of both qualitative and quantitative impact data collected within the MEMA kwa Vijana randomised controlled trial, which had an extraordinarily large qualitative research component. From 1998–2002, the trial evaluated an adolescent sexual and reproductive health programme that was implemented in 62 primary schools, 18 health facilities, and the broader community in rural Mwanza, Tanzania.

The MEMA kwa Vijana programme

The MEMA kwa Vijana programme was designed for low-cost implementation through existing government education and health systems, to maximise the possibility that it could be scaled up and sustained. At the time of the trial, the Tanzanian education and health systems were some of the most disadvantaged in the world, characterised by extremely limited resources and professional capacities (Cooksey and Riedmiller 1997, Changalucha et al. 2002). Delays in children starting and completing school meant that, at the time of the study, over half of Tanzanian Year 7 pupils were 15–17 years old, and only 19 per cent went on to secondary school (United Republic of Tanzania 2003, Palmer et al. 2007).

The MEMA kwa Vijana programme consisted of four interrelated components: community mobilisation; a teacher-led, peer-assisted primary school curriculum; training of health workers to provide youth-friendly services; and the promotion and distribution of condoms by out-of-school youth (Obasi et al. 2006). The school curriculum was the largest programme component, consisting of 10–11 40-minute sessions per year for pupils in Years 5–7. The programme was based on two behavioural theories: the Social Cognitive Theory and the Theory of Reasoned Action. Those theories identify largely overlapping factors that are believed to determine behaviour, including knowledge of the risks and benefits of behaviours; perception of personal risk; anticipated outcomes; intentions or goals; sense of self-efficacy or control; observational learning or modelling; and contextual facilitators and impediments. The programme aimed to influence those determinants in order to reduce high-risk sexual practices and promote low-risk sexual behaviours including abstinence, being faithful (partner reduction, monogamy) and condom use. The initial draft of the MEMA kwa Vijana school curriculum drew on adolescent interventions and epidemiological studies in Mwanza and other parts of Africa; guidelines from the Tanzanian Ministries of Health and Education and Culture; international 'best practice' reviews and recommendations; and extensive consultations with parents, youth, and local government, health, and education representatives. From 1997–1998, the draft school curriculum and other programme components were developed, pretested, pilot tested, and modified in Mwanza.

The MEMA kwa Vijana programme addressed its behavioural goals in different ways within each programme component, and the extent to which they were addressed also varied over the course of the trial. For example, representatives of the Tanzanian Ministry of Education and Culture instructed programme developers that abstinence promotion must be the main focus of the school curriculum. Abstinence before marriage was thus strongly promoted in every school year, and the curriculum could be categorised as an 'abstinence-plus' rather than a 'comprehensive' curriculum (Dworkin and Santelli 2007). Tanzanian government guidelines expressly forbade condoms to be visually depicted or shown in primary schools. In order to teach pupils how to use condoms correctly, programme developers provided step-by-step verbal instructions about how to use a condom in a preliminary draft of the curriculum. When this draft was reviewed by the Mwanza Region Education Officer, he specified that the condom use instruction must be removed.

The version of the curriculum used during the first year of the trial only superficially addressed condom use. Process evaluation findings and intensive advocacy with government authorities during the trial led to increased attention to fidelity and condom use for sexually active youth in later versions of the curriculum, although even this was limited. Given government restrictions about teaching condom use in schools, programme teachers were instructed to schedule visits to government health facilities with their classes, where programme health workers showed condoms to young people, provided condom demonstrations, and explained that condoms were available there for free. In addition, an out-of-school youth condom distribution component was designed at the end of the first year of the trial specifically to improve youth awareness of and access to condoms.

The MEMA kwa Vijana research

Quantitatively, the impact of the programme was evaluated through a trial in which 20 communities were randomly assigned to either an intervention or control group (Hayes et al. 2005). Each community consisted of five or six villages, five or six primary schools, one or two government health facilities, and an average population of 17,000 people. Between 1998 and 2002, three trial surveys were conducted with 9,645 young people in intervention and control communities. Trial participants were 14 years old or older at recruitment, and 94 per cent were 14–17 years old in the first year of the programme. At each survey, trial participants were asked to provide serum, urine, and/or vaginal swab specimens which were tested for HIV, herpes, syphilis, Chlamydia, Gonorrhoea, Trichomonas (females only), and/or pregnancy (females only) (Ross et al. 2007). Survey interview methods included both face-to-face questionnaire interviews and assisted self-completion questionnaire interviews that focused on participants' knowledge, attitudes and self-reported behaviours.

Qualitative formative, process and impact evaluation of the programme was based on participant observation, in-depth interviews, group discussions and simulated patient exercises (Plummer and Wight 2011, Plummer 2012). Preliminary data analysis early in the trial suggested that participant observation was the most useful method for understanding the nature, complexity and extent of youth sexual behaviour. Recognising this, the length, geographic range, and diversity of researchers involved in participant observation were increased to maximise the quantity and representativeness of the participant observation data collected. Participant observation took place in 17 host households in nine villages (four intervention, five control), and was conducted by six young East African researchers for a total of 158 person-weeks. The villages and host households were selected to represent the range of socio-demographic conditions within the study area (i.e. primarily agricultural or fishing; entirely Sukuma ethnicity or multiethnic; dispersed/remote or large villages). During participant observation visits, each researcher lived in a village household and accompanied young people in diverse daily activities (e.g. fetching water, preparing meals, going to market, working and socialising) and at special events (e.g. funerals, drumming–dancing events, video shows and public holidays). Each day, researchers spent one to two hours writing field notes in Swahili or English. Over the three year research period, 927 people of all ages were identified as participant observation informants, including 118 trial participants.

Qualitative researchers also conducted 186 two-hour in-depth interviews with 92 trial participants or their surviving family members (49 intervention, 43 control). These semi-structured interviews were designed to collect general background information on respondents (e.g. family, school experiences, friendships and work), as well as attitudes towards young people's sexual activity, in-depth information about their own sexual history, and (for programme participants) their experiences and opinions related to the programme. Of these 92 trial participants, 76 were randomly selected from the broader trial population in order to increase the possibility that they represented typical adolescents. Three others were girls who had been pregnant in primary school and 13 were HIV-positive; those 16 were selected to gain a better understanding of the experiences and needs of high-risk youth. In total, 73 trial participants were interviewed in 1999–2000, of whom 71 (or a surviving family member) were re-interviewed at the end of the trial in 2002, and 23 were interviewed again during long-term follow-up research in 2009. Nineteen trial participants were interviewed only once, at the end of the trial in 2002.

Qualitative researchers also conducted two series of focus group discussions during the trial. Generally, focus group discussions are used to examine participants' beliefs and norms, not intimate, personal experiences, so their interpretive value is limited in the study of sensitive behaviours. The first series consisted of eight discussions with MEMA kwa Vijana class peer educators and other programme participants. Those focused on pupil experiences and impressions of the in-school component of the programme. In the second series, 21 focus group discussions were conducted with six groups of out-of-school young adults in trial control communities. These were designed to explore unusual and sensitive sexual topics (e.g. induced abortion, anal sex), because researchers had found those topics difficult to investigate through participant observation or in-depth interviews with school pupils. Researchers conducted 50 15–30 minute individual unstructured interviews with two or three participants immediately after each discussion. These interviews focused on salient topics that had arisen during the group discussion and that warranted further private exploration.

In order to evaluate the quality of sexual health services for adolescents in health facilities (e.g. the extent to which consultations were comprehensive, confidential, respectful and private), qualitative researchers trained rural adolescents to conduct simulated patient exercises. In such exercises, trained local community members visit health facilities in the assumed role of clients, and then report on their experiences to researchers afterwards (Boyce and Neale 2006). Simulated patient research has the potential to be more objective and less biased than some other methods, such as clinician interviews or formal observation, because clinicians may not report or follow their normal practice in such conditions (O'Hara et al. 2001). In this study, six months before the simulated patient exercises took place, all trial intervention and control health facilities were informed of, and agreed to, the possibility of such visits, and all health workers were subsequently reminded of it by a letter from the Regional Medical Officer. Two male and two female 15–17 year olds were selected to be simulated patients from 84 young applicants in a village outside the study area. They were trained to present themselves at health facilities as patients seeking condoms, contraception or advice about a possible sexually transmitted infection. Simulated patient exercises were attempted in one randomly selected facility in each of the intervention and control communities. Immediately after each exercise, a clinical supervisor debriefed the simulated patient using a semi-structured questionnaire.

In-depth interviews, group discussions and simulated patient exercises were audio-recorded. Those recordings and the participant observation field notes were transcribed verbatim in their original Sukuma, Swahili or English. The Sukuma and Swahili transcripts were translated into English for formal analyses.

Concerns with the validity of self-reported data

Assessment of data validity is necessary, because if data are not valid, they cannot accurately estimate a programme's impact. In this study, the validity of self-reported sexual behaviour was evaluated by comparing the consistency of individuals' reports within and between surveys and in-depth interviews. In addition, across all research methods, reported experience of sex (or lack thereof) was triangulated with biomedical test results, as detailed below.

In the 1998 trial survey, 9,283 trial members participated in a face-to-face questionnaire survey, and a sub-set of 4,958 boys (average age 16) and girls (average age 15) also completed an assisted self-completion questionnaire survey on the same day. For that sub-set, overall reports of sexual experience appeared very similar in both surveys. In the face-to-face and assisted self-completion questionnaire interviews, 52 per cent and 56 per cent of boys reported having had sex, respectively, while 23 per cent and 22 per cent of girls reported the same (Plummer et al. 2004a). However, when each individual's responses were compared between the two surveys, 40 per cent of boys and 59 per cent of girls who had reported sex only did so in one of the questionnaires, and not in the other questionnaire. In addition, 1 per cent (12 males, 49 females) of the sub-set tested positive for one or more biological markers, but only seven (58 per cent) of those boys and 14 (29 per cent) of those girls reported ever having had sex in both interviews (Plummer et al. 2004b). Most of the remaining youth with biological markers denied ever having had sex in both surveys.

The in-depth interview respondents provided an opportunity for comparison of data validity across both qualitative and quantitative research methods. From 1998–2000, 73 trial members participated in as many as five research activities, including face-to-face questionnaire and assisted self-completion questionnaire interviews in 1998 and 2000, and in-depth interviews in 1999–2000. Twenty-four (33 per cent) of those individuals provided invalid responses, either because they reported ever having had sex in one interview and then denied it in a later one, or because they consistently denied ever having had sex, but tested positive for pregnancy or a sexually transmitted infection (Plummer et al. 2004b). Generally there was greater reporting of sexual experience in the in-depth interviews than in either type of survey interview. For example, only one of the six females with a biological marker reported ever having had sex in any of the four surveys, while five reported it in in-depth interviews that took place contemporaneously or prior to survey interviews.

These findings raise concerns about the accuracy of self-reported adolescent sexual behaviour in general, and particularly in structured, quantitative interviews. Other studies scrutinising the consistency and validity of adolescent sexual behaviour reports in surveys in sub-Saharan Africa have identified similar problems (e.g. Palen et al. 2008, Beguy et al. 2009). Nonetheless, the vast majority of evaluations of adolescent sexual health programmes assess impact based on such self-reported survey information (Michielsen et al. 2010).

Preliminary qualitative impact assessment

A preliminary qualitative impact assessment was carried out prior to the trial impact analyses to ensure that qualitative researchers were not biased by knowledge of the trial's biomedical or other results. To conduct this assessment, the lead qualitative principal investigator, the social science research coordinator, and five qualitative field researchers wrote independent responses to a series of questions related to programme process and impact, without discussing them with other team members until they had finished. All the researchers then reviewed and gave feedback on one another's responses, and the combined responses were integrated into a final report. There were few discrepancies of opinion between the researchers.

The preliminary qualitative impact assessment predicted that sexual and reproductive health knowledge had improved greatly among intervention programme participants during the trial, and those participants were likely to have significantly greater knowledge than their control counterparts. The report found much less evidence of genuine change to programme participants' attitudes and skills in the targeted areas. The assessment noted, however, that many programme participants were aware of promoted attitudes and behaviours, and thus might falsely report them, even at a statistically significant level. The report predicted that significant positive programme impact on actual sexual behaviours (i.e. abstinence, partner reduction, monogamy and condom use) and biological markers (i.e. pregnancy, HIV or other sexually transmitted infections) was very unlikely.

These preliminary qualitative impact findings were highly consistent with subsequent trial analyses, as well as subsequent in-depth qualitative analyses. The 2001–2002 trial impact survey found that intervention programme participants had significantly better sexual health knowledge, and were significantly more likely to report several desirable attitudes and behaviours, than control participants (Ross et al. 2007). However, 14 per cent of males (average age 19) and 45 per cent of females (average age 18) tested positive for Trichomonas, herpes, syphilis, Chlamydia, Gonorrhoea, and/or HIV, and there was no statistically significant and positive programme impact on those sexually transmitted infections or pregnancy (Weiss 2010).

In-depth qualitative impact evaluation

Analysis of the five million-word, English qualitative dataset took place using a thematic grounded theory approach (Charmaz 2000, Ryan and Bernard 2000). Anticipated codes were developed from research objectives, prior knowledge and early analysis, and these were refined in light of further data. Grounded codes were developed during a thorough reading of the field notes and transcripts. For analysis of most topics, data organised under specific codes (e.g. condom use) were summarised within a few dozen pre-identified themes, as well as themes that emerged during analysis. Additional analysis often included: triangulation and comparison of findings with field summary reports; direct searching of the original transcripts using key words; and/or reading all data for people mentioned within particular incidents or topics. This latter step was often critical to obtain a nuanced and full understanding of individuals and their behaviour over the three years of the trial.

The in-depth qualitative impact evaluation found that the MEMA kwa Vijana programme had varying impacts on the pre-identified theoretical determinants of low-risk sexual behaviour (i.e. knowledge of the risks and benefits of behaviours; perception of personal risk; anticipated outcomes; intentions or goals; sense of self-efficacy or control; observational learning or modelling; contextual facilitators and impediments). Generally, the impacts were only mild for most programme participants, and only great for a few. Ultimately, the programme effect on behavioural determinants was not sufficient to result in significant and sustained impact on the trial population's behaviour, unintended pregnancy and/or sexually transmitted infections. The qualitative findings for the abstinence, partner reduction, fidelity and condom use behavioural goals are summarised below.

Abstinence

At the end of the trial, the vast majority of programme participants understood that unprotected vaginal intercourse could result in pregnancy, infection and other reproductive health problems, and that abstinence was the only certain way to avoid these consequences. The programme successfully influenced a small minority of adolescents to actively set abstinence as a personal goal. For example, some youth who were highly motivated to finish school, or to establish financial independence before starting a family, believed that abstinence would help them achieve their ambitions because they would not be distracted by sex, or would not have to leave school due to pregnancy. Some girls had a goal to abstain to maintain their reputations, as this had implications for their self-esteem, community regard and future marriage prospects.

However, the qualitative research found that most programme participants did not consider abstinence to be a feasible goal in either the short or long term. The programme participants who had the greatest perceived self-efficacy to be abstinent – adolescents who believed they could control themselves and successfully abstain – were almost always those who had never had sex. Nonetheless, widespread and persistent pressures and temptations for young people to have sex often wore down the resistance of all but those who were most highly motivated to abstain.

A number of other qualitative findings illustrate the challenge of promoting abstinence among young people in the trial. For most, the immediate benefits of sex outweighed the risk of pregnancy or other negative consequences later. The programme acknowledged and addressed some motivations to have sex, including peer pressure, coercion, curiosity and desire for material goods. However, the programme only superficially addressed the two motivations that the qualitative research found to be the most common reasons why youth had sex, namely sexual desire for boys and material need for girls (Plummer and Wight 2011). The qualitative study further found that, when programme participants' main incentives to have sex were not well addressed, some distrusted the programme and felt its goals were unrealistic.

It was very rare for pupils to give plausible reports of intentionally abstaining after sexual debut (i.e. secondary abstinence) in order to avoid infection or pregnancy. When they did, this almost always resulted from a frightening personal experience of negative consequences of sexual activity (e.g. a symptomatic sexually transmitted infection, or almost being expelled from school for impregnating a girl). In contrast, most sexually experienced adolescent boys believed they had a natural, biological drive that they could not overcome, so it was not possible or desirable for them to abstain. Similarly, once adolescent girls had had sex, it quickly became the main way for them to obtain basic needs and small luxuries, and very few perceived abstinence as a feasible option.

Within the school curriculum, abstinence was modelled in stories and dramas in which abstinent characters remained in school and healthy while some pupils who had sex became pregnant, contracted an infection, and/or dropped out of school. However, the programme did not have much success in modelling abstinence in real life (i.e. providing new opportunities for pupils to learn how to abstain by observing others). Class peer educators were intended to be such role models, but the qualitative research suggested that only a small minority of them practised lower risk behaviours than other pupils, including abstinence.

Many social, economic and cultural influences on young people's sexual behaviour were contextual impediments of abstinence, and the programme had very little impact on them. This included girls' low and subservient social status, which made it difficult for them to resist pressure from men who approached them for sex. Girls' economic dependence on boys and men was also a great impediment to abstinence, because it contributed to sex being an important source of cash and goods for them. For boys, contextual impediments to abstinence included the widespread beliefs that sexual activity was central to masculine identity, and that continued sexual activity was inevitable once a boy had experienced sex. The programme's promotion of abstinence was in line with some contextual facilitators of abstinence, such as the common adult ideal that school pupils should abstain, especially pupils who hoped to go further in formal education. However, most sexually experienced adolescents did not share that ideal, and for those who did, the programme was not able to strengthen or reinforce such beliefs by making them more feasible to achieve. This was largely due to structural impediments such as poverty and gender inequality. For example, although programme teachers repeatedly encouraged pupils to abstain so they could pursue further schooling, programme participants knew that only a minority of Year 7 pupils ever won a place in secondary school, and that few girls who achieved this were supported by their parents to pursue secondary education.

Low partner number and/or fidelity

The qualitative research found that young people's knowledge of the risks and benefits of having few sexual partners and/or being faithful improved with programme participation. For example, at the end of the trial, programme participants generally understood that they could contract a sexually transmitted infection from a sexual partner who began a relationship already infected, or who contracted it from other partners during the relationship. Programme participants generally had a more favourable attitude towards fidelity than abstinence or condom use, because they perceived fidelity as involving less sacrifice and thus being more feasible and desirable. Unlike other promoted behaviours, partner reduction and/or monogamy could satisfy the main motivations youth had to have sex (i.e. the pleasure of unprotected intercourse for boys, the receipt of money or gifts for girls). Both allowed for pregnancy, if desired. Fidelity was also a social ideal in rural Mwanza, and as such, it was reinforced positively by sexual partners and the broader community, especially for girls. Thus, programme participants often expected some positive personal, physical and social outcomes related to partner reduction and monogamy.

In practice, the programme only seemed to influence a small minority of pupils, particularly males, to become concerned about risk related to their multiple partnerships, or those of a partner. The qualitative research found that such individuals typically tried to reduce their risk by being mutually monogamous in their premarital relationships, and then marrying and having a long-term, mutually faithful relationship. Some of these young people also tried to be selective in who they chose as sexual partners, studying potential partners before choosing one who they believed had had few prior sexual relationships and would be faithful to them. This attempt to reduce risk depended on subjective impressions and imperfect risk assessment, but nonetheless sometimes may have been protective.

Although most programme participants' general understanding of the risk of multiple partnerships improved during the trial, personal risk perception remained limited for most, for several reasons. First, few villagers had ever had any biology education, and it was commonly believed that illnesses were cured once symptoms were gone. Although programme participants developed a basic understanding that some infections can be asymptomatic for a long period, most still felt they were not at risk if a sexual partner appeared healthy and they had agreed to be faithful to one another. Second, concurrent sexual partnerships were fairly common but well hidden, so it was difficult to know when a partner had other partners. Third, while adolescents typically expected their partners to be faithful – and ended relationships if a partner's infidelity was discovered – they often did not hold themselves to the same standard, and were not as concerned by the risk posed by their own infidelity. Fourth, many young people considered themselves to be safely monogamous, even if they had a series of monogamous relationships with only short gaps in between them over a period of months or years.

The qualitative research also found that some young people perceived immediate, positive benefits to having multiple partners, and the programme did not have much impact on those expectations. Many young men sought new partners to maximise their sexual pleasure. Some young women took new sexual partners to maximise what they received in exchange for sex, because men typically offered the most money or gifts for sexual encounters early in a relationship. Such outcome expectations contributed to opportunistic sexual relationships (particularly when travelling or attending special events), serial monogamy and concurrency.

As was the case with abstinence, some social, economic and cultural norms and expectations were barriers to partner reduction and/or fidelity, and the programme did not seem to have an impact on them. Many programme participants continued to manage contradictory social norms and expectations by hiding their sexual relationships from adults. This practice often concealed an individual's partners from one another, helping to maintain concurrency and inhibiting realistic risk perception. The programme was not able to enhance adolescent girls' limited alternatives to sex to obtain basic supplies, and this economic dependence sometimes contributed to girls seeking new serial or concurrent sexual partners. Among adolescent boys and young men, the programme only superficially addressed a common belief that seducing new and/or multiple partners demonstrated masculinity. It also did not promote alternative ways to establish masculinity, such as through sports, disciplined employment or entrepreneurship. Finally, in rural Mwanza several contextual facilitators encouraged low partner numbers, particularly for women, but they mainly related to adulthood and marriage. By primarily promoting abstinence until marriage and fidelity after marriage, the programme was broadly in line with social ideals related to marriage. However, such ideals may not have seemed immediately relevant to school pupils who were at an exploratory stage of their sexual lives and whose premarital sexual relationships were hidden.

Condom use

The qualitative research found that, at the end of the trial, the vast majority of intervention programme participants had better knowledge of the risks and benefits of condom use than their control counterparts. Health workers played an important role in teaching pupils correct information about condom use, for several reasons. Their prior training and experience made them unusually aware of youth sexual health needs and confident in teaching about condom use. Other adult community members were usually comfortable with health workers in that role. Finally, health workers were typically not constrained from engaging in explicit sexual discussion in their work.

Educational authorities did not allow condoms to be shown or visually depicted within the school curriculum or the class peer educator trainings. Educational authorities allowed condom use to be explained verbally in detail only in the last year of the trial, but only in the last curriculum session of Year 7 if schools and teachers elected that option. Class visits to health facilities were strategic in enabling many pupils to see condoms and a condom demonstration. However, most pupils only participated in these visits once or twice, and some never did. Programme participants' understanding of condom use varied greatly, with many having a positive but somewhat confused and incomplete comprehension of it.

During the qualitative research, a very small number of young people gave plausible reports of having used condoms. Those individuals were typically extraordinarily fearful of infection or pregnancy, such as out-of-school male youths who had experienced symptoms of a sexually transmitted infection, or school girls who were unusually determined to further their education. The in-depth interviews and participant observation found that, after leaving school, a small minority of male programme participants sometimes used condoms with women who they considered to be high risk (e.g. bar maids, guest house workers), but they rarely continued to use condoms beyond their first few sexual encounters with those women.

At the end of the trial, most programme participants believed that condom use was safe and protective against pregnancy and sexually transmitted infections. However, most male participants, like other rural men and boys, continued to believe widely reported rumours that condom use reduces sexual pleasure. As noted earlier, sexual pleasure was hardly discussed within the school programme, even though this was the main motivation for male youth to have sex. By only marginally addressing boys' and men's central concern about the possibility of reduced pleasure during condom use, male programme participants may have felt the programme was out of touch with their reality and their concerns.

There were other ways in which the programme was limited in its promotion of condom use. Some programme teachers felt a conflict between the promotion of abstinence and the promotion of premarital fidelity or condom use for sexually active pupils. It was not unusual for teachers to manage this by insisting that pupils abstain, but also telling them that, once they left school and became adults, they could marry and/or use condoms to protect themselves during sex outside marriage. Some other school-based HIV prevention programmes in sub-Saharan Africa have encountered similar conflicts (e.g. UNESCO 2008). Even in optimal circumstances within this programme, when teachers taught the detailed condom session at the end of Year 7, practical instruction and exercises related to condom use only addressed how to obtain, put on and dispose of condoms, not broader behavioural issues, such as negotiation with a partner, or strategies to use condoms consistently.

Poor access to condoms was also an obstacle for condom promotion within the programme. Prior to the programme, condoms were entirely unavailable in some villages, and in others they were only available in very small numbers in a few village kiosks. The programme team ensured condoms were available in both intervention and control health facilities during the trial, and intervention health workers were more likely than control health workers to promote and distribute condoms to unmarried young people, but the numbers of condoms distributed at facilities remained extremely low (Larke *et al.* 2010). The condom distribution initiative was intended to improve condom access for sexually active adolescents, but in practice most youth condom distributors established very small clienteles that mainly consisted of out-of-school male youths and adults. Programme developers had hoped that those condom distributors would not only educate youth and promote condom use for those who were sexually active, but also use condoms themselves and acknowledge this openly and positively with their peers, in this way becoming role models. It seems likely that most, if not the vast majority, of condom distributors tried using condoms after receiving their brief programme training. However, many of them found that condom use reduced their pleasure to an unacceptable extent, so they soon stopped completely or only used condoms in certain circumstances, such as when they considered a sexual partner to be high risk.

Conclusion

This study demonstrated that in-depth, well-structured qualitative research can evaluate a programme's impact effectively, whether as a robust, stand-alone assessment, or complementing a biomedical or interview survey evaluation. The interactive and interpretive nature of participant observation and in-depth interviews was particularly effective in collecting in-depth, nuanced and valid information about young people's everyday lives, values, perspectives and sensitive behaviours. The variety, duration and geographic range of those two methods as employed in this study also contributed to extraordinarily representative qualitative data. Triangulation and interpretation of all qualitative methods illuminated the sociocultural logic determining young people's decision making, enabled clear distinctions between common and uncommon attitudes and behaviours, provided great insight into the particular ways that the programme did and did not influence behaviour change over time, and accurately predicted the programme's biomedical outcomes. In contrast, triangulation of qualitative, survey interview, and biomedical data raised serious concerns about the accuracy of self-reported adolescent sexual behaviour in general, and particularly in structured, quantitative interviews. Those findings suggest that interview surveys focused on highly sensitive topics may not be representative, because widespread bias can lead to consistent under- or over-reporting across a population.

The qualitative study also revealed how implementation of a low-cost, large-scale programme in a 'real world' scenario may necessarily involve critical compromises, and those compromises may have substantial detrimental effects on the programme and its potential impact. Examples include compromises between national policies and international best practice recommendations, between the most desirable programme design and one that is affordable and sustainable at a large scale, between optimal teaching methods and real-world teaching capacity, between ideal curriculum content and what is acceptable to the local community, and between adults' values and youths' realities. In summary, this study demonstrates that interpretive qualitative research, particularly carefully designed and conducted ethnographic research, can provide nuanced, valid and representative findings that evaluate and explain a programme's impact effectively, and also provide valuable evidence to improve programme design and implementation in the future.

References

Agadjanian, V. (2005) 'Fraught with ambivalence: reproductive intentions and contraceptive choices in a sub-Saharan fertility transition', *Population Research and Policy Review*, 24: 617–645.

Beguy, D., Kabiru, C.W., Nderu, E.N. and Ngware, M.W. (2009) 'Inconsistencies in self-reporting of sexual activity among young people in Nairobi, Kenya', *Journal of Adolescent Health*, 45: 595–601.

Boyce, C. and Neale, P. (2006) *Using Mystery Clients: A guide to using mystery clients for evaluation input*. Pathfinder International Tool Series: Monitoring and Evaluation – 3. Watertown: Pathfinder International.

Changalucha, J., Gavyole, A., Grosskurth, H., Hayes, R. and Mabey, D. (2002) 'STD/HIV intervention and research programme Mwanza Region, NW Tanzania', *Sexually Transmitted Infections*, 78(Suppl. 1): ii91–ii96.

Charmaz, K. (2000) 'Grounded theory: objectivist and constructivist methods', in N.K. Denzin and Y.S. Lincoln (eds) *Handbook of Qualitative Research*, London: SAGE, pp. 509–535.

Cooksey, B. and Riedmiller, S. (1997) 'Tanzanian education in the nineties: beyond the diploma disease', *Assessment in Education*, 4: 121–135.

Devine, O.J. and Sevgi, O.A. (2004) 'The impact of inaccurate reporting of condom use and imperfect diagnosis of sexually transmitted disease infection in studies of condom effectiveness', *Sexually Transmitted Diseases*, 31(10): 588–595.

Dworkin, S.L. and Santelli, J. (2007) 'Do abstinence-plus interventions reduce sexual risk behavior among youth?', *PLoS Medicine*, 4(9): e276.

Fenton, K.A., Johnson, A.M., McManus, S. and Erens, B. (2001) 'Measuring sexual behaviour: methodological challenges in survey research', *Sexually Transmitted Infections*, 77: 84–92.

Hayes, R.J., Changalucha, J., Ross, D.A., Gavyole, A., Todd, J., Obasi, A.I.N., Plummer, M.L., Wight, D., Mabey, D.C. and Grosskurth, H. (2005) 'The MEMA kwa Vijana Project: design of a community-randomised trial of an innovative adolescent sexual health intervention in rural Tanzania', *Contemporary Clinical Trials*, 26: 430–442.

Larke, N.L., Cleophas-Mazige, B., Plummer, M.L., Obasi, A.I., Rwakatare, M., Todd, J., Changalucha, J., Weiss, H.A., Hayes, R.J. and Ross, D.A. (2010) 'Impact of the MEMA kwa Vijana adolescent sexual and reproductive health interventions on use of health services by young people in rural Mwanza, Tanzania: results of a cluster randomised trial', *Journal of Adolescent Health*, 47(5): 512–522.

Michielsen, K., Chersich, M.F., Luchters, S., De Koker, P., Van Rossem, R. and Temmerman, M. (2010) 'Effectiveness of HIV prevention for youth in sub-Saharan Africa: systematic review and meta-analysis of randomized and nonrandomized trials', *AIDS*, 24: 1193–1202.

Obasi, A.I., Cleophas, B., Ross, D.A., Chima, K.L., Mmassy, G., Gavyole, A., Plummer, M.L., Makokha, M., Mujaya, B., Todd, J., Wight, D., Grosskurth, H., Mabey, D.C. and Hayes, R.J. (2006) 'Rationale and design of the MEMA kwa Vijana adolescent sexual and reproductive health intervention in Mwanza Region, Tanzania', *AIDS Care*, 18(4): 311–322.

O'Hara, H.B., Voeten, H.A.C.M., Kuperus, A.G., Otido, J.M., Kusimba, J., Habbema, J.D.F., Bwayo, J.J., and Ndinya-Achola, J.O. (2001) 'Quality of health education during STD case management in Nairobi, Kenya', *International Journal of STD & AIDS*, 12: 315–322.

Palen, L., Smith, E.A., Caldwell, L.L., Flisher, A.J., Wegner, L. and Vergnani, T. (2008) 'Inconsistent reports of sexual intercourse among South African high school students', *Journal of Adolescent Health*, 42(3): 221–227.

Palmer, R., Wedgwood, R. and Hayman, R., with King, K. and Thin, N. (2007) *Educating Out of Poverty? A synthesis report on Ghana, India, Kenya, Rwanda, Tanzania and South Africa*. Department for International Development: Educational Paper No. 70. Edinburgh: Centre of African Studies, University of Edinburgh.

Plummer, M.L. (2012) *Promoting Abstinence, Being Faithful, and Condom Use with Young Africans: Qualitative findings from an intervention trial in rural Tanzania*, Lanham, MD: Lexington Books.

Plummer, M.L. and Wight, D. (2011) *Young People's Lives and Sexual Relationships in Rural Africa: Findings from a large qualitative study in Tanzania*, Lanham, MD: Lexington Books.

Plummer, M.L., Wight, D., Ross, D.A., Balira, R., Anemona, A., Todd, J., Salamba, Z., Obasi, A.I.N., Grosskurth, H., Changlucha, J. and Hayes R.J. (2004a) 'Asking semi-literate adolescents about sexual behaviour: the validity of assisted self-completion questionnaire (ASCQ) data in rural Tanzania', *Tropical Medicine & International Health*, 9: 737–754.

Plummer, M.L., Ross, D.A., Wight, D., Changalucha, J., Mshana, G., Wamoyi, J., Todd, J., Anemona, A., Mosha, F., Obasi, A.I.N. and Hayes, R.J. (2004b) '"A bit more truthful": the validity of adolescent sexual behaviour data collected in rural northern Tanzania using five methods', *Sexually Transmitted Infections*, 80(Suppl. 2): ii49–ii56.

Pool, R. (1997) 'Anthropological research on AIDS', in J. Ng'weshemi, J.T. Boerma, J. Bennett and D. Schapink (eds) *HIV Prevention and AIDS Care in Africa: A district level approach*, Amsterdam: Royal Tropical Institute.

Prowse, M. (2007) *Aid Effectiveness: The role of qualitative research in impact evaluation*, London: Overseas Development Institute.

Ross, D.A., Changalucha, J., Obasi, A.I., Todd, J., Plummer, M.L., Cleophas-Mazige, B., Anemona, A., Everett, D., Weiss, H.A., Mabey, D.C., Grosskurth, H. and Hayes, R.J. (2007) 'Biological and behavioural impact of an adolescent sexual health intervention in Tanzania: a community-randomized trial', *AIDS*, 21(14): 1943–1955.

Ryan, G.W. and Bernard, H.R. (2000) 'Data management and analysis methods', in N.K. Denzin and Y.S. Lincoln (eds) *Handbook of Qualitative Research*, London: SAGE, pp. 769–802.

UNESCO (2008) *Review of Sex, Relationships and HIV Education in Schools: Prepared for the first meeting of UNESCO's Global Advisory Group, 13–14 December 2007*, Paris: UNESCO.

United Republic of Tanzania (2003) *Basic Statistics in Education 2003: Regional data*, Dar es Salaam: United Republic of Tanzania.

Weiss, H. (2010) 'Re: Question about any STI at MkV final survey'. E-mail (24 May 2010).

Index

Please note: locators in **bold type** indicate figures or illustrations, those in *italics* indicate tables.

abstinence, adolescents in Tanzania 239–40 (*see also* MEMA kwa Vijana adolescent sexual health programme)
accountability: and emphasis on the need to generate evidence 34; funding and 2, 32, 33–5; implicit dominance of the function in conventional approaches to evaluation 33, 34; monitoring for reasons of 32; and Oxfam's effectiveness reviews 220–1 (*see also* Oxfam's effectiveness reviews); as reason for monitoring and evaluation 2; and the status of money in public decision-making 143
adequacy evaluations 43
adolescent sexual behaviour, value of qualitative research in studying 232
anthropology, associations with ethnography 99
antiretroviral therapy: client approaches to adherence 74–6; discrimination and access to 66–7; eligibility criteria 66; importance of adherence 66; improving adherence to 72; *see also* HIV treatment
Audit Cultures 220
Avahan programme, for HIV prevention in India 39–42

behavioural psychology 154
Beyond Zero Campaign, Kenya 52
Bolivia: effectiveness review survey 230; use of Photovoice 25

Central American countries, using consumer insight to improve HIV treatment adherence in *see* combination prevention programme for HIV
child abuse: FGM as form of 211; teenage pregnancy and early motherhood as 111
child health: 'the 1000 days window of opportunity' 48–9; availability of effective interventions globally 47–8
circumcision, female *see* FGM
climate change resilience: Pakistan study 221–5; Ruti Irrigation Project, Zimbabwe 225–9
Cochrane Collaboration 35
combination prevention programme for HIV: client approaches to treatment adherence 74–6; design implications 77–8; framework for treatment adherence 70; HIV diagnosis findings 71–2; intervention packages 67; need for consumer insight 67–8; social media strategy 77; study findings 69–76; study methodology 68–9; target populations 67; targeted groups 67; treatment initiation and adherence 72–4
communication, as barrier to health education 166
community-based organisations, theory and interpretation in intervention design/evaluation 40–2
complex interventions, evidential challenges for the evaluation of 32–44
complexity, taking complexity seriously 194–5
complexity-aware options for evaluation, necessity of 188

condom use, adolescents in Tanzania 242–3 (*see also* MEMA kwa Vijana adolescent sexual health programme)
consumer focus, as basis of social marketing 65
consumer insight, and HIV treatment adherence 65–79 (*see also* combination prevention programme for HIV)
context, defining levels of 103
contraception: simulated patient exercises 236; traditional and alternative methods 121; young women's experiences in Sierra Leone 115, 117, 120–1
conversation starters, examples of 167
critical consciousness, Freire's concept 20
cultural relativism 18

Dalits: household survey findings 180–1; position in the caste system 95
data collection: ensuring high quality 193; ethical perspective 199; influence of social values on 28–9; interpretive approach 5; modality analysis 199; validity concerns regarding self-reported data 236–7; value judgement and 22
data validity, necessity for assessment 236
development studies, use of ethnography in 5
dietary management of diarrhoea, example of rapid ethnographic assessment 6
discrimination, likely impact on adherence to HIV treatment 67

early pregnancy and motherhood: causes of 115–17; girls' interpretation of 90–1; impact on girls' education 111; impact on young women's lives 118–19; risk levels in Sierra Leone 111
early sexual initiation: pressure on vulnerable young women for 111; as risk factor for HIV 127
'effectiveness auditing' 220
emic understanding, development difficulties 6
Empowering Girls at Risk: data collection and analysis 113–14; ethnographic approach to programme design 112–14; findings from formative research 115–22; project goal 112; recruitment and training of peer researchers 113; reflections and conclusion 123; stakeholder consultation 114; transitioning from research to the girls' programme 122–3; young women's views on access to information, health and support services 119–22
Engel curves 178–9
environmental management, monitoring and improving volunteering for sustainability 143–57
ESSENCE (Enhancing Support for Strengthening the Effectiveness of National Capacity Efforts) 33
ethical challenges, for evaluation research 36
ethnographic methods: analytic tools 86–7; generating local knowledge through 84–5; improving programme design through 79; Nastasi and Berg on the benefits of 19; project ethnography 51; reasons for usefulness in evidence-based programming 85; use of in Baltimore's 'STEP Into Action' programme 161 (*see also* STEP into Action HIV prevention programme)
ethnographic process evaluation: defining 160; evaluation findings 163–8; overview 159–61; requirements for success 161
ethnographic research: common methodology 99; informing principles 84–5; key principles 5–6; methods 6; potential value for the design of programmes 41; rapid approaches 6–7; sensitivity to local subjectivities 129; similarities between evaluation and 33; using to inform design of girl empowerment programmes 85 (*see also* Empowering Girls at Risk)
ethnography: associations with anthropology 99; definition and role of 5–6; overview 84; research practice 99–100; types of 84; use of in development studies 5; use of in health service programming 129
evaluation: accountability, implicit dominance of the function in conventional approaches to 33, 34; categories of 160; commensurability between different regimes 42–3; distinction between research and 34; instruments/methods selection

Index

33; qualitative research and the character of 33–5; similarities between anthropologically informed ethnographic research and 33; tension between inward- and outward-facing modes of 36–7; tripartite characterisation 42–3
evaluation of complex interventions, evidential challenges 32–44
evaluation research: function of 159–60; value of methodological pluralism 183
evidence, the political economy of (*see also* LNG Project impact assessment)
'evidence pyramid' 35
evidence transfer, and the limitations of RCTs 35–6
evidence-based global health, Vincanne Adams on 47
evidence-based programming: designing for success from the perspective of recipients 85; 'inspiration' vs 'information' 83; local knowledge and 81–5; political perspective 82; popularity of the term 81; problems with 82–3; and quality of evidence 82–3; reasons for the usefulness of an ethnographic approach 85; and upward accountability 83

female genital mutilation *see* FGM
FGM (female genital mutilation): FORWARD's focus on 110–11; legal status in the UK 211; peer outreach initiatives 123, 211–16 (*see also* FGM Special Initiative); rite of as sex education opportunity 120
FGM Special Initiative: aim 211; cultural perspective 214–15; funding 211; generational perspective 214; mixed methodology 211–12; questions included 212–13; religious perspective 213, 215; training regime 212
Freire, P. 20
funding, accountability and 2, 32, 33–5

Geertz, C. 54, 83, 146, 196
gender-based power relations, and sexual/reproductive health 204
Ghana: girls' network 123; mixed methods evaluation project 177–80 (*see also* Reality Check Approach)

girl empowerment programme: analytic tools 86–7; comparison of programme goals and girls' goals 88, **89**; ethnographic approach to design 85–93; girl-led research approach 85–6; importance of local knowledge 57–60; and local knowledge about marriage 89–90; and local knowledge about pregnancy 90–3; research locations 85; research theories and methodologies 85; stages of research 86; understanding girls' daily lives through a local lens 87–9; use of discourse analysis 87
girls and young women: challenges for in developing countries 110; education of *see* girls' education; empowerment programmes (see Empowering Girls at Risk; girl empowerment programme); impact of early pregnancy and motherhood on the lives of 118–19; impact of economic dependence on boys and men 240; importance of securing the rights of 110; increasing recognition of the value of investing in 110; and pregnancy outside marriage 92; pressure on for sex 91; responsibility for contraception 91; *see also* early pregnancy and motherhood
girls' education: Ghana 179; impact of early pregnancy on 111, 118; lack of value placed on 116; support recommendations 122
global theory of change 148, 153

harm reduction, encouraging injecting drug users towards 163 (*see also* STEP into Action HIV prevention programme)
health: communication as barrier to education 166; examples of social interventions which can have important effects on 36
health interventions, tripartite characterisation of evaluation 42–3
health service programming, use of ethnography in 129
HIV infection: 'corridors' of risk 130; discrimination and access to treatment 66–7; inadequacy of standard intervention categories 134, 136; injection risk ladder 167–8; populations at special risk of 37; using

consumer insight to influence national treatment policy 78; vulnerable communities 42, 67
HIV prevention: as aim of *Tokaut na Tokstret* marital training programme 206 (*see also* Tokaut na Tokstret marital training programme); the Avahan approach 39; combination prevention programme 67–8 (*see also* combination prevention programme for HIV); community engagement 37; comparison of two community-based programmes in India 37–40; and consumer insight 67–8; ethnographic process evaluation 159–69 (*see also* STEP into Action HIV prevention programme); examples of interventions 39; STEP into Action programme *see* STEP into Action HIV prevention programme; Tingim Laip STEPs Model 134, **135** (*see also* Tingim Laip, HIV prevention and care project)
HIV treatment: adherence framework 70; factors influencing treatment access and adherence 66–7; improving adherence using consumer insight 65–79 (*see also* combination prevention programme for HIV); *see also* antiretroviral therapy
homophobia: and adherence to HIV treatment 66; importance of recognising 29

immersion approach, to research 173
inclusive business measurement, impact areas 189
India: community-based HIV prevention programmes comparison 37–40; example of rapid ethnographic assessment 7; safe sex negotiation skills provision for sex workers 38
indigenous researchers, requirements for training 20
injecting drug users: conversation starters 167; harm reduction as step towards getting clean 164; HIV prevention programme evaluation 159–69 (*see also* STEP into Action HIV prevention programme); injection risk ladder 167–8; safe drug-splitting procedures 165, 167–8; tension between 'getting clean' and 'harm reduction' 163

integrated mixed methods research, challenges for 230
international development sector, nature of evaluation 187
interpretation, and levels of context 103
interpretative turn 18
interpretive and ethnographic approaches: barriers 6; benefits of to HIV and sexual health fields 1; documenting of success 1; to monitoring and evaluation 6–7; overview 4–6; sidelining of in contemporary evaluation work 1; skills requirements 6
interpretive approaches: benefits of using in structured cycles of action and learning 154; an examination of 18–20; the 'interpretive turn' in social science 4, 18; personal reflections on the value of 17–29 (*see also* LNG Project impact assessment); shift towards 4; vs statistical approaches 25
interpretive research: goal of 5; Oxfam's effectiveness reviews 220–1 (*see also* Oxfam's effectiveness reviews); vs positivist 4–5
intervention design and evaluation, theory and interpretation 40–2
inward-facing modes of evaluation: examples of 36; tension between outward-facing modes and 36–7

Kenya: Beyond Zero Campaign 52; maternal, newborn and child health project 47–61 (*see also* maternal, newborn and child health project)

learning, emphasis of bilateral agencies on 33
listening, importance of as basic premise of the Reality Check Approach 173
LNG Project impact assessment: changing outcomes 22–3; funding issues 23–4; gender issues 21–3, 24–5; and the importance of an interpretive approach 28–9; location 24; need for understanding and sensitivity 21–2; overcoming the influence of Christianity 21; politics of evidence 19–20; 'significant change' stories 20–3, 24–5; use of visual methodology 25–7

local knowledge: the concept 54, 83; contrasted with authoritative knowledge 47–8; distinguished from local-level knowledge 84; and evidence-based programming 81–5; generating in Rwanda 85–7 (*see also* girl empowerment programme); generating through an ethnographic approach 84–5; impact of standardisation on 59; importance of 57–60, 87–93; interaction of universalistic knowledge with 54; knowing 'what does not work' 47; meaning of local knowledges 48
local misconceptions, dispelling 49
local perspectives, understanding change and impact from 181–3

maternal, newborn and child health project: background to project 48–51; community suspicions 56–7; contexts and practices 51–3; enumerator training 57–60; importance of local knowledge 57–60; intervention targets 49; location 52–3; mismatch in expectations 56; monitoring and evaluation system 50–1; project ethnography approach 51; project logic 49; project partners 49; survey tool question on ante-natal clinic attendance **58**; volunteer training 49–51, 53
maternal mortality, in Taita Taveta County, Kenya 52
MEMA kwa Vijana adolescent sexual health programme: abstinence findings 239–40; components 233; condom use findings 242–3; in-depth qualitative impact evaluation 238–43; number of sexual partners and/or fidelity findings 240–2; preliminary qualitative impact assessment 237–8; the research 234–6
men who have sex with men: HIV prevalence rate in Central American countries 65–6; and HIV prevention 37, 39, 42, 67–8, 132; living with HIV 77–8
'methodological triumphalism' 2
mixed methodology: challenges for integrated mixed methods research 230; evaluation project in Ghana 177–80 (*see also* Reality Check Approach); FGM Special Initiative 211–12 (*see also* FGM Special Initiative); longitudinal evaluation in Nepal 176–7; Oxfam's exploration of integrated mixed methods research 230 (*see also* Oxfam's effectiveness reviews)
monitoring and evaluation: failings of traditional frameworks 187; practical assumptions 194; rationales for 32

narrative, as method of evaluation 188 (*see also* SenseMaker; storytelling)
Nepal: cardamom production as driver of change in 181–2; mixed methods longitudinal evaluation in 176–7; neonatal mortality reduction initiative 35; opium cultivation in 180; public poverty levels 180; surprise living standards findings 172, 181
NGOs (non-governmental organisations), accountability function, implicit dominance 33
Nicaragua: decline between eligibility for HIV treatment and adherence 66; eligibility for antiretroviral therapy 66; HIV prevalence 65–6
Nigeria, example of rapid ethnographic assessment 6
nutrition, as focus of maternal, newborn and child health initiative in Kenya 48–9

open-ended questions, usefulness for impact evaluation 189
outcome measurement: adoption of rigorous approaches to 34; emerging options 187; impact of a rigid focus on 203
outsider-led quantitative studies, drivers of current preference for 2
outward-facing modes of evaluation: examples of 36; perceptions of generalisability 37; risks of relying exclusively on 41; tension between inward-facing modes and 36–7
Oxfam: exploration of the use of integrated mixed methods research 230; introduction of a 'Global Performance Framework' 220; structure 220; use of interpretive research 219–30

Oxfam's effectiveness reviews: Disaster Risk Management and Livelihoods Programme, Pakistan 221–5; Ruti Irrigation Project, Zimbabwe 225–9

Pakistan, climate change resilience study 221–5
Papua New Guinea (PNG): HIV prevention and care project *see* Tingim Laip, HIV prevention and care project; Tingim Laip, social mapping study; LNG Project impact assessment *see* LNG Project impact assessment; main transport corridor 130; resource development and human well-being research *see* LNG Project impact assessment
participant observation: benefits of 52; effectiveness for studying sensitive behaviours 232
Participatory Ethnographic Evaluation Research (PEER) approach, Price and Hawkins' publication 203 (*see also* Rapid PEER approach)
participatory monitoring 22, 40
participatory research, description of SAR as 146 (*see also* systemic action research (SAR))
peer educators: peer-led health education 39; as role models 240; sex workers engaged as 38
peer outreach, benefits of 138–9
Peru, example of rapid ethnographic assessment 6
Photovoice research method 25
plausibility evaluations 43
positivist research: goal 4; influence of in current monitoring and evaluation practice 1; vs interpretive 4–5; methodological character 4; problems with 1–2
poverty: levels of in Nepal 180; as risk factor for teenage pregnancy 115; in Taita Taveta County, Kenya 52
pregnancy, early *see* early pregnancy and motherhood
process evaluation: the concept 160; ethnographic approaches, usefulness of 159 (*see also* Ethnographic process evaluation); importance of 159
programme evaluation, primary purposes 19

programme improvement, evaluating for 32
prostitution 88, 90, 116, 119
public engagement, funders' expectations of researchers 34

qualitative enquiry, definition 203
qualitative perspectives, marginalisation 2
qualitative research: assumptions about 232–3; and the character of evaluation 33–5; merits of well-conducted 232; self-reported data, validity concerns 236–7; suitability for impact assessment 232–44 (*see also* MEMA kwa Vijana adolescent sexual health programme); valuable attributes 232
quantitative approaches to evaluation, assumptions about 2
quantitative methods, historic dominance of in medicine and public health assessment, planning and evaluation 129

rapid ethnographic approaches, growing literature 6
rapid ethnographic assessment, examples of 6–7
Rapid PEER approach: benefits of the method 206; case studies 206–16; development and aims of the PEER methodology 203–4; FGM initiative 211–16 (*see also* FGM Special Initiative); marital training programme 206–11 (*see also* Tokaut na Tokstret marital training programme); methodology 205–6; reliance on story-telling 205; sociocultural perspective 203–4; third person data collection 205; training 205; usefulness of the methodology 204
RCTs (randomised controlled trials): adolescent sexual health programme in Tanzania *see* MEMA kwa Vijana adolescent sexual health programme; assumptions of generalisability in results 35; evidence transfer and the limitations of 35–6; favouring of systematic reviews and 34–5; and the polarisation of debate 219
Reality Check Approach: behavioural insights 179; criteria for team members 174; evaluation frameworks/

instruments, improving design 176–7; evaluation surveys, enriching findings from 177–81; experiences of using 175–83; Ghana Millennium villages project 177–80; guiding principles 173–4; immersive core 173; importance of listening 173; Indonesian study 174, **175**; local people's perspectives 181–3; Millennium villages project 177; Nepal household survey scoping study 176–7; Nepal survey findings explained 180–3; overview 172–5

reproductive health, impact of economic–rationalist models of human behaviour in 203–4

research, distinction between evaluation and 34

research paradigms, conventional 35

resource extraction, funding of health impacts studies 23 (*see also* LNG Project impact assessment)

rigorous impact evaluations, examples of 35

risk, environments of 138

risk sharing, 'stones' question about **191**

risk-reduction, community mobilisation and 37

safe sex negotiation: challenges for 166; skills provision for girls in Sierra Leone 119–20; skills provision for sex workers in India 38

self-reported data, validity concerns 236–7

SenseMaker: analysis and use 193; analytical steps 193; bias reduction 196; challenges of evaluation innovation 198–200; complexity, taking seriously 194–5; data collection issues 193, 199; 'disconfirming cherished expectations' 195–6; findings from pilot studies in Vietnam and Ecuador 196–8; interpretation process 194; interpretive and evaluative basis 194–6; issues of scale 195; modus operandi 189–94; overview 188; pattern detection 193; question framework design 189–92; shared decision making slider **191**; similar options 187; 'stones' question about risk sharing **191**; story collection and respondent self-coding 192–3; value chain autonomy question **190**

serodiscordant couples, eligibility for antiretroviral therapy 66

sex education, young women's experience of in Sierra Leone 119–20

sex work: criminalisation of and adherence to HIV treatment 66; and HIV prevention 37, 136; personal experiences 26; transactional sex vs 134

sex workers: community-based HIV prevention project in Kolkata 37–40; determinants of vulnerability to HIV infection 38; discriminatory banking policies 38; inadequacy of the term in PNG context 134; Kolkata HIV prevention project 38; peer education role 38

sexual and reproductive health programmes, Rapid PEER approach for the evaluation of *see* Rapid PEER approach

sexual and reproductive health research, debates about the role of naturalistic qualitative enquiry 203

sexual health, benefits of interpretive and ethnographic approaches 1

Sierra Leone: health and leadership programs for vulnerable young women *see* Empowering Girls at Risk; safe sex negotiation skills provision for girls in 119–20; social and economic impact of civil war in 111

signification frameworks 190, 192, 196

smallholder studies: connecting smallholders to inclusive markets 188–9; findings 196; pilot cases 189; question framework 189; sampling and training issues 193; stones question 192; story collection 192–3; story trends for production, trade and processing **196**

social development: action research approach 145 (*see also* systemic action research (SAR)); and the distinction between 'planning' programmes and 'designing' them 82; programme cycle stages **82**; rebalancing investment towards people and processes 156; role for ethnography in evidence-based programme design for 81–93 (*see also* girl empowerment programme; local knowledge)

social development programming: stages 81–2; typical approach 81
social interventions, examples of 36
social marketing: basis of 65; definition 65
social science, 'interpretive turn' 4, 18
Sonagachi project, for HIV prevention in India 38–9, 41–2
South Africa, use of Photovoice 25
STEP into Action HIV prevention programme 161, 169; communication issues 166–7; data collection and analysis 162–3; ethnographic approach to evaluation 161 (*see also* ethnographic process evaluation); harm reduction philosophy 163–4; harm reduction practices 167–8; importance of staying positive 165–6; inclusion criteria for participants 162; location 162; 'partner' and 'network member' terminology 164–5; study design 161
storytelling: harnessing the power of 205; 'significant change' stories 20–3, 24–5; story collection and respondent self-coding 192–3
systematic reviews 35, 245
systemic action research (SAR): evaluation of training 153–6; implementation, adapting 151–3; and its interpretive basis 145–8; principles 146; project activities, assessing appropriateness of 149–51; relationship building 153; social networks review 149; storyboard exercise 149–50, 152, 154; systems map 150; training tools and techniques 148; as volunteer action understanding/enhancement approach **147**; volunteer training 146–8
systems thinking 187

target setting, distorting effects 41
TB control: challenges for 97; communication issues 104; Directly Observed Treatment, Short-course (DOTS) strategy 96; ethnographic approach to strategy development 99–103; health provider issues **106**; Indian government's Tribal Action Plan 98–9; local strategy design 106–8; strategic framework **107**; study methods 101; and treatment costs 104–6; from tribal action plan to empirically grounded strategy 103–8; in 'tribal districts' in India 96–9
teenage girls, treatment of by government health workers 121
teenage pregnancy, Sierra Leone 111
'thick description' 18, 65, 146, 205
Tingim Laip: independent review and recommendations 134; meaning of 128
Tingim Laip, social mapping study: clarification of at-risk populations 134–8; context of HIV risk and impact along the Highlands Highway **137**; data collection, reflection and analysis 131–3; environments of risk 138; ethnographic approach 129; field work 131–2; group talk sessions 133; interview process 132; locations 130; mapping team selection and training 131; outreach workers, benefits of engaging peers 138–9; service provision and access findings 139–40; thematic focus 130; volunteer review 138–9
top-down quantitative studies, drivers of current preference for 2
traditional frameworks for monitoring and evaluation, failings 187
transactional sex: and HIV prevention 132, 134; pathways into **137**; as risk factor for HIV 127; vs sex work 134; and teenage pregnancy 115
trends in monitoring and evaluation, current trends 2–4
triangulation, achieving rigour through 173
tuberculosis, ethnographically inspired approach to strategy development for control of 95–108 (*see also* TB control)

Uganda, effectiveness review survey 230
United Kingdom (UK), female genital mutilation special initiative *see* FGM Special Initiative
United States (USA): example of rapid ethnographic assessment 7; HIV prevention programme with injecting drug users *see* STEP into Action HIV prevention programme

value chain development: autonomy in the value chain question **190**; complexity of the process 188; monitoring and evaluation requirements 188; *see also* SenseMaker; smallholder studies

value judgement, importance of 22

visual tools, importance of in research 25–7

volunteer activities, gaining insight into appropriateness and effectiveness of 149–51, 151–3

volunteer training: evaluation of 153–6; maternal, newborn and child health project 49–51, 53

volunteering: evaluation of as a force for social change 143–4; the ICS programme 144–5; supporting through action research 145 (*see also* systemic action research (SAR))

Vredeseilanden (VECO) 188; *see also* SenseMaker; smallholder studies

VSO (Voluntary Services Overseas) 144

WE-Care ('Women's Empowerment and Care'), Oxfam GB's initiative 230

well-being, and effectiveness 154

WHO (World Health Organisation) 47, 96

women: land ownership in Zimbabwe 227; unpaid care work study 230

Zimbabwe: land ownership by women 227; Ruti Irrigation Project 225–9

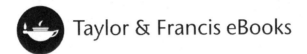

Taylor & Francis eBooks

Helping you to choose the right eBooks for your Library

Add Routledge titles to your library's digital collection today. Taylor and Francis ebooks contains over 50,000 titles in the Humanities, Social Sciences, Behavioural Sciences, Built Environment and Law.

Choose from a range of subject packages or create your own!

Benefits for you
- Free MARC records
- COUNTER-compliant usage statistics
- Flexible purchase and pricing options
- All titles DRM-free.

Benefits for your user
- Off-site, anytime access via Athens or referring URL
- Print or copy pages or chapters
- Full content search
- Bookmark, highlight and annotate text
- Access to thousands of pages of quality research at the click of a button.

REQUEST YOUR FREE INSTITUTIONAL TRIAL TODAY

Free Trials Available
We offer free trials to qualifying academic, corporate and government customers.

eCollections – Choose from over 30 subject eCollections, including:

Archaeology	Language Learning
Architecture	Law
Asian Studies	Literature
Business & Management	Media & Communication
Classical Studies	Middle East Studies
Construction	Music
Creative & Media Arts	Philosophy
Criminology & Criminal Justice	Planning
Economics	Politics
Education	Psychology & Mental Health
Energy	Religion
Engineering	Security
English Language & Linguistics	Social Work
Environment & Sustainability	Sociology
Geography	Sport
Health Studies	Theatre & Performance
History	Tourism, Hospitality & Events

For more information, pricing enquiries or to order a free trial, please contact your local sales team:
www.tandfebooks.com/page/sales

Routledge
Taylor & Francis Group

The home of
Routledge books

www.tandfebooks.com

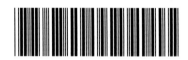